Praise for *Mastering Informa*...

"A fantastic book! This is a timely and needed healthcare informatics book that can help both practicing informaticians and students. It includes essential knowledge needed in the current healthcare environment and helpful tools that can be used for diverse health IT projects. I am very grateful for the authors' generous sharing of their expertise with others."

–Eun-Shim Nahm, PhD, RN, FAAN
Professor and Program Director
Nursing Informatics
University of Maryland School of Nursing

"The experience and diversity of the authors bring together a rich compendium of forward-thinking and practical advice that covers most aspects of the informatics lifecycle. I highly recommend this valuable resource for today's informaticians—from novice to experienced."

–Deborah Ariosto, PhD, RN
Director, Patient Care Informatics & CNIO
Vanderbilt University Medical Center

"*Mastering Informatics* provides a critical resource for those working to improve health and healthcare through the practice of informatics. The authors articulate a clear, well organized, pragmatic approach to the multiple challenges in this field. The chapters present the basics and then move beyond to offer application of principles, lessons learned by informatics experts, helpful tips, and a vision for future directions. This book offers outstanding support to facilitate and enhance the mastery of informatics practice."

–Carol A. Romano, PhD, RN, FAAN, FACMI
Rear Admiral (Ret), U.S. Public Health Service
Professor and Associate Dean, Uniformed Services University, Bethesda, Maryland
Former Senior Consultant for Clinical Research Informatics, National Institutes of Health

"Sengstack and Boicey have provided the necessary elements for mastering informatics for professionals engaged in the design and delivery of systems to support the changing model of care. This book presents emerging trends facing the delivery system and how informatics and informatics professionals can respond to the demands for consumer quality outcomes and experience of care."

–Andrea Mazzoccoli, PhD, RN, FAAN
Chief Nursing Officer, Bon Secours Health System
Center for Clinical Excellence and Innovation

"Sengstack and Boicey have compiled a very comprehensive resource for both practicing informaticists and those interested in nursing informatics. This is an excellent resource in all areas of nursing informatics."

–Mary Beth Mitchell, MSN, RN, BC, CPHIMS
CNIO, Texas Health Resources

"This is sure to become the 'go to' book for implementers of all types of health IT. The pragmatic lessons and practical examples will assist both those new to health informatics and those experienced who are looking for new ideas. This introspective text will help implementers understand informatics and how to use health IT to advance the vision of better health, better care, and lower costs."

–Judy Murphy, RN, FACMI, FHIMSS, FAAN
Chief Nursing Officer, IBM Healthcare

Mastering Informatics

A Healthcare Handbook for Success

Patricia P. Sengstack, DNP, RN-BC, CPHIMS
Charles M. Boicey, MS, RN-BC, PMP, CLNC, CPHIMS

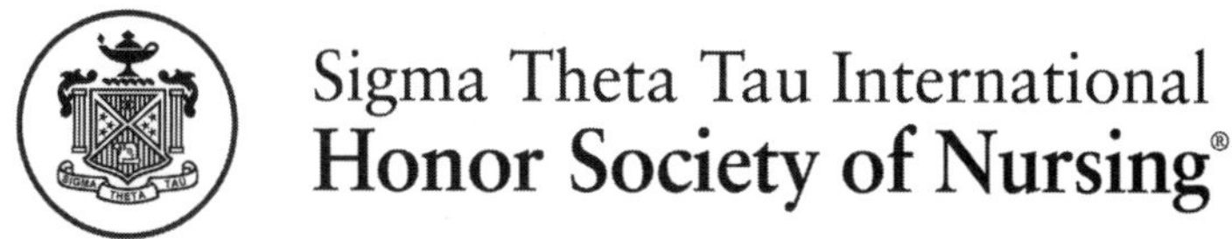

Copyright © 2015 by Sigma Theta Tau International

All rights reserved. This book is protected by copyright. No part of it may be reproduced, stored in a retrieval system, or transmitted in any form or by any means, electronic, mechanical, photocopying, recording, or otherwise, without written permission from the publisher. Any trademarks, service marks, design rights, or similar rights that are mentioned, used, or cited in this book are the property of their respective owners. Their use here does not imply that you may use them for similar or any other purpose.

The Honor Society of Nursing, Sigma Theta Tau International (STTI) is a nonprofit organization whose mission is to support the learning, knowledge, and professional development of nurses committed to making a difference in health worldwide. Founded in 1922, STTI has around 130,000 members in 86 countries. Members include practicing nurses, instructors, researchers, policymakers, entrepreneurs and others. STTI's 499 chapters are located at 695 institutions of higher education throughout Australia, Botswana, Brazil, Canada, Colombia, Ghana, Hong Kong, Japan, Kenya, Malawi, Mexico, the Netherlands, Pakistan, Portugal, Singapore, South Africa, South Korea, Swaziland, Sweden, Taiwan, Tanzania, United Kingdom, United States, and Wales. More information about STTI can be found online at www.nursingsociety.org.

Sigma Theta Tau International
550 West North Street
Indianapolis, IN, USA 46202

To order additional books, buy in bulk, or order for corporate use, contact Nursing Knowledge International at 888.NKI.4YOU (888.654.4968/US and Canada) or +1.317.634.8171 (outside US and Canada).

To request a review copy for course adoption, email solutions@nursingknowledge.org or call 888.NKI.4YOU (888.654.4968/US and Canada) or +1.317.634.8171 (outside US and Canada).

To request author information, or for speaker or other media requests, contact Marketing, Honor Society of Nursing, Sigma Theta Tau International at 888.634.7575 (US and Canada) or +1.317.634.8171 (outside US and Canada).

ISBN: 9781938835667

EPUB ISBN: 9781938835674

PDF ISBN: 9781938835681

MOBI ISBN: 9781938835698

Library of Congress Cataloging-in-Publication Data

Mastering informatics : a healthcare handbook for success / [edited by] Patricia Sengstack, Charles Boicey.
p. ; cm.
Includes bibliographical references and index.
ISBN 978-1-938835-66-7 (print : alk. paper) -- ISBN 978-1-938835-67-4 (EPUB) -- ISBN 978-1-938835-68-1 (PDF) -- ISBN 978-1-938835-69-8 (MOBI)
I. Sengstack, Patricia, 1959- , editor. II. Boicey, Charles, 1959- , editor. III. Sigma Theta Tau International, issuing body.
[DNLM: 1. Medical Informatics--methods. 2. Electronic Health Records. 3. Health Information Management. 4. Telemedicine. W 26.5]
R855.3
610.285--dc23

2014039190

First Printing, 2015

Publisher: Dustin Sullivan
Acquisitions Editor: Emily Hatch
Editorial Coordinator: Paula Jeffers
Cover Designer: Michael Tanamachi
Interior Design/Page Layout: Rebecca Batchelor
Illustrator: Clint Lahnen

Principal Book Editor: Carla Hall
Development and Project Editor: Brian Walls
Copy Editor: Teresa Artman
Proofreaders: Erin Geile and Barbara Bennett
Indexers: Joy Dean Lee and Larry Sweazy

Dedication

I dedicate this book to my father, Dr. Donald Keith Pumroy, who taught me to be a lifelong learner, to mentor others, to focus on the behavior, and to always wear a grin.

–Patricia Pumroy Sengstack, DNP, RN-BC, CPHIMS

Acknowledgments

First, we would like to thank Sigma Theta Tau International for providing the opportunity to author this book on informatics. Such a book is something we knew was needed, but we didn't have a publisher to make it happen—until now.

A huge thank you to all our contributing authors who put in a significant effort to develop chapters that reflect more than just textbook information, but content infused with both evidence and experience to give readers some great tools.

I would like to acknowledge the support from the Bon Secours Health System in the writing and editing of this book—in particular, my boss, Andrea Mazzoccoli, RN, PhD, FAAN, who supported me by giving me the time and encouragement to make this possible. I would also like to acknowledge my wonderful husband, Glenn J. Sengstack, who had to take over cooking, laundry, and sundry other tasks, so I could disappear for a few months and dedicate my time to this effort, and to my comedic son, Donald G. Sengstack, for his constant reminders to "quit procrastinating."

–Patricia P. Sengstack, DNP, RN-BC, CPHIMS

I would like to acknowledge Patty Sengstack for providing me the opportunity to play a role in the production of this manuscript as well as authoring a chapter. It was an excellent learning experience. Special acknowledgements to my family, Ana and Bryan, for their patience over the years and for being cool with late nights, early mornings, and weekends at work. I would also like to acknowledge Dr. Howard Belzberg; Dr. William Shoemaker; Emma Farmer, RN; Jim Murry; Lisa Dahm, PhD; Carol and Carolyn Bloch, RN, for giving me inspiration and the freedom to take the road less traveled; and to Patricia Ramos, RN, for traveling with me on that road for 10 years.

–Charles M. Boicey, MS, RN-BC, PMP, CLNC, CPHIMS

30+ Hours of CNE Available With This Book

Congratulations! By purchasing a new copy of Mastering Informatics, you can complete all of the continuing nursing education (CNE) units required for the nursing informatics exam from one product.

WHAT DOES THIS MEAN FOR YOU?

- The content in this book and the additional online information will help prepare you for the ANCC board certification exam in nursing informatics (RN-BC).
- Written by the top informaticists in healthcare, the book covers everything from planning and analysis to designing, testing, training, implementing, maintaining, evaluating, security, patient safety, analytics, mobility, and much more.
- When you use the unique discount code from the affixed card in the front of the book to purchase the *Mastering Informatics* course from www.nursingknowledge.org/educationalproducts.html, you get 30+ hours of CNE—a $250 value—for only $50!

HOW DO YOU ACCESS THE ONLINE CNE?

- Tear out the affixed card from the front of your new book and uncover the unique discount code in the scratch-off box. IMPORTANT—YOU MUST FIRST REGISTER OR SIGN IN TO YOUR NURSING KNOWLEDGE INTERNATIONAL ACCOUNT BEFORE ENTERING THE UNIQUE DISCOUNT CODE.
- Then simply go to www.nursingknowledge.org/educationalproducts.html to purchase the Mastering Informatics-ONLINE COURSE.
- Proceed to checkout, enter the unique discount code in the Discount Codes box, and click Apply Coupon. When the coupon code has been accepted, you will see the discount in your Shopping Cart Totals.
- Once your purchase is complete, your online course is available. Go to My Accounts (top right of the page) and select CNE from the left-hand side of your screen. You will then be routed to our e-learning platform, where you can access Mastering Informatics-ONLINE COURSE.

WHAT IF YOU BOUGHT THIS BOOK USED OR DO NOT HAVE AN ACCESS CODE?

If you do not have an access code, you can still obtain the CNE. However, you will have to pay full retail price. You can access the CNE by going to www.nursingknowledge.org/educationalproducts.html and selecting Mastering Informatics-ONLINE COURSE.

For questions or additional help, please email us at solutions@nursingknowledge.org.

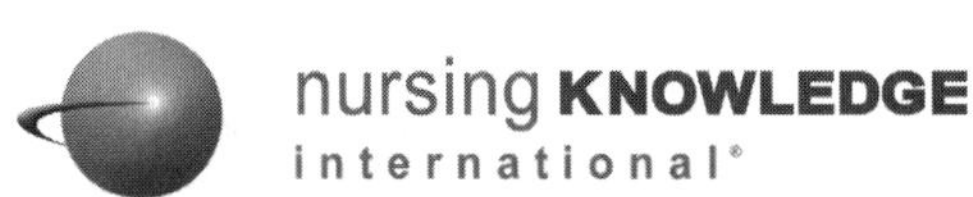

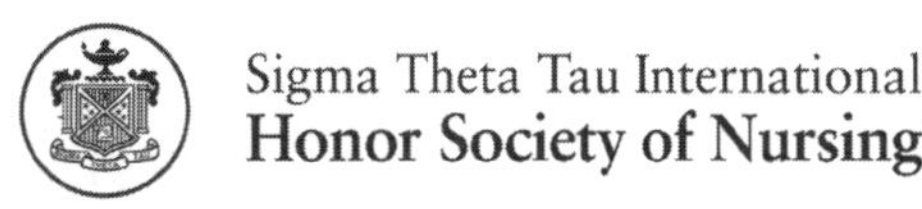

Sigma Theta Tau International is an accredited provider of continuing nursing education by the American Nurses Credentialing Center (ANCC) Commission on Accreditation.

About the Authors

Patricia P. Sengstack, DNP, RN-BC, CPHIMS

Patricia Sengstack is the Chief Nursing Informatics Officer for the Bon Secours Health System based in Marriottsville, MD, and is the former Deputy CIO and Chief of Clinical Informatics at the National Institutes of Health, Clinical Center in Bethesda, Maryland. Prior to holding these positions, she worked for Computer Sciences Corporation and was on the leadership team that implemented the Clinical Research Information System at the NIH Clinical Center.

Sengstack received her BSN from the University of Maryland and went on to receive her master's degree in Healthcare Administration and a post-master's degree in Nursing Informatics, also from the University of Maryland. She now serves on the curriculum advisory Board for the University of Maryland's Nursing Informatics program. She received her doctor of nursing practice degree from Vanderbilt University in Nashville, Tennessee, and now serves on that faculty and instructs informatics students at both the master's and doctoral levels. In May 2014, she received the Dean's Award for Recognition of Faculty Achievement in Informatics from the Vanderbilt University School of Nursing. She is now the President of the American Nursing Informatics Association and has served on its board of directors since 2012. Her nursing background includes working as an ICU Nurse and a Clinical Nurse Specialist in the Washington, D.C. metropolitan area. She has multiple publications, most recently in the *Journal of Healthcare Information Management* on the configuration of safe CPOE systems. She has presented at the national level in multiple venues, including the 2014 HIMSS and AONE annual conferences. She is board certified in Nursing Informatics and has been certified as a professional in health information management (CPHIMS) since 2008. Her focus over the last several years has been health IT's impact on patient safety as well as building a program to improve the evaluation process of healthcare IT systems.

Charles M. Boicey, MS, RN-BC, PMP, CLNC, CPHIMS

Charles Boicey is the Enterprise Analytics Architect for Stony Brook Medicine. In his role, he is developing the analytics infrastructure to serve the clinical, operational, quality, and research needs of the organization. Prior leadership roles include: Informatics Solution Architect, University of California, Irvine; Chief Informatics Officer, Riverside County Regional Medical Center; Senior Project Manager, City of Hope; Nurse Manager,

Nursing Information Systems, LAC + USC Medical Center; and Nurse Manager, Trauma/Surgical Intensive Care Unit, LAC + USC Medical Center.

Boicey received his diploma in Nursing from the Los Angeles County General Hospital School of Nursing, his BS in Business Administration from the University of Phoenix, and his master's degree in Technology Management from Stevens Institute of Technology, Hoboken, New Jersey. He is the vice president of the American Nursing Informatics Association and has served on its board of directors since 2010. He is a member of the HIMSS National Innovation Committee, a former member of the HIMSS National Nursing Informatics Committee, and the former Chair of the HIMSS SoCal Chapter Clinical Informatics Committee. He has given more than 50 national/regional presentations and webinars to such professional organizations as HIMSS, AORN, ANIA, and AMIA. He is board certified as an Informatics Nurse and holds certifications as a Project Management Professional (PMP), Certified Legal Nurse Consultant (CLNC), and Certified Professional in Healthcare Information and Management Systems (CPHIMS).

His work for the past 4 years has centered on bringing the Big Data technologies that power Yahoo!, Facebook, LinkedIn, and Twitter to healthcare. He was a founding member of the team that developed the Health and Human Services award-winning application "MappyHealth" and he developed "Saritor," which is a novel Big Data healthcare data platform for advanced healthcare analytics.

Contributing Authors

Maria Arellano, MS, RN

Maria Arellano is the Clinical Product Manager for American Healthtech, a post-acute care information technology company. She has 30 years experience in nursing specializing in long term post-acute care (LTPAC), and has served roles in nursing administration, consulting, and teaching. Arellano has assisted nursing homes across the country with regulatory compliance and quality improvement activities and is a frequent presenter of national and statewide workshops on clinical and leadership topics. Prior to her current role, Arellano worked on telehealth research projects involving veterans with PTSD, medication management, and heart failure. She also designed software applications for clinicians in LTPAC settings.

Arellano received her nursing degree from Arapahoe Community College, a BS in business from the University of Phoenix, and a master's degree in Health Care Informatics from the University of Colorado, School of Nursing. Arellano served on technical expert panels for CMS and is currently serving on the Nursing Informatics Committee for HIMSS.

Melissa Barthold, MSN, RN-BC, CPHIMS, FHIMSS

Melissa Barthold is the Senior Clinical Solutions Strategist at the University of Mississippi Medical Center, in Jackson, Mississippi. She has more than 25 years of nursing practice, with more than an additional 15 years practice as a nursing informaticist. She obtained her master's in Nursing Informatics in 1999 from Loyola University of Chicago's Niehoff School of Nursing where she is currently completing her doctor of nursing practice degree. She has served on the HIMSS Nursing Informatics Taskforce and Committee as the Chair of both the HIMSS Annual Conference Education Committee (2010) and the Distance Education Committee (2011). She has chaired the NI Taskforce's Standard Practices Forum for the last several years. Melissa has served as adjunct faculty at Loyola University of Chicago and Barry University, Miami Shores, Florida, as a faculty facilitator at Excelsior College, and was appointed as adjunct faculty at Nova Southeastern University School of Nursing. She holds certifications from HIMSS (CPHIMS) and Board Certification from the American Nursing Credentialing Center, where she is serving her second term on the Content Expert Panel: Nursing Informatics.

Lisa Anne Bove, DNP, RN-BC

Lisa Anne Bove is currently a Senior Manager with Leidos Health. Lisa Anne is a nursing informatics specialist focused on improving health using electronic information and improving nurses and physicians work processes using technology in healthcare. Lisa Anne has worked in healthcare informatics for more than 25 years in a variety of positions and has been certified by the American Nurses Credentialing Center in Nursing Informatics since 1986. Lisa Anne functioned as the CNIO of a major multi-system hospital system, as a program manager for larger clinical design and implementation projects, and as an educator for continuing education and college-level classes.

Bove received her DNP from Duke University in North Carolina in 2013, focusing on informatics and the value of bedside documentation. Lisa Anne was also on the American Nursing Informatics Association Board of Directors from 2005–2012 and was Conference Co-Chairperson from 2010–2012. Lisa Anne is an active conference planning committee member of the Delaware Valley Nursing Computer Network (DVNCN). Lisa Anne has published and spoken on numerous topics, including informatics and project management.

Seth D. Carlson, BS

Seth D. Carlson has more than 16 years experience in the field of Information Technology, with the past 9 years in healthcare IT. He currently works as a principal business analyst and integrator of new IT systems. In a former position, he served as a Testing Lead for several years and specialized in the testing of Clinical Health Systems, HL7 interfaces, and databases. He received his bachelor of science degree in Computer Science in 1997 from the University of Maryland in College Park. He is currently enrolled in the master of science in Business and Management, Information Systems program at the University of Maryland in College Park.

(*Disclaimer:* The views and opinions of the author expressed in "Testing in the Healthcare Informatics Environment," Chapter 4, do not necessarily state or reflect those of the U.S. government.)

Lincoln S. Farnum, MS, RRT, CPHIMS

Lincoln Farnum is a health IT consultant living in the Tampa Bay, Florida area. A registered respiratory therapist (RRT) with experience in both neonatal/pediatrics and adults ranging from pulmonary lab and polysomnography to intensive care, Mr.

Farnum brings his clinical experience to improving healthcare IT system usability and intelligence. He received his master's degree in Medical Informatics degree from the Northwestern University' Feinberg School of Medicine. He has been implementing information systems, developing clinical decision support and business intelligence features, and working to improve the experiences of clinicians for more than two decades.

Rick Gagnon, RN, FNP

Rick Gagnon is a registered nurse and a family nurse practitioner. As a clinician, he has a valuable perspective on clinical operations with expertise in public health, acute care, and home healthcare agency operations and management. In the home care arena, he specializes in agency startups and consulting for certified and private duty agencies. As a business and leadership coach, Mr. Gagnon illuminates the notion of possibility through his passion for helping others develop their full potential. He also possesses valuable experience as a private business owner.

Gagnon has been a nurse for 30 years and has worked both as a clinician and in leadership positions in acute care, public health, and home healthcare, as well as corporate positions in healthcare and IT. For the past 15 years, Mr. Gagnon has focused his professional attention on home healthcare, in operations, startups, and informatics. He has been a certified agency administrator, a branch manager, and a private duty manager, and also served as the director of operations for private duty for one of the largest home care companies in the United States, with 55 agencies reporting to him. He has worked in a variety of healthcare software settings, including hospital IT and informatics, enterprise patient access, scheduling, and physician orders management, in implementation, education, and systems analytics roles.

Daniel Gracie, DNP, RN-BC

Daniel Gracie received his bachelor of science in Nursing from Mountain State University in Beckley, West Virginia. In 2007, he began work on his master of science in Nursing in Administration at the Medical University of South Carolina. In 2010, he returned to the Medical University of South Carolina and completed his doctor of nursing practice in 2012. During this time, he focused his time on the implementation of informatics competencies into the curriculum of baccalaureate nursing students.

Currently, Gracie leads his team in the build of CPOE with the Epic project at the Medical University of South Carolina. In this role, he also serves as a project lead for the Meaningful Use and Regulatory Reporting planning and implementation. Prior to this, he served in roles that focused on the implementation of healthcare IT solutions and frontline staff support at the Medical University of South Carolina. Gracie also teaches informatics and healthcare quality and leadership as adjunct faculty at a number of nursing schools.

As a board member of the American Nursing Informatics Association, Gracie has served as the social media liaison and a member of the conference planning committee, and has lead the conference planning committee for the past 3 years.

Susan M. Houston, MBA, RN-BC, PMP, CPHIMS, FHIMSS

Susan is the Chief Portfolio Officer at the National Institutes of Health Clinical Center where she is responsible for the full lifecycle management of the clinical and administrative applications. She has extensive clinical, informatics, and project management experience with a variety of healthcare-related organizations. Susan has taught project management at the University of Maryland School of Nursing Masters of Informatics program and has presented at local and national conferences. She has co-authored a number of informatics articles and the book *Project Management for Healthcare Informatics* (Springer publishing). She has authored a number of courses in the HIMSS eLearning Academy as well as *The Project Manager's Guide to Health Information Technology Implementation* (HIMSS).

Susan C. Hull, MSN, RN

Susan Hull is a nursing executive and national thought leader who is passionate about co-creating technology-enabled innovations, transforming health and care eco-systems to dramatically improve population health and wellbeing, with national and international reach. Susan believes we can achieve an affordable, sustainable learning health system where consumers, providers, and communities are dynamically engaged and thriving, with personalized health solutions achieving the Triple Aim.

With more than 30 years experience, Susan has served in a variety of roles transforming health and improving health of populations, including nursing and health system executive, new healthy community partnership and community health information network (CHIN) executive, clinical informatics and decision support executive, consultant and action researcher, and designing and managing a new Children's Hospital Emergency Service. Susan is the founder and CEO of WellSpring Consulting, supporting healthcare organizations and communities in the United States and Canada since 1994 to strengthen their capacity for innovation in services, products, and impact. She recently served as the chief health informatics officer for Diversinet and the vice president of the Elsevier CPM Resource Center, has served on the NeHC Consumer e-Health Advisory Board and the ONC FACA Consumer Technology Standards Workgroup, and serves on the Tiger Initiative Foundation board.

Amy K. Jacobs, MSN, RN-BC

Amy K. Jacobs is a terminology specialist at Medicomp Systems, Inc. She has 28 years of nursing experience and has been actively involved in nursing informatics for the last 12 years. She is board certified in nursing informatics by the American Nurses Credentialing Center. She previously provided medical expertise for the National Library of Medicine (NLM) Unified Medical Language System (UMLS) and the National Cancer Institute (NCI) Enterprise Vocabulary Services (EVS). She also has extensive system analysis and system testing and evaluation experience. She served on the board of the American Nursing Informatics Association (ANIA) in the role of treasurer and job bank liaison. She currently is a member of ANIA, HIMSS, and AMIA. She holds a post-master's certificate in Nursing Informatics from the University of Maryland, School of Nursing, a MSN from Georgetown University, School of Nursing, and a BSN from Pensacola Christian College in Pensacola, Florida.

Brenda Kulhanek, PhD, MSN, MS, RN-BC, CPHIMS

Brenda Kulhanek is the Corporate Director for Clinical Practice and Education at Adventist Health in California where she works with hospital, clinic, and home care leaders to increase the performance of healthcare staff within their organizations. She received her PhD in Training & Performance Improvement from the School of Education at Capella University. She is a registered nurse, and is board certified in both nursing informatics and health information management systems. Kulhanek has served as a contributing faculty member for the School of Nursing at Walden University since 2011, serves on the board of the American Nursing Informatics Association, and is a frequent presenter at nursing informatics conferences throughout the country.

Susan Martin, RN, BSN, JD

Susan Martin is chief of the Security & Privacy Office at the National Institutes of Health (NIH) Clinical Center (CC). As part of the senior leadership team in the Department of Clinical Research Informatics, she is responsible for ensuring that the clinical information systems, networked medical devices, and mobile technology supporting clinical care and research are secure and compliant with the Federal Information Security Management Act (FISMA) and the Privacy Act. Her interest in privacy law and the protection of health information in clinical IT systems developed while implementing a new electronic medical record system, a surgery and anesthesia information system, a clinical barcode application, and two-factor authentication for access to networked information systems at the Clinical Center. She serves on the NIH Privacy Incident Response Team, reviewing security and privacy incidents involving sensitive information. She is also a staff nurse at Suburban Hospital, a Johns Hopkins Health System affiliate hospital in Bethesda, Maryland. In this role, she is reminded of the informatics professional's delicate balance to improve the user interface with clinical IT systems and provide timely access to the patient's data in acute care settings while satisfying requirements for security.

Theresa (Tess) J. Settergren, MHA, MA, RN-BC

Theresa (Tess) Settergren is the director of nursing informatics in the Enterprise Information Services department at Cedars-Sinai Health System in Los Angeles, California. Tess directed several ambulatory electronic medical record implementations for Cedars-Sinai, and helped to enable integrated enterprise workflows for computerized physician order management at Cedars-Sinai Medical Center. Tess has more than 18 years of experience implementing and optimizing clinical systems and technologies. She was director for more than 200 clinical applications, including the enterprise electronic health record (EHR), in her position prior to Cedars-Sinai. Tess has been board certified in Nursing Informatics since 1997.

Tess earned her MHA from University of Minnesota Carlson School of Business, and her MA in Nursing (CNS) from the College of St. Scholastica. She was co-founder and president of the MInnesota Nursing INformatics Group (MINING) from 2000–2007, where Tess established an annual nursing informatics conference program featuring internationally recognized informaticists, and collaborated to launch the first and second Minnesota T.I.G.E.R. conferences. She has served on boards of directors for Alliance for

Nursing Informatics, Center for Healthcare Innovation, Minnesota Epic User Group, and Community Health Information Collaborative (Minnesota), and served on the management committee for the Minnesota Center for Health Electronic Commerce.

Christy St. John, MSN, RN-BC

Christy St. John is the associate chief nursing informatics officer for the Bon Secours Health System. Bon Secours is a large integrated health system with 14 acute care hospitals, ambulatory practices, home health, and long-term care facilities across seven states. She holds an MSN in Nursing Informatics from Walden University and a Nursing diploma from Bon Secours School of Nursing. She is a board-certified informatics nurse and a member of Sigma Theta Tau. Her experience includes bedside practice in cardiopulmonary care, nursing leadership, and informatics leadership. Christy has led multidisciplinary teams of health professionals in designing, promoting, and facilitating evidence-based, patient-focused content within the EHR. She is an expert in all phases of the clinical system development lifecycle, including design, build, test, train, implement, and evaluate. She has led and supported go-live efforts across the system at each of the 14 acute care hospitals. Christy has presented at the national level on a variety of topics related to informatics and nursing practice, including strategies for developing evidence-based care plans and clinical pathways within the EHR and early recognition of deterioration. Her focus over the last year has been elevating and integrating nursing practices and workflows within the EHR. Additionally, Christy continues to focus on how technology and informatics can best support care delivery at each phase of the patient's journey.

Marcy Stoots, DNP, MS, RN-BC

Marcy Stoots has more than three decades of strategic and operational leadership experience in healthcare informatics and nursing. She has specific expertise in clinical adoption and optimization of EHRs to promote evidence-based practice and improved clinical outcomes. Stoots recently led the clinical adoption team through a successful large-scale, multi-facility EHR implementation at BayCare Health System in Clearwater, Florida. She received her MS in Nursing Informatics from the University of Maryland, and is currently pursuing her DNP with a focus in nursing and clinical informatics from Vanderbilt University. She is board certified in nursing informatics and a frequent speaker at industry conferences.

Luann Whittenburg, PhD, RN-BC, FNP-BC, CPHQ, CPHIMS

Luann Whittenburg is the chief nursing informatics officer at Medicomp Systems, Virginia. Luann is an RN and board-certified Family Nurse Practitioner who has authored several chapters and publications on nursing informatics, data quality, metadata, and terminology. Her healthcare informatics experience is in information operations for large healthcare delivery systems. She is a United States delegate from the American National Standards Institute to the International Organization for Standardization (ISO) Technical Committees on Health Informatics (TC215) and Traditional Chinese Medicine (TC249). Luann is board certified by the ANCC in Nursing Informatics, HIMSS health information management systems, and NAHQ healthcare quality. Whittenburg volunteers with the Virginia Medical Reserve Corp and is a member of the National Capital Area HIMSS Chapter, the American Nurses Association; American Academy of Nurse Practitioners; and board member of the ICNP National Scientific Advisory Board and the Clinical Care Classification System. She holds a PhD from George Mason University; master's of science in Nursing and a post-master's certificate from Marymount University, Virginia; and bachelor of science in Nursing from George Mason University; and is a member of Sigma Theta Tau, Epsilon Zeta Chapter.

Table of Contents

Foreword .... **xxvi**
Introduction .... **xxviii**

1 **The Widening Field of Healthcare Informatics** **1**
Patricia P. Sengstack, DNP, RN-BC, CPHIMS

Introduction to Informatics 1
History of Informatics 2
The Growing Need for Informaticists 2
The Various Informatics Domains 3
Nursing Informatics *4*
Clinical Informatics *5*
Pharmacy Informatics *7*
Dental Informatics *8*
Informatics in Other Disciplines *8*
Healthcare Informatics Certifications for All Disciplines *9*
Core Elements for All Informatics Disciplines 11
Planning and Analysis *11*
Design and Usability *12*
Testing *13*
Training *14*
Implementation *15*
Maintenance *15*
Evaluation *15*
Project Management *16*
Security and Privacy *16*
Clinical Decision Support *16*
Emerging Trends in Informatics 17
Conclusion 18
References *18*

2 **Healthcare Informatics Planning and Analysis** **21**
Marcy Stoots, DNP, MS, RN-BC

Critical Success Factors 22
Vision and Guiding Principles *22*
Leadership Engagement and Executive Sponsorship *24*
Governance and Decision-Making *24*
Bidirectional Communication *26*
End-User Engagement *26*
Benefits Measurement and Value Realization *27*
Workflow-Based Training and Ongoing Support *28*

Leading Practices: System Selection, Readiness, and Workflow 30
System Selection *30*
Readiness Assessment *32*
Workflow, Workflow, and More Workflow *32*
Measuring Success *36*
Future Directions 37
Conclusion 38
References *39*

3 Designing a Usable Healthcare Information System 41
Christy St. John, MSN, RN-BC
Assessing Usability 42
Applying Usability Evidence 44
Simplicity *45*
Naturalness *47*
Consistency *48*
Minimizing Cognitive Load *49*
Efficient Interactions *50*
Forgiveness and Feedback *52*
Effective Use of Language *53*
Effective Information Presentation *54*
Preservation of Context *56*
Usability Testing for Your EHR 57
Future Directions 58
Conclusion 59
References *59*

4 Testing in the Healthcare Informatics Environment 61
Seth D. Carlson, BS
Testing in Clinical Systems 62
The Phases of Testing 63
Unit Testing *63*
Function Testing *64*
Integration Testing *68*
Performance Testing *70*
User Acceptance Testing *71*
Regression Testing *72*
What Helps Testing Run Efficiently? 73
The Testing Process 74
Identify the requirements to be tested, the key stakeholders, and the business processes involved. *75*
Identify the relevant types of testing to be performed. *75*

Engage your clinical users in the process. 75
Identify key requirements (both functional and technical) to be tested.. 75
Identify key business processes/scenarios to be tested. 75
Define criteria on whether a test script passes or fails. 76
Define how issues/bugs are identified, prioritized, and followed up on with the developer and determine whether software will be used to document each issue. 76
Define when you will know that testing is completed for a given phase. 76
Create a testing timeline. 77
Define reporting metrics.. 77
How Much Testing Is Enough? 77
Applying the Technology 78
Testing Commercial Off-the-Shelf Applications 78
Testing Custom Applications 79
Testing Web-Based Applications 80
What Software Tools Can Assist with Testing? 81
Future Directions 82
Including the Underlying Architecture/Authentication Mechanisms in Testing 83
Testing in the Cloud. 84
Testing for Mobile Devices 84
The Importance of Understanding Enterprise Architecture for Testing 85
Conclusion 85
References 86

5 Delivering Healthcare Informatics Training 87
Brenda Kulhanek, PhD, MSN, MS, RN-BC, CPHIMS

Assessing Training 87
Applying the Technology: Tools and Evidence 90
A Training Development Model 92
Analysis 92
Design 96
Development 97
Implementation 98
Evaluation 100
Future Directions 104
Critical Training Elements 105
Cost-Effectiveness 105
Relevant Evaluation 105
Learner Characteristics 105
Using Learning Theory to Improve Acceptance 106

Design to Increase Engagement *106*
Improving the Performance Gap *106*
Conclusion 107
References *107*

6 Healthcare System Implementation 109
Susan M. Houston, MBA, RN-BC, PMP, CPHIMS, FHIMSS

Activation Planning 110
Communication 112
Plans and Lists 115
Activation Checklist and Rehearsals 122
Activation 127
Support 127
Conclusion 128
References *129*

7 Maintaining and Optimizing a Healthcare Information System 131
Theresa (Tess) J. Settergren, MHA, MA, RN-BC

System Maintenance Components 133
Change and Configuration Management *134*
Downtime and Business Continuity *138*
Enhancement Request Management *143*
Optimization 145
Goals of Optimization *150*
Resource Considerations *155*
Conclusion 156
References *156*

8 Conducting Quality Healthcare IT Outcome Evaluations: Guidelines and Resources 159
Patricia P. Sengstack, DNP, RN-BC, CPHIMS

The Healthcare IT Climate 160
Assessing Healthcare IT Outcomes 161
Steps, Tools, and Resources to Evaluate Healthcare IT Outcomes 164
Step 1: Determine What Will Be Evaluated *164*
Step 2: Determine the Question *169*
Step 3: Conduct a Literature Search *171*
Step 4: Determine the Needed Data *172*
Step 5: Determine the Study Type *173*
Step 6: Determine the Data Collection Method and Sample Size *174*
Step 7: Collect, Analyze, and Display Data *175*
Step 8: Document Your Outcome Evaluation *177*

Future Directions....179
Conclusion....180
References.... *180*

9 Essential Tools for Project Management....181
Lisa Anne Bove, DNP, RN-BC

The Focus of Project Management: Projects....182
Project Management....183
Phases of a Project.... *185*
Applying Project Management Skills.... *187*
Stakeholder Management.... *187*
Project Management Tools....191
Project Charter.... *191*
Scope Management Plan.... *194*
Work Breakdown Structure and Timeline.... *197*
Communication.... *199*
Dashboards.... *199*
Status Reports.... *201*
Future Directions....203
References.... *203*

10 Security and Privacy Concepts in Healthcare IT....205
Susan Martin, RN, BSN, JD

Protecting Medical Information....206
Network Administrator....207
System Administrator.... *208*
Application Administrator.... *209*
Information Security Official.... *209*
Privacy Official.... *210*
Security and Privacy Regulatory Frameworks....210
Fair Credit Reporting Act.... *211*
Privacy Act.... *212*
Federal Information Security Management Act.... *212*
Health Insurance Portability and Accountability Act.... *213*
Basic Safeguards of IT Security....214
Administrative Safeguards.... *215*
Physical Safeguards.... *216*
Technical Safeguards.... *217*
IT Security and Privacy Professionals Jargon....218
Recommended Best Practices and Checklist....222
References.... *227*

11 **Healthcare Clinical Decision Support** **229**
Lincoln S. Farnum, MS, RRT, CPHIMS

Background 231
Uses and Types of CDS 233
Usability Issues and CDS Frameworks 237
The Five Rights of CDS *238*
The Ten Commandments of CDS *240*
Convene a CDS Committee 242
Specification Form for CDS Intervention Design 243
Tasks Checklist for CDS Implementation 245
Conclusion 249
References *251*

12 **Use of Standard Terminologies in Healthcare IT** **253**
Luann Whittenburg, PhD, RN-BC, FNP-BC, CPHQ, CPHIMS
Amy K. Jacobs, MSN, RN-BC

HIRS Implementation 254
Structured Data *254*
Nursing Data Systems *255*
Use of Standard Terminologies 255
American Nurses Association Committee for Nursing Practice Information Infrastructure *259*
Clinical Care Classification System™ *261*
International Classification for Nursing Practice (ICNP®) *261*
NANDA International *262*
Nursing Interventions Classification (NIC) *262*
Nursing Outcomes Classification (NOC) *263*
Omaha System *263*
Perioperative Nursing Data Set (PNDS) *263*
Nursing Minimum Data Set (NMDS) *263*
Nursing Management Minimum Data Set (NMMDS) *264*
Alternative Billing Codes (ABC) *265*
Logical Observation Identifiers Names and Codes (LOINC®) *265*
Systematized Nomenclature of Medicine Clinical Terms (SNOMED CT) *266*
How to Incorporate Standard Terminologies 267
How to Incorporate the Nursing Process 272
Data Collection *274*
Data Tree Build *274*
Data Management *276*
Nursing Plan of Care *277*
Future Directions 287
References *288*
Recommended Reading *290*

13 Patient Safety and Healthcare IT 291
Patricia P. Sengstack, DNP, RN-BC, CPHIMS

Background... 292
Institute of Medicine – Health IT and Patient Safety Report *293*
ONCs Safety Plan *296*
Health IT Safety Tools and Resources 298
AHRQ Guide to Reducing Unintended Consequences of Electronic Health Records *299*
AHRQ Common Formats.. *300*
AHRQ Hazard Manager.. *301*
Institute for Safe Medication Practices................................. *302*
SAFER Guides.. *304*
ECRI Institute... *307*
CPOE Design Checklist and the Pick-list Checklist *309*
Future Directions... 312
Conclusion 314
References *314*

14 Patient Engagement in Healthcare IT.......................... 317
Daniel Gracie, DNP, RN-BC
Melissa Barthold, MSN, RN-BC, CPHIMS, FHIMSS

Assessing Patient Engagement.. 320
Provider Driving Forces *320*
Health Consumer Driving Forces *324*
Applying the Technology: Some Tools and Growing Evidence.............. 326
Social Media, Healthcare, and Patient Engagement......................... 327
The Future Is Now: Patient-Provided Data................................ 330
Hardware and Software *331*
Wearable Devices.. *332*
PulsePoint.. *334*
Google Glass and CHaRM... *335*
Conclusion 337
References *337*

15 Informatics in Non-Acute Care Settings....................... 341
Maria Arellano, MS, RN
Rick Gagnon, RN, FNP

Health Information Technology in Non-Acute Settings 343
Ambulatory Care *343*
Skilled Nursing and Long-Term Care Facilities............................ *345*
Home Healthcare.. *348*

Telehealth ... 350
Long-Term Acute Care Hospitals and Inpatient Rehabilitation Facilities ... 353
LTPAC Provider Recommendations to the ONC ... 354
LTPAC Industry-Led Initiatives and Priorities for Action ... 357
References ... 359

16 Healthcare Analytics ... 361
Charles M. Boicey, MS, RN-BC, PMP, CLNC, CPHIMS

Assessing Healthcare Analytics ... 361
Best Practices, Applications, and Resources for the Application of Healthcare Analytics ... 363
Science of Sight ... 364
Data Visualization Techniques ... 368
Data Visualization for Clinical Practice ... 370
Infographics ... 370
Big Data ... 372
Future Directions ... 376
References ... 378
Recommended Reading ... 378

17 Connected and Mobile Health's Promise for the Triple Aim ... 379
Susan C. Hull, MSN, RN

Mobile Health Is a Disruptive Innovation ... 381
Mobility Is a New Care Model ... 382
mHealth Enables Co-producing Individualized and Personalized Health ... 385
mHealth's Potential to Impact the Triple Aim ... 387
Current Experience ... 397
Patient and Consumer Apps ... 397
Clinical Care and Coordination ... 400
Pilots, Interoperability, Clinical Trials, Research, and FDA Regulation ... 401
mHealth Evaluation ... 403
Future Directions ... 404
A Global, Immersive, Invisible, Ambient Networked Sensing Environment ... 404
Portable High Resolution Diagnostics ... 405
Embedded Nanosensors with Signals to Smart Phones ... 406
The Intelligent Home ... 406
Conclusion ... 406
References ... 407

Index ... 411

Foreword

In my era, none of us even thought about the possibility of nursing informatics as a career option. Yet, as our careers progressed, we recognized the deficiencies in our healthcare and educational systems and could envision possible technological solutions. The process of making sense out of our data, translating that data into information, and beginning to build knowledge bases for our practice seemed to have no limits when new technologies emerged. I remember spending an entire week with Dr. Judith Graves in 1999. She was determined that, before her retirement, she would pass along her passion for data organization and knowledgebase building to those coming behind her. We were just beginning to gather those tools that could help us, but we certainly shared her passion!

As new nursing informaticists, we recognized along the way that we were in uncharted territory. Not only did we need to seek recognition from the nursing profession for this specialty, but we had to progress the science of nursing informatics at the same time. Through successes and failures, we continued to seek new knowledge and varying ways to support the informatics process in a variety of settings. We discovered a younger group of nurses who had no problem accepting the informatics challenge and taking it on with renewed passion and interest.

These nurses weren't afraid to accept the challenge of translating informatics to others, particularly in relation to contributing to improved patient care. They were the ones spending unmentionable hours at "go-lives" for their projects, or arguing daily for improved user interfaces, or using new technologies for lifelong learning. The authors and editors of this book are extraordinary examples of informaticists in the era I describe. They have years of on-the-job experience, coupled with advanced education that allows them to explore applications of informatics concepts in practical ways. This book is their gift to the rest of us.

Those of us in educational informatics have often had a difficult time proving our value when promoting the informatics agenda. I would argue that our best outcome measurement would be the contributions of our graduates. I am honored to say that both Patty Sengstack and Marcy Stoots have been my DNP advisees (both would have been a joy for any advisor). I first met Patty at a HIMSS conference, where she spent 45 minutes convincing me that the advanced degree she wanted to seek was a DNP and not a PhD. Given that she was employed at that time at the NIH Clinical Center, I wasn't convinced that a research-oriented PhD wasn't what she needed. I will never forget the convincing argument she delivered—that spunky "ball of fire" who knew that she could make a difference in nursing informatics and that the DNP was just the applied vision she needed to push her horizons. She was impatient to start on her agenda, and as her advisor, I remember telling her that the committee appointments and leadership positions she wanted would come in time. I have only met Charles Boicey on a few American Nursing Informatics Association (ANIA) occasions, but he is well-equipped to serve as coeditor on this book. Informatics has always been an active participant in Big Data, even before the terminology was used.

As I acknowledged in my opening paragraphs, advancing the message of nursing informatics is an ongoing battle. As a nursing informatics pioneer, I continue this battle and dedicate my endowed chair funds to promote that agenda. One of our greatest challenges has been simplifying our message about what nursing informatics is and what added value it provides. *Mastering Informatics* provides a comprehensive testimonial view to that agenda from a variety of authors who have been active players in many settings. Its content represents more guideposts along the way to the never-ending battle of helping nurses and the public better understand the contributions of nursing informatics. For those of us considered pioneers in this specialty, it has been a long journey! I hope you enjoy this book as much as I did, and I encourage you to congratulate all those in our next generation of nursing informatics.

–Betsy Weiner, PhD, RN-BC, FACMI, FAAN
Senior Associate Dean for Educational Informatics
Centennial Independence Foundation Professor of Nursing
Professor of Biomedical Informatics
Vanderbilt University

Introduction

Welcome to *Mastering Informatics: A Healthcare Handbook for Success,* written by a team of professionals who are passionate about what they do—and it shows in the chapters that follow. The authors are on the front lines performing the work they write about, and they have the experience to know what works, what does not work, and what to avoid while implementing evidence-based best practices. The science and evidence surrounding the use of clinical systems is still relatively young but growing. Informatics began within the lifetime of most of us currently working in the healthcare field, driven by the invention and implementation of the electronic health record (EHR). In this book, the authors combine the available evidence with their experience in order to disseminate best practices. Contained within these chapters are concepts that lay the foundation for strong informatics practice, and content that covers several emerging trends. The primary goals for this book are to:

- Provide readers with an understanding of the essential concepts of informatics in the healthcare environment
- Provide readers with an understanding of emerging trends in healthcare informatics
- Provide readers with resources, guidelines, ideas, and tools that can be applied to current informatics practice

Although EHRs and clinical systems in general have been in existence for decades, their use has been limited to the larger, more-affluent healthcare systems and academic medical institutions. With the signing of the Health Information Technology for Economic and Clinical Health (HITECH) Act in 2009, however, EHRs have seen a significant increase in adoption. Many organizations have already benefited from the CMS incentive program and have received millions of dollars for the meaningful adoption of these systems. With increasing adoption, the need for informatics resources has also increased. Many nursing and clinical informaticists transitioned into their positions from super-user roles during or after a system implementation. They proved themselves during the process and found themselves enjoying the work. These informatics workers possess "on the job" experience, but lack the applied science that exists in the field of informatics. Informatics has evolved into a specialty that possesses a unique body of knowledge backed by science, and this book provides an essential guide to surviving in many of these new and emerging roles. The emphasis here is on practical application of informatics concepts, an area where current literature is still evolving.

An estimated 8,000 nursing informatics specialists are practicing in the United States, but this is more than likely an underestimation. Nursing informatics specialists—whether a new informatics nurse receiving on-the-job training or an experienced nursing informaticist looking for the latest evidence and experience to improve practice—will find this book's tools and practical information helpful. Additionally, this book will be helpful for the hundreds of newly emerging healthcare IT professionals moving into the field of informatics as a result of the funding from the HITECH Act. The Office of the National Coordinator for Health Information Technology (ONC) Workforce Development Program has conducted multiple initiatives to increase the training capacity within a network of more than 90 academic institutions. More than 17,000 healthcare IT professionals have now graduated from the Community College Consortia, and another 1,747 from university-based training programs (ONC, 2013). This book focuses on key informatics concepts to increase knowledge and credibility as informaticists grow in their roles. The core concepts in this book transcend care settings and clinical disciplines. The information is intended to assist nurses, physicians, pharmacists, and other clinicians who are employed in informatics roles at primarily operational levels and are responsible for the management of clinical systems across all care settings—acute care, ambulatory settings, and home health, among others.

The book begins with the components or phases of the system development lifecycle (SDLC). These phases include Planning and Analysis, Design and Usability, Testing, Training, Implementation, Maintenance, and Evaluation. Each phase is defined, described, and explored. Ensuring a solid foundation of knowledge of each phase provides the best chance of success throughout the life of any clinical system. A firm grasp in each of these areas is essential regardless of whether you are an informatics nurse, physician, pharmacist, dentist, dietician, or other clinical professional. With a sound working knowledge of each phase, your value to the organization only increases.

As the chapters progress from planning to evaluation, it may appear that systems follow a linear path as they proceed through their lifecycle. The truth is that although a system generally follows this pathway, it can go backward or forward to any phase, depending on the scenario. For example, in a system that has been in place for years, you may go back to the design phase to improve usability and streamline a process that takes a user multiple clicks with navigation through many screens. Or, it becomes apparent that education needs to be reinforced in a particular area, and end users are re-trained. Or, after an unexpected downtime, the system needs to be tested to ensure appropriate functioning. To add complexity, you may be dealing with several of these phases concurrently. The bottom line is that each phase is essential to your informatics practice. The first eight chapters will help develop your background knowledge in these areas and provide multiple resources to use as your skills continue to develop.

Following the SDLC content, chapters address informatics infrastructure essential to the optimization, maintenance, and safety of clinical systems. For example, Chapter 9 covers evidence-based guidelines for success that include information adopted from the principles supported by the Project Management Institute (PMI). Chapter 10 covers key concepts to ensure that these systems are secure and backed up appropriately, and provides best practices in the area of ensuring privacy and appropriate access to clinical systems. Chapter 10 also addresses system interruptions, a hot topic today, as organizations look for guidance on how to negotiate the dreaded system downtime.

The introductory chapter (Chapter 11) on clinical decision support (CDS) provides definitions and descriptions of how it can be used to impact care delivery. This broad topic can encompass many things and truly does include a wide array of concepts, many proven to be successful. In this chapter, CDS is defined along with examples for implementation and evaluation. Chapter 12 discusses the importance of integrating standard terminologies into the EHR. We are at a point in EHR evolution where this is important, but lack the knowledge on where to start. This chapter provides methods for informaticists to begin to incorporate standard terminologies into their systems. The final chapter in this section (Chapter 13) discusses healthcare IT and patient safety, which has received increased attention recently. After the Institute of Medicine report was published in November of 2011, the ONC developed and published the *Health IT Patient Safety Action & Surveillance Plan*. Components of this plan are presented, along with tools to use during configuration that can assist in the improvement of patient safety. The chapter also covers methods that informaticists can implement that have proven to increase patient safety that pen-and-paper charts were just not able to do.

The final chapters include some of the newer and still emerging informatics concepts, also known as "hot topics." With the increasing availability of personal health records (PHRs), we are seeing a push for improving consumer engagement. These tools are being supported by the ONC in the form of the "Blue Button," where consumers can download their healthcare data in electronic form. Chapter 14 on patient engagement covers these concepts and provides tools to inform our patients as we encourage access to personal data. Other trends in healthcare IT are covered that include technology training for our healthcare workforce in general, not just training for our informatics specialists. Additionally, healthcare is seeing a trend toward less of a focus on acute care, and more of a focus on care outside the walls of the hospital. Clinical information systems are now being used in ambulatory care settings as well as home care, long-term, and hospice care. With limited evidence and knowledge in this area, as well as limited software vendor focus, we had difficulty finding an informatics subject matter expert to write Chapter 15, but we finally succeeded! The resources, links, and subject matter unique to the non-acute setting in this chapter will prove to be very helpful as we all attempt to transform our informatics practices to incorporate population-based care, changing payment models, and care across the continuum. Chapter 16 covers the concept of data analytics, population health, or predictive analytics—referred to as Big Data. A key underpinning for the informatics specialist is the ability to manage data. We have never had the capacity to acquire and manipulate data like we have today. The promise of Big Data is overwhelmingly seen as key to making improvements in a learning health system. This chapter addresses how informatics specialists can take advantage of data to improve care to patients both in acute care settings and throughout the entire care continuum. Chapter 17 covers mobile technology and access to data anywhere, anytime. With the ubiquitous nature of smart phones and tablets, we are slowly seeing these devices infiltrate the healthcare world. How this is occurring successfully is presented, along with ideas on how informaticists may take advantage of these technologies in their workplace.

This book is not intended to be put on a shelf to collect dust, but instead have pages that have dog-eared corners and stains as readers find the tools useful enough to reference again and again. We hope readers will find it useful and practical, and will recommend it to colleagues as they continue to advance their own informatics practice.

Suggested Reading

The Office of the National Coordinator for Health Information Technology (ONC) (2013). *Update on the adoption of health information technology and related efforts to facilitate the electronic use and exchange of health information: A report to Congress.* Retrieved from http://www.healthit.gov/sites/default/files/rtc_adoption_of_healthit_and_relatedefforts.pdf

"We have the greatest hospitals, doctors, and medical technology in the world—we need to make them accessible to every American."

–Barbara Boxer

1 The Widening Field of Healthcare Informatics

Patricia P. Sengstack, DNP, RN-BC, CPHIMS

OBJECTIVES

- Describe the need for healthcare informatics specialists.
- Highlight disciplines in the field of healthcare informatics.
- Discuss professional certifications available for practitioners of healthcare informatics.
- Identify core concepts of healthcare informatics pertinent for all disciplines.
- Reveal emerging trends in healthcare informatics.

Introduction to Informatics

The word *informatics* was introduced around 1957 and was believed to be Russian (from *informatika*) in origin (Informatics, n.d. c; Informatics, n.d. a). Other sources have postulated that it was coined in the 1960s and was influenced by the combination of the words *information* and *automatic* (Informatics, n.d. b). Regardless of its origin, informatics has come to represent a growing field with a focus on the use of technology and data to improve patient care.

The more formalized role of informatics that we see today emerged with the implementation of the electronic health record (EHR). As advancements in technology continue at a record pace and more organizations adopt EHRs, informatics continues to evolve. Several disciplines (nursing, medicine, pharmacology, nutrition, and dentistry) have developed informatics expertise within their respective domains, each adding their skills and knowledge to a dynamic field.

Informatics is not just about the EHR, though. Although the EHR remains at the core of informatics practice, many areas within informatics' scope deal with things peripheral or tangential to the EHR: for example, telehealth, use of mobile devices, patient portals, data analytics, use of technology for education, and conducting health IT research. Much of the focus of informatics work between 2003 and 2013 has clearly revolved around the EHR in the inpatient setting, but with changing payment models and care delivery systems consolidating and converging, informatics practice has begun to migrate outside the walls of the hospital and infiltrate new areas of practice.

This chapter introduces informatics within the domains of nursing, medicine, pharmacy, dentistry, and others, along with educational and certification efforts to ensure competency of this new field. It also provides an overview of the core elements of informatics practice as well as emerging trends.

History of Informatics

One might assume that the practice of informatics began in the 1960s; one could also argue, however, that at its core, informatics has been around for centuries. The medical record dates back to Hippocrates in the fifth century B.C. He noted that the patient's record should accurately reflect the course of the disease and indicate the probable cause of the disease—not too different from today's goals (National Institutes of Health National Center for Research Resources [NIH NCRR], 2006). Many have documented that the first informatics nurse was Florence Nightingale as she compiled and processed data to improve sanitation conditions in military hospitals during the Crimean War in the 1850s (Betts & Wright, 2006).

Fast-forward to the 1960s when the first electronic health records (EHRs) began to emerge. Most of this pioneering work occurred at our nation's academic medical centers and at major government clinical care organizations. Even in hospitals prior to the 1960s, personnel collected data and looked at trends to make inferences and improvements in care delivery. These practitioners were not "informaticists," nor did they have the advantage of the technology we have today, but they often served such a role within their quality control, risk management, and even administrative positions.

The Growing Need for Informaticists

The need for expertise in the field of informatics has undoubtedly increased since the signing of the American Reinvestment and Recovery Act (ARRA) in 2009. The ARRA included the authorization of the Health Information Technology for Economic and

Clinical Health (HITECH) Act, which allocated more than $17 billion to stimulate the adoption of quality health IT systems or EHRs that demonstrate meaningful use (Office of the National Coordinator for Health Information Technology [ONC], 2009). Organizations have become increasingly eager to adopt EHRs and receive sizeable incentive payments. In fact, the percentage of hospitals with certified EHR technology increased from 72% to 85% between 2011 and 2012. In 2012, nearly three-quarters of office-based physicians (72%) had adopted an EHR system, up from 42% in 2008 (ONC, 2013).

Meaningful Use

The phrase *meaningful use* was tagged to an initiative that the Office of the National Coordinator for Health Information Technology (ONC) introduced as part of the Health Information Technology for Economic and Clinical Health (HITECH) Act signed in 2009. This act, through the Centers for Medicare and Medicaid, provides incentive payments for hospitals and eligible professionals if they configure and use their EHR so that it meets a strict set of guidelines developed by the ONC that represent the best available evidence in the configuration of EHRs. The guidelines are being developed in three stages, with stages 1 and 2 focusing on processes and stage 3 targeting clinical outcomes resulting from EHR use.

As use of technology in healthcare becomes more and more pervasive, the need for a workforce that possesses the expertise necessary to successfully guide healthcare organizations to improve patient care increases. We have seen an emergence of informatics education and training at varying levels across domains, with each domain striving to build a profession with the right expertise.

The Various Informatics Domains

The nursing profession holds the longest track record of formal training using standard core competencies within the field of informatics. In 1992, the American Nurses Association (ANA) recognized informatics as a unique specialty and offered board certification (ANA, 2008). In 2013, the medical profession offered the first examination for board certification in the subspecialty of Clinical Informatics to primarily a physician group. Pharmacists, dentists, and other clinicians continue to evolve in their domain specialties. The following section will review the status of informatics practice among the various disciplines as well as the impact that the ARRA has had on the informatics profession as whole.

Nursing Informatics

As technology becomes increasingly pervasive, our nation's 3 million nurses are interacting with varying modes of hardware and software on a routine basis, and the need for nurses trained in informatics has become stronger than ever. To educate these specialists, universities began offering graduate education in Nursing Informatics, first at the University of Maryland and the University of Utah beginning in the 1980s. More than 40 Nursing Informatics graduate programs are now available across the United States, including several that are completely available online. Typical Nursing Informatics education is a Master's degree program, although some universities offer a post-Master's program for those who already possess another graduate degree. Post-Master's programs focus solely on informatics content and are typically of shorter duration than a full Master's degree.

Recognizing that the field of Nursing Informatics (NI) possesses a unique body of knowledge, the ANA recognized NI as an official specialty in 1992. The ANA published the *Nursing Informatics: Scope of Practice* in 2004, followed by *Standards of Practice* in 2005. Combined and updated versions were published in 2001 and again in 2008 (ANA, 2008). Another update is scheduled to be published. This document contains standards of professional practice for informatics nurses: 16 standard categories of informatics practice, with each including measurement criteria that describe the expected knowledge, skills, and abilities necessary to meet each standard. The ANA defines nursing informatics as:

> "A specialty that integrates nursing science, computer science, and information science to manage and communicate data, information, knowledge, and wisdom in nursing practice. Nursing informatics facilitates the integration of data, information, knowledge, and wisdom to support patients, nurses, and other providers in their decision-making in all roles and settings. This support is accomplished through the use of information structures, information processes, and information technology. The goal of nursing informatics is to improve the health of populations, communities, families and individuals by optimizing information management and communication" (ANA, 2008, p. 1).

With recognition as a specialty, the ANA, in conjunction with their subsidiary organization, the American Nurses Credentialing Center (ANCC), developed board certification in Nursing Informatics also beginning in 1992. In order to sit for the certification examination, several eligibility criteria must be met. These include (ANCC, 2014):

- Hold a current, active RN license within a state or territory of the United States or the professional, legally recognized equivalent in another country
- Hold a bachelor's or higher degree in nursing or a bachelor's degree in a relevant field
- Have practiced the equivalent of 2 years full-time as a registered nurse
- Have completed 30 hours of continuing education in informatics nursing within the last three years
- Meet one of the following practice hour requirements:
    - Have practiced a minimum of 2,000 hours in informatics nursing within the last 3 years
    - Have practiced a minimum of 1,000 hours in informatics nursing in the last 3 years and completed a minimum of 12 semester hours of academic credit in informatics courses that are part of a graduate-level informatics nursing program
    - Have completed a graduate program in informatics nursing containing a minimum of 200 hours of faculty-supervised practicum in informatics nursing

Upon successful completion of the Nursing Informatics certification exam, a nurse is eligible to add RN-BC (Registered Nurse – Board Certified) to her/his title designations.

Clinical Informatics

Physicians have also been practicing in the area of clinical informatics for several decades, but until recently, a core curriculum had not been formalized, standardized, or officially recognized as a board-certified subspecialty. Recognizing the need for physician leadership with the implementation of EHRs and computerized provider order entry (CPOE) systems in the 1990s, organizations began to recruit physicians into roles to help with design and workflow of these new systems (Friedman, 1990). Physicians serving in healthcare IT roles were typically those who showed technical savvy and felt comfortable in the use of technology but did not necessarily possess formal computer science or informatics training.

Informatics training was conducted in a variety of venues without a uniform curriculum. Most of the training was obtained on the job. One exception to this since the 1970s was the National Library of Medicine (NLM) support and funding of medical informatics post-doctoral fellowships. It was not until 2007, with financial support from the Robert Wood Johnson Foundation, that the American Medical Informatics Association (AMIA) began an initiative to identify and define the core content of the subspecialty of Clinical Informatics and determine the training requirements for proposed fellowships (AMIA, 2014a; Detmer, Lumpkin, & Williamson, 2009). The American Board of Preventive Medicine (ABPM) sponsored an application in 2009 for the new subspecialty of Clinical Informatics; and after an extensive review by the American Board of Medical Specialties (ABMS), the proposal was approved in September of 2011. The first Clinical Informatics board examination was conducted in the fall of 2013. Preparation and training for the exam and competency in Clinical Informatics is now available via the AMIA face-to-face Clinical Informatics Board Review Courses or its distance learning programs, called "10 X 10." These online training courses are conducted in collaboration with key academic partners in the biomedical and health informatics education community.

AMIA describes Clinical Informatics as the transformation of healthcare by analyzing, designing, implementing, and evaluating information and communication systems that enhance individual and population health outcomes, improve patient care, and strengthen the clinician-patient relationship. Clinical informaticists use their knowledge of patient care combined with their understanding of informatics concepts, methods, and tools to (AMIA, 2014b):

- Assess information and knowledge needs of healthcare professionals and patients;
- Characterize, evaluate, and refine clinical processes;
- Develop, implement, and refine clinical decision support systems; and
- Lead or participate in the procurement, customization, development, implementation, management, evaluation, and continuous improvement of clinical information systems, such as electronic health records and order-entry systems.

To be eligible to take the Clinical Informatics certification, the following criteria must be met (ABPM, 2013):

- Current certification by at least one of the Member Boards of ABMS is required.
- Graduation is required from a medical school in the United States.
- Unrestricted and currently valid license(s) to practice medicine is required.
- Completion of one of the following:
  - Three years of practice in Clinical Informatics
  - Fellowship program of at least 24 months in duration

Pharmacy Informatics

Given that EHRs with CPOE are becoming increasingly prevalent, it only makes sense that pharmacists develop expertise in informatics. The medication-ordering process is complex and nonlinear with the potential for errors always a risk, and that's with or without technology. The American Society of Health-System Pharmacists (ASHP) recognizes Pharmacy Informatics as a unique subset of medical informatics with a focus on the use of information technology and drug information to optimize medication use (ASHP, 2007). ASHP uses the term "Medical Informatics" (MI) and states that MI in pharmacy is focused on safe and effective medication selection and prescribing, verification, dispensing, administration, and monitoring of medication therapy (ASHP, 2007). As this discipline has evolved, the development of core competencies has been documented and disseminated throughout the Pharmacy Informatics community. At the core, ASHP states that pharmacists must use their knowledge of information systems and the medication-use process to improve patient care by ensuring that new technologies lead to safer and more effective medication use (ASHP, 2007; Fox, Thrower, & Felkey, 2010).

Formal training via ASHP–accredited informatics residency training programs are few, but the numbers are growing. Pharmacists interested in formal training programs have gone outside the pharmacy profession and obtained a Master's degree in Healthcare Informatics. As of this writing, board certification in Pharmacy Informatics does not exist.

Dental Informatics

Another evolving discipline is Dental Informatics. The clinical systems used in dentistry today are sophisticated, complex, and graphic-laden. Educating professionals with skills in not only the practice of dentistry but also the application and management of technology is increasingly important. If practicing dentists wish to qualify for the EHR adoption meaningful use incentive program under the HITECH Act, there is a clear need for trained informatics expertise to facilitate implementation of certified EHRs, capture data for data analysis, and track patient outcomes.

As early as 1996, the NLM and the National Institute of Dental and Craniofacial Research (NIDCR) funded Dental Informatics training programs at three universities. Funding continues to increase for these programs which train both predoctoral and postdoctoral trainees. Despite this growth, dentistry has been slow to develop and define a standard set of dental informatics competencies for predoctoral students and dental informaticists (Zimmerman, Ball, & Petroski, 1986).

Pioneers in the field of Dental Informatics continue to formalize their approach and strategy to define, train, and ensure competence for professionals serving in these roles (Zimmerman & Ball, 1992). As Dental Informatics evolves, consensus on core competencies will develop, with the potential for providing certification.

Informatics in Other Disciplines

As EHR adoption increases, the need for trained professionals to design, build, test, train, implement, maintain, and evaluate these clinical systems becomes increasingly apparent. Clinicians in fields other than nursing, medicine, pharmacy, and dentistry have made transitions to the world of informatics. Many respiratory therapists, physical therapists, medical technicians, dietitians, and others have made the move to the field of informatics. To prepare and train this workforce, the Office of the National Coordinator for Health Information Technology (ONC) has provided expertise and funding to community colleges and universities across the nation at the undergraduate and graduate levels as they support the training mission. As part of the HITECH Act, ONC Workforce Development Programs have built a solid foundation of complete curricula, adaptable curricula materials, and training capacity within a network of more than 90 of the nation's community colleges and universities (ONC, 2014). More information and informatics training opportunities can be found on the ONC website at

http://www.healthit.gov/providers-professionals/workforce-development-programs

As a result of the work of ONC, the opportunities for formal education have grown nationwide for both onsite and remote classroom training. In fact, 81 colleges in five regions have collectively trained more than 17,000 professionals since the launch of the Community College Consortia Program. The University-Based Training Program exceeded its enrollment goal of 1,685 students. As of February 2013, 1,747 students had enrolled in one of these informatics programs, and an Internet search using the term, "healthcare informatics training programs" yields thousands of results (ONC, 2013).

Healthcare Informatics Certifications for All Disciplines

Informatics professionals interested in becoming certified in the field of informatics but who do not meet the eligibility criteria for ANCC (nurses) or ABMS (physicians) exams have other options for certification that are offered through professional organizations.

American Health Information Management Association (AHIMA)

The Commission on Certification for Health Informatics and Information Management (CCHIIM) is an AHIMA commission dedicated to ensuring the competency of professionals practicing healthcare informatics. CCHIIM establishes, implements, and enforces standards and procedures for certification and recertification of health informatics professionals. More information on this certification can be found on the AHIMA website (AHIMA, 2014) at

http://www.ahima.org/certification/cchiim

Health Information and Management Systems Society (HIMSS)

HIMSS has offered certifications in the field of healthcare informatics for several years. This examination can be taken by clinical and nonclinical professionals. Its Certified Professional in Healthcare Information & Management Systems (CPHIMS) credential is felt to be a designation that distinguishes informatics workers in an increasingly competitive workplace and demonstrates one's commitment to continuing professional development. Eligibility requirements for the CPHIMS exam include:

- Baccalaureate degree from an accredited college or university plus 5 years of information and management systems experience, 3 of those years in a healthcare setting
- Graduate degree or higher from an accredited college or university plus 3 years of information and management systems experience, 2 of those years in a healthcare setting

HIMSS also offers the Certified Associate in Healthcare Information & Management Systems (CAHIMS). This credential is for emerging informatics professionals with less than 5 years of experience in healthcare IT. Eligibility for the CAHIMS examination requires a high school diploma or equivalent. Information on both of these certifications can be found at

http://www.himss.org/health-it-certification

American Society of Health Information Managers (ASHIM)

ASHIM offers the Certified Health Informatics Systems Professional (CHISP) credential to its members indicating that a professional has met a defined set of skills-based competencies believed to be needed by professionals working in the healthcare IT field, regardless of their discipline. Rooted in informatics core competencies to reflect the nature of the field, it is designed to validate the dedication and professionalism of those who successfully complete it. Eligibility requirements to sit for the CHISP exam include:

- Member of ASHIM and one of the following:
  - Successful completion of the ASHIM Health IT Professional online training program
  - Three years working IT experience

More information on this certification can be found at

http://www.ashim.org/health-it-certification

Core Elements for All Informatics Disciplines

Despite the fact that unique discipline-specific areas of informatics expertise are needed as technology evolves and is used by multiple types of end users, a core set of concepts provide the foundation of informatics practice. These concepts encompass some of the essential knowledge areas regardless of discipline that span the field of informatics, beginning with the components of the system development life cycle (Planning and Analysis, Design and Usability, Testing, Training, Implementation, Maintenance, and Evaluation). These components or phases represent the "must-knows" for anyone serving in an informatics role, and an overview of each will be presented here. Additionally, the key areas of project management, security and privacy, and clinical decision support are covered, and then followed by some of the latest emerging trends. Subsequent chapters provide a deeper look into tools, resources, and reference materials to allow practical application to the practice setting.

Planning and Analysis

Whether you are planning for the initial implementation of an EHR, an addition of a module to a current EHR, or even just a slight enhancement to your current system, the planning and analysis phase lays the foundation for the entire project. The initial planning for any health IT project requires more than just ensuring that the technology will function properly within the current IT infrastructure. Before the project even starts, there are multiple considerations to ensure success. Assessing organizational readiness and looking at such considerations as current workflow, organizational policies/procedures, consensus from key stakeholders, culture and politics, and the people involved are all aspects of a project that need attention. Multiple tools are available with which to assess an organization's readiness for IT implementation; Chapter 2 describes several of these tools. Using these tools along with a framework, such as the Sittig and Singh (2010) socio-technical model for health IT, the planning phase can be more robust than ever. Answer the following questions as you begin the planning phase of any health IT project:

- What is the problem you are trying to solve?
    - Answering this question helps lay the foundation for the metrics that you want to consider collecting as part of your evaluation: for example, *We want to reduce medication errors; We want to be made aware of when the patient has an abnormal lab value; We want to save paper*; or *We want to spend less time documenting.*
    - Sometimes technology is not the right answer to the particular problem. If you begin with a dysfunctional process and then you add technology, guess where blame is pointed?
- What is the current workflow for this process?
    - Mapping workflow will help identify those dysfunctional processes.
    - Mapping workflow will also help determine opportunities for streamlining processes and potentially eliminating duplication.
- Have you identified all the key stakeholders for the proposed project?
    - Without all the right people at the table from the project's inception, success will be a challenge.
    - Ensure that you have strong administrative support.

CAUTION

Never forget to include the people who will be using the system (or system change) in your planning.

Design and Usability

Determining what the screens will look like as well as how they will link to one another and how the end user will navigate between them, all comprise the human-computer interface. It is imperative that end users assist in the design. This point cannot be over emphasized. If the end users do not assist with the design of something they will be using, the chances of success become less and less probable. There has been a significant amount of work and research in the field of usability in the healthcare IT arena (HIMSS, 2009). We have learned that there are some key concepts to keep in mind when designing the human-computer interface. Some of these concepts are listed here, with more details available in Chapter 3:

- Consistency
  - On medication ordering screens: The location of the drug name, dose, frequency, and route should always be in the same place for every drug.
  - The Save button should always be located in the same place on the screen: for example, not on the bottom right for some screens, and the top right for others.
- Forgiveness and feedback
  - Any warning messages that appear should give the user instructions on how to fix the issue: for example, *Must enter value in dose field.*
  - Provide users the ability to go back (move to an earlier screen) without losing any of their work.
- Minimize cognitive load
  - Develop workflows to reduce the number of screens (or clicks) a user must go through to get to what they need.
  - Do not require users to have to remember something several screens back when entering data. Provide all the relevant information on the current screen.
- Simplicity
  - Less is best. Display only what is needed to accomplish the particular task.
  - Keep the screens as uncluttered as possible. Make good use of onscreen space.

Testing

Software testing for health IT projects is often not given the attention and rigor that it should. Many of you reading this can attest to the fact that testing is sometimes cut short to save time in order to get the system or the change into the production environment in the promised time frame. Additionally, time is saved by having the person making the system changes also be the person to conduct the testing.

CAUTION

The person building the software and the person testing the software should be two different people.

There are several types of testing designed to cover the key functions and scenarios or use cases in a healthcare IT environment. For each project, the testing plan should be developed early in the lifecycle. But face it—there are far too many individual logistical pathways to ensure testing of every possible combination. For that reason, a sound testing methodology is needed that includes the following types of testing (as described in Chapter 4):

- Unit testing
- Functional testing
- Integration testing
- Regression testing
- Performance testing
- User acceptance testing

Training

Effective end-user training is a key element to an implementation's success. The type of training required depends on the implementation project. For the installation of a new EHR, a classroom model of education will most likely be needed. If you are adding only a new module to a current system, computer or web-based training may be adequate. If the change is a simple addition to current functionality, a "cheat sheet" or just-in-time training may suffice. An organization's training team now has tools, models, and frameworks available from which to develop materials and deliver content to system users. Chapter 5 describes these resources and includes case examples.

TIP

Never underestimate the value of a well-trained end-user community.

Implementation

Preparations for a system activation or a "go-live" take a considerable amount of planning, right down to the very minute in some cases. It is never just a case of flipping a switch or popping in a CD. The planning for a system's actual implementation requires a multidisciplinary approach, with a team that must work in concert to ensure that events occur in the right sequence and at the right time. Events that occur during a go-live include minute-by-minute instructions, such as blocking end users from accessing the system, stopping interface messages, updating security components, starting interface messages—the list goes on for pages. The level of detail needed during implementation is probably more than any other phase of the system lifecycle, and attention to each of the events that occur during go-live will lead to the best chance of a smooth roll out. Chapter 6 presents strategies, tools, and checklists that help coordinate activities surrounding implementation.

Maintenance

After a system is up and running, it does not simply go on autopilot. Care and maintenance are required to keep it functioning properly. Routine software updates, security updates, and enhancements to the system itself are constantly needed. Using best practice methodologies to develop a maintenance plan to handle system changes is essential to a highly functioning system. The processes to support configuration and change management after a system is implemented should be evidence-based. These practices or processes may have their roots in industries outside healthcare, but they provide sound approaches that can help avoid some common pitfalls of system management. Chapter 7 describes components of the IT Infrastructure Library (ITIL) framework and maintenance of clinical systems.

Evaluation

Technology is advancing faster than organizations can consume it and develop the processes and policies to support it. Given this, we find it hard to stop and take the time to allocate the resources needed to conduct evaluations on the outcomes of our work. Did the technology meet the desired need? Did the CPOE system reduce medication errors? Did the patient portal increase patient engagement and reduce readmissions? Was the alert to reduce the number of days a urinary catheter stayed in place effective? We have found that evaluation studies of the highest quality have traditionally been conducted at the larger academic medical centers and required grant money to bring in resources with the right skill set. Chapter 8 provides tools and guidelines to conduct a straightforward quality outcome evaluation study that can provide information regarding the effectiveness your organization's EHR.

Project Management

A 2012 global survey conducted by PricewaterhouseCoopers (PricewaterhouseCoopers, 2012) on the current state of project management reported that as many as 97% of respondents believe that project management is critical to business performance and organizational success. Not only is it essential for organizations to manage their projects effectively and strategically, but poor execution can lead organizations down a path of disappointment. Interestingly, a subsequent Project Management Institute (PMI) study found that since 2008, the percentage of projects that project managers say have met their original goals and business intent has declined from 72% in 2008 to 62% in 2012 (PMI, 2013). This speaks to the importance—especially in healthcare IT—for the use of evidence-based principles when managing projects. Healthcare IT projects are complex, costly, and integral to an organization's care delivery processes as well as the bottom line. Informatics professionals working in project-management roles can find effective and essential project-management skills described in Chapter 9.

Security and Privacy

The buzz of security and privacy in health IT has been getting louder and louder as technology expands outside the walls of the hospital and becomes increasingly more mobile. News of vulnerabilities of health-system technology are being exposed and publicized at a rate that is making the buzz even louder. Changes to the Health Insurance Portability and Accountability Act (HIPAA) rules that influence how we manage our clinical systems are challenging to keep up with and operationalize. Chapter 10 presents foundational concepts of health IT security and privacy that informaticists can use to evaluate their systems and help keep personal information where it belongs.

Clinical Decision Support

HIMSS defines *clinical decision support (CDS)* as "a process for enhancing health-related decisions and actions with pertinent, organized clinical knowledge and patient information to improve health and healthcare delivery" (HIMSS, 2011, p. 1). Other definitions—and there are several—are equally vague. Type "definition of clinical decision support" into your search engine, and you will get myriad hits.

Thinking of CDS as an umbrella concept that comprises a number of methods or operations that can be configured into an EHR is helpful. CDS is using technology to get the right information to the right provider, at the right time, for the right patient. It can include access to information from within the EHR (links to PubMed or drug databases), evidence-based order sets, alerts and reminders, and various reports. Chapter 11 reviews several types of CDS so you can explore how they may apply to your setting and evaluate their effectiveness.

Emerging Trends in Informatics

The concepts discussed in this chapter represent foundational knowledge in the field of informatics. Elevating your informatics practice to the next level is difficult without a firm understanding of these concepts. With technology continually advancing and applications of technology expanding, it becomes imperative to develop a firm grasp on these foundational concepts so they can be applied to the many emerging trends that we are seeing today. The following list contains the topics becoming increasingly prevalent in today's healthcare IT environment. The last seven chapters of this book provide you with more resources, tools, and ideas to help your organization tackle some of these significant technology initiatives.

- Chapter 12, "Use of Standard Terminologies in Healthcare IT": Ensuring use of standard terminologies in the EHR to improve the ability to evaluate and assess effectiveness of care
- Chapter 13, "Patient Safety and Health Information Technology": Assessing the ability for your EHR to improve the safety of care delivery as well as ensuring that your EHR is not the cause of medical errors
- Chapter 14, "Patient Engagement in Healthcare IT": Getting the patient involved, using a patient portal or personal health record (PHR)
- Chapter 15, "Informatics in Non-Acute Care Settings": Increasing your knowledge of emerging technologies in settings such as ambulatory care, home health, hospice, and long-term care

- Chapter 16, "Healthcare Analytics": Covering data analytics/big data/population management; effectively managing the geopbytes of data out there lurking in our electronic records (one of the hottest topics in the field of informatics today)
- Chapter 17, "Connected and Mobile Health's Promise for the Triple Aim": Providing care and entering data in real time from anywhere using a tablet, smartphone, or laptop

Conclusion

The adoption of healthcare IT across the nation is in its infancy. Several hundred hospitals, ambulatory practices, long-term care facilities, and home health and hospice agencies have still not yet adopted electronic records. The trend to do so is increasing, but the fact is clear that the work ahead will continue to need resources with the right skills. Informatics specialists can help drive the work of the nation to ensure as we move forward that evidence-based best practices be used in designing, building, testing, training, implementing, maintaining, and evaluating our clinical systems. Building that solid knowledge base upon which to grow starts with the key concepts offered in this book.

References

American Board of Preventive Medicine (ABPM). (2013). *Clinical informatics requirements for board certification*. Chicago, IL: The American Board of Preventive Medicine. Retrieved from http://www.theabpm.org/abpm_clinical_informatics.pdf

American Health Information Management Association (AHIMA). (2014). *Certification*. Chicago, IL: American Health Information Management Association. Retrieved from http://www.ahima.org/certification/cchiim

American Medical Informatics Association (AMIA). (2014a). *Clinical informatics board review course*. Bethesda, MD: American Medical Informatics Association. Retrieved from http://www.amia.org/clinical-informatics-board-review-course/history

American Medical Informatics Association (AMIA). (2014b). *The Science of informatics*. Bethesda, MD: American Medical Informatics Association. Retrieved from http://www.amia.org/about-amia/science-informatics

American Nurses Association (ANA). (2008). *Nursing informatics: Scope and standards of practice*. Silver Spring, MD: American Nurses Association. Retrieved from http://nursesbooks.org/

American Nurses Credentialing Center (ANCC). (2014). *Informatics nursing certification eligibility criteria*. Silver Spring, MD: American Nurses Credentialing Center. Retrieved from http://www.nursecredentialing.org/Informatics-Eligibility.aspx

American Society of Health-System Pharmacists. (2007). ASHP statement on the pharmacist's role in informatics. *American Journal of Health-System Pharmacy, 64*(2), 200–203.

Betts, H. J., & Wright, G. (2006). Lessons on evidence-based practice from Florence Nightingale. In C.A. Weaver, C. W. Delaney, P. Weber, & R. L. Carr, (Eds.), *Nursing informatics for the 21st century: An international look at practice, trends and the future*, 1st ed. (pp. 285–289). Chicago, IL: HIMSS.

Detmer, D., Lumpkin, J., & Williamson. J. (2009). Defining the medical subspecialty of clinical informatics. *Journal of the American Medical Informatics Association, 16*(2), 167–168.

Fox, B., Thrower, M. R., & Felkey, B.G. (2010). *Building core competencies in pharmacy informatics.* Washington, DC: American Pharmacists Association; Pharmacy Library. Retrieved from http://pharmacylibrary.com/resource/19

Friedman, B. A. (1990). The potential role of physicians in the management of hospital information systems. *Clinics in Laboratory Medicine, 10*, 239–250.

Healthcare Information and Management Systems Society (HIMSS). (2009). *Defining and testing EMR usability: principles and proposed methods of EMR usability evaluation and rating.* HIMSS EHR Usability Task Force. Chicago, IL: Healthcare Information and Management Systems Society. Retrieved from http://www.himss.org/files/HIMSSorg/content/files/himss_definingandtestingemrusability.pdf

Healthcare Information and Management Systems Society (HIMSS). (2011). *Clinical decision support. What is clinical decision support?* Chicago, IL: Healthcare Information and Management Systems Society. Retrieved from http://www.himss.org/library/clinical-decision-support

Informatics. (n.d. a). In *American Heritage Dictionary* online (4th ed.). Retrieved from http://www.yourdictionary.com/ics-suffix

Informatics. (n.d. b). In *Merriam-Webster online dictionary* (11th ed.). Retrieved from http://www.merriamwebster.com/dictionary/informatics

Informatics. (n.d. c). In *Oxford Dictionaries* online (4th ed.). Retrieved from http://www.oxforddictionaries.com/definition/english/informatics

National Institutes of Health National Center for Research Resources (NIH NCRR). (2006). *Electronic health records overview.* McLean, VA: The MITRE Corporation (contractor). Retrieved from http://www.himss.org/files/HIMSSorg/content/files/Code%20180%20MITRE%20Key%20Components%20of%20an%20EHR.pdf

Office of the National Coordinator for Health Information Technology (ONC). (2009). *Certification and EHR incentives, HITECH Act 2009.* Washington, DC: The Office of the National Coordinator for Health Information Technology. Retrieved from http://www.healthit.gov/policy-researchers-implementers/health-it-legislation-and-regulations

Office of the National Coordinator for Health Information Technology (ONC). (2013). *Update on the adoption of health information technology and related efforts to facilitate the electronic use and exchange of health information: A report to Congress.* Washington, DC: The Office of the National Coordinator for Health Information Technology. Retrieved from http://www.healthit.gov/sites/default/files/rtc_adoption_of_healthit_and_relatedefforts.pdf

Office of the National Coordinator for Health Information Technology (ONC). (2014). *Workforce development programs.* Washington, DC: The Office of the National Coordinator for Health Information Technology. Retrieved from http://www.healthit.gov/providers-professionals/workforce-development-programs

PricewaterhouseCoopers. (2012). *Insights and trends: Current portfolio, programme, and project management practices.* New York, NY: PwC. Retrieved from http://www.pwc.com/en_US/us/public-sector/assets/pwc-global-project-management-report-2012.pdf

Project Management Institute, Inc. (2013). *PMI's pulse of the profession: The high cost of low performance.* Newtown Square, PA: Project Management Institute. Retrieved from http://www.pmi.org/~/media/PDF/Business-Solutions/PMI-Pulse%20Report-2013Mar4.ashx

Sittig, D., & Singh, H. (2010). A new socio-technical model for studying health information technology in complex adaptive healthcare systems. *Quality and Safety in Health Care, 19*(Suppl 3), i68–i74.

Zimmerman, J. L., Ball, M. J., & Petroski, S. P. (1986). Computers in Dentistry. *Dental Clinics of North America, 30*(4), 739–743.

Zimmerman, J. L., & Ball, M. J. (1992). Model for informatics knowledge and informatics in the dental curriculum. In L. Abbey & J. L. Zimmerman (Eds.), *Dental informatics: Integrating technology into the dental environment* (pp. 165–177). New York, NY: Springer.

"By failing to prepare, you are preparing to fail."

–Benjamin Franklin

Healthcare Informatics Planning and Analysis

2

Marcy Stoots, DNP, MS, RN-BC

Healthcare IT projects are often large and complex. They involve a variety of stakeholders, including clinicians, IT staff, various organizational executives and boards, patients, and (in today's era of healthcare reform and population health management) even communities at large. Cost-containment initiatives, such as value-based purchasing and pay-for-performance, are driving tighter fiscal organizational constraints. Worse, many headlines and stories are circulating about healthcare IT projects failing, monies being wasted, and clinicians who are very frustrated because they cannot use the system as intended.

Although large-scale projects of this magnitude might sound overwhelming, adequate planning and a sharp focus on critical success factors can mitigate the feeling. Informaticists need to execute strong planning and quality readiness assessments for new technology initiatives. The goal is to deliver clinical technology on time, within budget, and with high rates of clinical adoption and clinician satisfaction that demonstrate value and quality.

OBJECTIVES

- Develop an understanding of critical success factors that are essential for planning successful healthcare informatics initiatives.
- Develop an understanding of the necessary key components to consider when conducting system selection and readiness assessments.
- Describe the importance of defining future state workflows and consider imperative planning factors to ensure successful adoption and hardwiring of the change.
- Describe ongoing system support and optimization considerations as part of effective planning along with their rationale.

The role of the informaticist is threefold:

- Understand the critical factors for success.
- Continually communicate and execute the factors for success.
- Be certain the factors for success are woven into the fabric of every planned healthcare IT initiative.

Critical Success Factors

Numerous factors play a role in successful healthcare IT implementations. These factors represent a combination of experience from numerous lessons learned and evidence in helping to prepare organizations for challenging and large-scale healthcare IT projects. These essential planning ingredients boil down to seven critical success factors:

- A clearly defined vision with guiding principles
- Adequate leadership engagement and executive sponsorship
- Robust governance and decision-making
- Effective and bidirectional communication with all stakeholders
- Adequate end-user engagement
- Baseline and ongoing benefits measurement and value realization
- Comprehensive workflow-based training and adequate "at the elbow" support

Health IT project success starts and ends with these success factors in mind. They should be built into every project's checklist during the initiation phase. Establish open communication with the project sponsor about these factors from the very beginning. The following section will review each of these factors and provide examples for informatics specialists to lay the foundation for success.

Vision and Guiding Principles

Without a clear path to a goal and a clear understanding of what you are trying to accomplish, project teams often flounder when attempting to establish a successful endpoint. It is therefore absolutely essential to have a clear vision defined from the start. Bring together key stakeholders and facilitate a discussion until everyone agrees on the vision of the initiative. It may take some conflict-negotiation skills to get everyone to agree to a common vision, but the effort is well worth taking the time to do this at the start. Everything you do afterward will be based upon this common vision: It is, therefore, mission critical to get this right. All projects that are undertaken should be linked to an organization's strategic goals, so make sure the project's vision statement aligns with the organization's strategic goals. An example vision statement follows.

> (Insert name of project) will provide (insert name) health system with reliable and actionable point-of-care data to generate information for timely decision-making in order to reduce costs, improve clinical outcomes, and generate new market growth.

After you define the vision, the next step is to establish guiding principles. Guiding principles are foundational in supporting the vision and project objectives. Their purpose is to get all stakeholders on the same page: If someone wants to veer course or change direction, the guiding principles can be reviewed and revisited to keep the project on track.

Informatics in Action

While implementing computerized provider order entry (CPOE), a health system established a guiding principle that all order sets would be standardized across the enterprise. Two weeks before going live, yielding to intense physician pressure, the Chief Medical Officer (CMO) decided the surgeons needed individual and highly customized order sets. This would have taken the project off track and put it behind schedule. Additionally, the customized order sets were not evidence-based. The project sponsor brought the executive leadership team together and reminded them of the guiding principles they had agreed to—specifically, that all order sets would be standardized and evidence-based. As a result, and after some discussion, the CMO changed course and agreed (with full support from the executive team) to move forward without individual customized order sets for surgeons.

Some example guiding principles for an analytics project:

- The electronic health record (EHR) is the source of truth for all clinical data.
- Accurate and high quality data will be available to the right people and at the right time for point-of-care decision-making across the continuum of care.

- Documentation will take place in real time, in the right format, and in the right location in the EHR.

Leadership Engagement and Executive Sponsorship

Every project needs an executive sponsor, period. Without an executive sponsor to support the team during challenging times and to help you clear hurdles and negotiate political landmines, the project will be more than frustrating and perhaps even fail. The role of a project sponsor includes acting as the champion, providing clear direction, facilitating the securing of adequate funding and resources, and working with the project team to resolve high priority issues. This sponsor can also help get other leaders on board.

Remember, though, that you are working on clinical IT projects. And even though they are based on technology, and IT drives the installation of the hardware and software, these projects absolutely should not have an IT executive as the project sponsor. Operational leaders need to own these projects from the beginning, because these are projects that impact and drive clinical care. For example, a physician documentation project typically should have the Chief Medical Officer (CMO) as the project sponsor; and a Meaningful Use project should have an operational leader as a project sponsor; such as a Chief Clinical Officer (CCO) or Chief Quality Officer (CQO).

Governance and Decision-Making

Effective decision-making coupled with strong governance to manage issues and variations in practice is mission critical. Every organization has its own version of a governance model. However, Davis and Stoots (2012b) claim the most effective models employ a three-tiered approach, as depicted in Figure 2.1

With this three-tiered model:

- The highest level of governance answers the questions of *what* will be done and *who* will do it.
- The middle layer determines *how* it will get done.
- The lowest level designs the details.

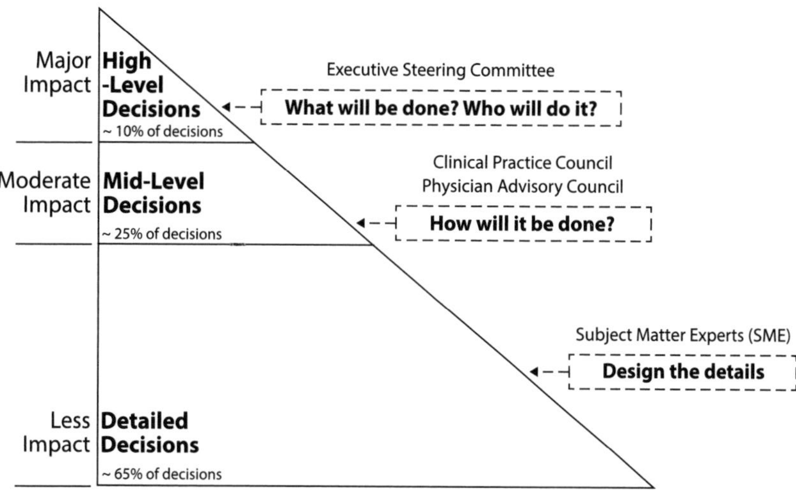

FIGURE 2.1 Three-tier governance model. Reprinted with permission from Davis, C. and Stoots, M. *A Guide to EHR Adoption: Implementation Through Organizational Transformation*. Chicago: HIMSS; 2012.

Typically, the highest level of governance comprises executives and senior leaders, the middle level consists of directors and managers, and the lowest level consists of subject matter experts (SMEs). Many organizations define these SMEs as "super users" or "end user champions." Often, these SMEs or super users will stay engaged with the system long after it is implemented to ensure ongoing support and optimization.

It is important to use these governance groups to manage variations. For example, suppose that you are designing an analytics project with the guiding principles described earlier, and the Quality Management SMEs decide that they want to use data from a separate system versus the EHR. This variation could impact the quality and accuracy of the data. Leveraging your governance groups to decide whether this variance is acceptable (or not) is an excellent way to manage these kinds of issues. Ask the Quality Management SMEs to present their rationale to the middle tier of governance: If they cannot decide or not agree, take it to the top tier of governance for a final decision.

Bidirectional Communication

Have you ever thought you were working on the right things and trying to fix the right issues for clinical end users, and then you find out that it is not at all the actual problem that needs to be solved? Hence, having effective *bidirectional communication*—that is, understanding what the end users are actually experiencing or expect to experience as a result of project decisions—is an essential planning component.

As an informaticist, you can lead efforts to communicate in a variety of ways. One, having standardized messaging is important so that everyone affected by the project hears the same message and has the same understanding of what is happening. Messages can be delivered via email; by attendance at departmental meetings; in town hall meetings; or in today's era of technology, via the Internet or social media (if your organization's policy permits this type of venue for communication).

Second, from a planning perspective, make sure you have someone designated as part of the project team to focus on communication. You must constantly communicate what you are working on and the value it brings, as well as the benefits to the clinicians and patients.

Leverage your super users and SMEs to achieve bidirectional focus and to clearly understand the true impact of the design to those who will be using it every day as part of the patient-care delivery process.

End-User Engagement

The most successful projects engage the people that are impacted the most from the project's implementation in the design. How many times have you heard, "We can't pull the nurses to help with the design—they are too busy taking care of patients." As an informaticist, your role is to work with the project sponsor in obtaining funding, as part of the project start up, to ensure that there are funds to backfill clinicians and SMEs to participate in the design so the system is designed right the first time. There are numerous examples where projects failed and enormous amounts of money were wasted because a system was designed without the right people at the table.

Securing support and funding for backfilling may be a hard selling point, especially in today's economic climate. One way to garner support for this is to do a cost-benefit analysis. Are there other projects in the organization that have failed because end users were not fully engaged? What did it cost the organization to rework these projects in the past? By examining lessons learned from other projects and quantifying the costs, you may be more successful in securing adequate funding for backfilling end users so they can fully participate in design, testing, training, and ongoing support.

Benefits Measurement and Value Realization

In today's era of cost constraints, measuring benefits and demonstrating value with every clinical IT initiative is essential from the start and on an ongoing basis. Have you ever been on a diet and lost some weight, only to find a few months later that you gained it all back? You probably went back to some old bad habits. The same thing happens with newly designed workflows and processes.

To ensure measuring benefits and demonstrating value is consistent and continual:

- **Engage stakeholders to define and *own* baseline metrics and ongoing measurements.** Ask them *how* they will define success. Get them to own the metrics—meaning that if it is a quality metric, have a discussion with the CQO to define the metric and ask for support in ongoing monitoring and adoption of the tools and processes to support the metric. Get them to validate the baseline metrics as well as ongoing measurements.
- **Consider surveying clinicians and patients about their satisfaction with the system as part of your measurements.** Often the loudest voices will be heard the most, and if you have surveys with results that do not match the same sentiment as the "squeaky wheels," it will go a long way in supporting appropriate system improvements. It will also help you get some factual data as to how the system is actually perceived by the people that are using it on a day-to-day basis, so that, if necessary, you can put an action plan around improving usability and the overall user experience.
- **Engage the finance team in your organization.** You need to constantly evaluate what you are working on and how it will reduce costs and improve efficiency and outcomes.

- **Focus on metrics that go outside the four walls of the hospital.** How will the project improve care across the continuum?

Examples of metrics are shown in Table 2.1.

Table 2.1 Example Benefit Realization Metric for a Patient Portal Project

Metric	*Organization Owner*	*Baseline Target*	*(Monthly) Actual*
Patient satisfaction with 24-hour access to personal health information via the patient portal	CQO	4.0 on a Likert scale of 1–5	4.2
Reduce denials due to improved accuracy of documentation of medications administered via the eMAR	CFO	25% reduction in denials	15% reduction in denials
Reduce number of physician call backs for medication reconciliation issues during first homecare visit post discharge	CMO	30% call back rate reduction	20% call back rate reduction

Workflow-Based Training and Ongoing Support

One of the hardest things to do with any project is to provide high-quality workflow-based training. Keep these factors in mind as you prepare for training that will ensure success:

- It is never too early to start working on training materials. Engage the training team or those responsible for training from the start.

- Competencies must be measured. Give some thought to how you will measure that users truly understand how to use the system *safely*. As an example, physicians should be assessed for competency, as part of their training, in their ability to enter complex orders, such as titratable drips or sliding scale insulin dosages.
- Always design training from a clinical workflow perspective versus simply "point-and-click" functionality. Having SMEs engaged in designing this will steer you along the right path. For example, instead of showing users how to navigate a screen or a form, show them how to admit a patient to the unit, incorporating the system into their workflow, versus just showing them how to use a form on a screen.
- Set expectations as to what you will train on specifically. There are many examples of doomed training where end users assume training will teach "everything." This is just not possible. Get agreement from your sponsor and governance regarding the amount of training, including how much time it will take, as well as exactly what will be trained. Develop training objectives and a training strategy and get your executive sponsor and governance group to sign off on the strategy and objectives.
- Remember that training should be just in time: meaning, not too far ahead of the go-live date, and ideally no more than four to six weeks in advance of a system implementation, lest clinicians forget what they have been taught. Also, training should be mandatory. Otherwise, clinicians will not find the time to attend training.
- Plan for training space and logistics. Often, training space and equipment are at a premium. If you need to train a large number of clinicians, determine costs and reserve space well in advance of training events.
- Post workflow-based training materials on the intranet with some frequently asked questions (FAQs) that end users can access quickly when they have a question.
- Training never ends. Plan for ongoing training including upgrades and advanced functionality.

Think broadly, not just about go-live support, but ongoing support. This is where having SMEs engaged from the beginning in designing the workflows and communicating with them routinely will be beneficial. Having super user SMEs who are "go-to" experts at the unit level will help ensure that knowledgeable, ongoing support is available. However, an additional support area to plan for is "at-the-elbow" support, meaning support in the setting where clinicians are practicing and at the time they need it. The IT department will provide help desk support that resolves technical issues, password resets, and so on. However, you will need workflow and system experts to support the clinicians at the time they need support and in their care-delivery settings. The number of staff required for ongoing at-the-elbow support is dependent upon the amount of change being implemented and the impact to operations.

Be sure to measure what type of at-the-elbow support you are providing: In other words, understand what the issues and questions are and how the team is supporting end users. You must demonstrate the value of the resources, what they are working on, and how they help clinicians.

Look for patterns and trends in this data as you collect it. Bring variations in practice to the attention of governance and safety issues to your risk management department. Provide the team with rounding topics for issues that frequently come up or particularly challenging workflows. Be proactive versus reactive.

Leading Practices: System Selection, Readiness, and Workflow

This section introduces leading practices on selecting clinical systems, determining and measuring readiness for implementations, and the importance of workflow analysis. The role of an informaticist in these activities, along with some helpful tools and tips, will be discussed.

System Selection

As a healthcare informatics expert, you will be asked to engage and work with operational leaders and teams on system selection. Your focus should be on analyzing the proposed technology for how it can be best leveraged to align with strategic initiatives and working with stakeholders to determine the requirements.

First, understand the problem to be solved. You will need to serve in a role of "translator": that is, translating the clinical requirements into technical capabilities of the system. Clinical needs should drive the technology, not the other way around.

Think broadly. In other words, ask questions such as these:

- Is a "best of breed" application with minimal integration the best choice to manage care across the continuum?
- Is it better to leverage existing vendors with fewer interfaces?
- How will discrete data be captured and available to ends users at the point of care?

Oftentimes, clinicians and executives will go to conferences or get calls from vendors about some late-breaking, trail-blazing technology, and they may call asking your opinion or asking you to participate in an analysis of new technology. Your role is to fully analyze the impact and value of new technology and advise on the best course of action. One tool that can help you do this is a key decision document that can be brought to governance for a decision. An example of a key decision document can be found in Table 2.2.

Table 2.2 Key Decision Document for System Selection

Benefits	***Implications***	***Culture***	***Cost***	***Recommendation***
Describe the benefits and value of the proposed technology and how it supports strategic initiatives and how it solves the problem.	Describe the pros and cons.	Describe the culture of the organization and how willing users will be to embrace the new technology.	Describe the costs and include the total cost of ownership: not just software costs, but training and support costs as well.	State your professional opinion and why. As a healthcare informatics expert, do you recommend the technology? Include your rationale and involve other experts and stakeholders in this opinion.

Readiness Assessment

A key activity to undertake prior to any clinical system initiative is a readiness assessment. Ideally, this should be done during the initial project planning phase and again at 90 to 120 days prior to going live, 60 days prior to going live, and again at 30 days prior to going live; and reported to the governance and the executive sponsor(s) routinely. You can also use a readiness assessment as part of a "go/no-go" decision meeting with key stakeholders and your sponsor. This is typically done 30 days prior to going live, and serves the purpose of bringing all stakeholders to the table to assess their buy-in and readiness for the impending implementation, as well as provide transparency around critical issues that could affect go-live. Examples of areas that should be evaluated as part of a readiness assessment include:

- Hardware and software. For example, is there enough hardware to support implementation and ongoing support? Are there enough software licenses? What interfaces need to be considered and planned for?
- Technology infrastructure. For example, do you have adequate wireless capability?
- Number of high-priority open issues
- Testing status
- Training status
- Status of design, including end-user engagement and key decisions
- Communication status. For example, do you have in place key messaging and planning for communication to the end users about the impending changes?

Workflow, Workflow, and More Workflow

As you plan and design the future state, keep two very important factors in mind from a planning perspective. Including these elements as part of planning and designing a new system will help provide long-term value and lay a solid foundation for reporting, analytics, and EHR safety as well as help avoid future rework:

- Use of a standardized terminology as part of the design process. See Chapter 12.
- Consideration for EHR safety. See Chapter 13.

Think about the "end game" and how clinicians will report and analyze data to improve quality, generate information, and ultimately create new knowledge. Free-text data fields do not provide high-quality data and the necessary foundation for advanced analytics. Use discrete data as much as possible, and use a standardized terminology to truly understand practice and generate new knowledge.

Additionally, from a safety and planning perspective, a good framework to use is the sociotechnical model as described by Singh, Ash, and Sittig (2013). Operationalizing the use of EHRs in fast-paced and highly disruptive, complex systems such as healthcare requires a comprehensive and multidimensional sociotechnical framework in order to thoroughly analyze all facets that can affect safety (Sittig & Singh, 2010).

Sittig and Singh (2010) introduced a model for healthcare IT to view clinical systems from multiple dimensions. It specifically addresses eight dimensions: hardware and software computing infrastructure; clinical content; human/computer interfaces; people, workflow and communication; internal organizational polices and procedure; culture; external rules and regulations; and system measurement and monitoring.

What is most striking about this framework (compared with others used for healthcare IT analyses and research) is the recognition that these dimensions are not independent or sequential, but rather intertwined and connected (Singh et al., 2013). Sittig and Singh's sociotechnical model (2010, p. 69) emphasizes how these dimensions should be "studied in relation to each other" and can provide a solid framework for designing and evaluating healthcare IT. Figure 2.2 depicts the model and the interplay of the eight dimensions.

With any clinical technology initiative, the importance of evaluating workflow impact and identifying areas for operational efficiencies cannot be emphasized enough. It is essential to do this as part of a multidisciplinary team—that is, avoid the mistake of designing workflows in silos. Clinical technology implementations will affect many departments and users. After all, one design decision could have multiple downstream effects on other users and systems.

It is therefore imperative to understand and map out future state workflows with a multidisciplinary team of stakeholders, including physicians, nurses, quality, department managers, risk managers, finance experts, and other departments that may be impacted by the change. Be sure to include this as part of your communication strategy. It is not uncommon for end users to ask, "Who designed this? Why were we not included?" By being proactive and providing a list of who participated in the design decisions and what the decisions are, you can avoid this common pitfall. A good and simple format to use to help clinicians understand new workflows and the future state is a stop, start, continue format as shown in Table 2.3.

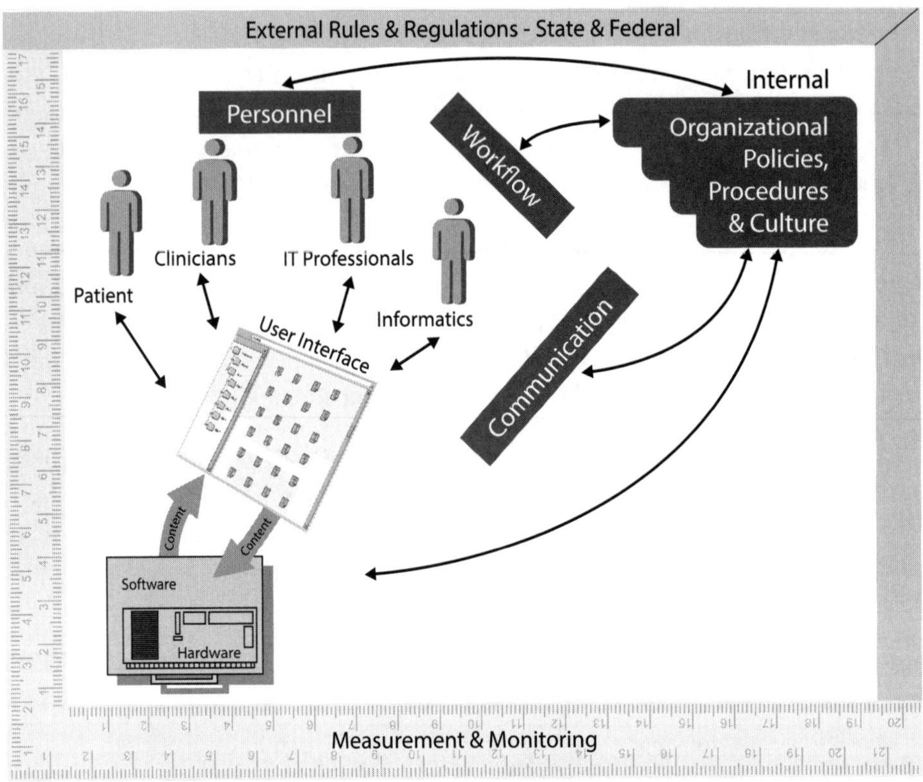

FIGURE 2.2 Sociotechnical Model. Sittig & Singh, 2010.

Table 2.3 Stop, Start, Continue Example

Role	*Process*	*Stop*	*Start*	*Continue*
Charge Nurse	Foley Day/ Urinary Catheter Monitoring	Collecting data manually	Using EHR "Catheter Days" Report to monitor and identify patients at risk of exceeding standard of care	Notifying physician to enter order to discontinue urinary catheters for patients with urinary catheters in place nearing or exceeding standard of care
Nurse	Heart Failure Education	Manually documenting heart failure education on paper form	Documenting heart failure education electronically on discharge education form	Documenting heart failure education prior to discharge

Reprinted with permission from Davis, C. and Stoots, M. A Guide to EHR Adoption: Implementation Through Organizational Transformation. Chicago: HIMSS; 2012a.

A word of caution: End users may want to automate bad processes. As a result of new technology and examining workflows, a flashlight will shine on bad processes and provide transparency around some of these processes. Be sure to drill down into every new workflow and look for opportunities to streamline processes and improve efficiencies. If you have workflow process improvement experts in your organization (such as Six Sigma Black Belts, or a performance improvement department), be sure to engage them in projects from the start and leverage their skills. They are often excellent resources to facilitate process improvement using Six Sigma, which is a methodology for process improvement that provides a set of tools to reduce variation and improve quality (American Society for Quality, n.d.).

How many times have you heard, "But we have always done it that way!" as the answer to why clinicians do things a certain way. By using experts in Six Sigma methodology as part of future state workflow design, you can break down the steps of a process and really determine what is adding value. As an informaticist, you should also consider getting Six Sigma certification as part of your career growth. With the emerging model of healthcare delivery focused on population health management, quality, cost reduction, value, and care across the continuum, having this type of skill set will be prove to be very valuable.

Finally, when it comes to workflows, remember that standardized workflows will simply not work everywhere. What works in the inpatient setting may not work in the ambulatory setting, and what works at an academic medical center will not work at a critical access hospital. So, it is important to standardize workflows across an enterprise and reduce variation as much as possible to drive quality improvements, and it is important to take the time to review and adjust these standardized workflows to meet local needs. This can best be accomplished by reviewing the future state workflows with a multidisciplinary, local team. If there are significant changes to workflows, they should be managed through governance. However, expect some variations given that it is often necessary to accommodate local practices and geographical differences.

And do not forget about the impact of new workflows to policies and procedures. Be sure to look at existing polices that may need updating as well as new policies that may need to be created as you plan for new technology. Governance is key in this respect as well, because it is very important to get both your executive sponsor and governance approval for any policy changes that need to be implemented as a result of technology initiatives.

Measuring Success

So how will you know you have succeeded in effective planning? Ask yourself the following questions as a guide to determine whether—as Benjamin Franklin noted—you are preparing to fail:

- Have you fully incorporated each critical success factor in planning the project?
- Do those impacted by the change understand the new processes, and have you won their hearts— meaning, are they excited and engaged with how the new technology will support them in delivering high-quality and efficient care?
- How have you demonstrated to the organization that the project has elevated quality and is truly making a difference in cost reduction and operational efficiencies?

Future Directions

From a planning perspective, it is important to note that a system implementation is just the beginning, not the end. As we note earlier, you must plan for ongoing support of optimization of any clinical system implementation. This should be planned for and budgeted up front, from the start. Table 2.4 lists some helpful hints and recommendations to plan for ongoing support and optimization. The overall message here is that after the system goes live, expect many requests for changes and enhanced functionality. Think of a system implementation as an ongoing journey that never ends.

Table 2.4 Tips for Ongoing Support and Optimization

Tip	*Rationale*
Do not make system changes for 60 to 90 days (unless they are safety or regulatory related).	Users require time to learn the new system and may want to go back to the old way of doing things because that is what they are used to.
Monitor new workflows for noncompliance and/or significant variations.	Bad habits are hard to break, and clinicians may not adapt to the new workflows.
Collect enhancement requests and requests for changes in a structured manner with a defined process.	This will allow for ongoing monitoring, tracking, and reporting.
Bring enhancement requests and changes to governance for approval.	Changes that affect practice or requests for enhanced functionality with training and workflow impacts should always go through governance to determine whether the requests align with practice and strategy.
Ask the governance oversight group to prioritize requests for changes and enhancements.	You will not be able to do everything, and there are limits to resources. Governance can help you prioritize and make sure you are working on the right things.

continues

Table 2.4 Tips for Ongoing Support and Optimization *(continued)*

Tip	*Rationale*
Communicate changes and enhancements made to the system on a routine basis and through a variety of venues.	Always close the loop with clinicians individually and through established broader communication channels on their suggestions and recommendations. Otherwise, they might think that their suggestion went unheard and into a "black hole."
Conduct ongoing workflow observations and concentrate on high risk areas (for example, medication reconciliation, shift handoff).	Complex processes designed before the system is live may not work so well after go-live. Measuring and monitoring processes will help you see where adjustments may need to be made to achieve project goals and benefits.
Routinely provide executives and managers talking points and questions to ask during rounding to assess workflow and compliance with new processes.	Keeping executive leadership and management engaged will help hard-wire the change.
Plan for downtime and ensure that super users and managers know what to do and how to do it when the system is not functional.	Users typically forget manual processes after a system goes live, which could significantly affect operations and patient safety.

Conclusion

In summary, ensuring use of the seven critical success factors as part of project planning, along with conducting a readiness assessment and engaging key stakeholders from the beginning, will help avoid a failed project. More importantly, approach healthcare IT initiatives as a journey and a means versus an end, and always keep a sharp focus on the problem(s) to be solved. By following these recommendations and using some of the tools outlined in this chapter, you will become a part of transforming healthcare by leveraging technology to promote quality, safety, cost reduction, and value for patients and communities.

References

Davis, C., & Stoots, M. (2012a). Stop, start, continue process analysis. In *A guide to EHR Adoption: Implementation through organizational transformation* (p. 65). Chicago, IL: HIMSS.

Davis, C., & Stoots, M. (2012b). Three-tier governance model. In *A guide to EHR Adoption: Implementation through organizational transformation* (p. 31). Chicago, IL: HIMSS.

Kubiak, T. M., & Benbow, D. W. (2009). *The certified Six Sigma Black Belt handbook,* (2nd ed.). (pp. 6-7). Milwaukee, WI: ASQ.

Singh, H., Ash, J., & Sittig, D. (2013). Safety assurance factors for electronic health record resilience (SAFER): Study protocol. *BMC Medical Informatics and Decision Making, 13*(46), pp. 1–8. doi:10.1136/qshc.2010.042085

Sittig, D., & Singh, H. (2010). A new sociotechnical model for studying health information technology in complex adaptive healthcare systems [Supplemental material]. *Quality and Safety in Health Care, 19*(3), 68–74. doi:10.1136/qshc.2010.042085

"Design is intelligence made visible."

–Alina Wheeler

3 Designing a Usable Healthcare Information System

Christy St. John, MSN, RN-BC

OBJECTIVES

- Define usability in the context of healthcare IT.
- Describe usability concepts through common clinical scenarios.
- Evaluate system usability using tools provided.
- Understand current state and future considerations of usability.

Healthcare leaders are increasingly expressing dissatisfaction with their clinical information systems, and often cite cost and difficulty of use as contributing factors (Gregg, 2014). Face it: Electronic health records (EHRs) and order-entry systems are complex and typically lack intuitiveness, and navigation does not always support a smooth workflow. The Healthcare Information and Management Systems Society (HIMSS) Electronic Health Record Usability Task Force report cited that usability was perhaps the most important factor that hindered the widespread adoption of EHRs prior to the signing of the Health Information Technology for Economic and Clinical Health (HITECH) Act in 2009 (Belden, Grayson, & Barnes, 2009). Since then, organizations have worked quickly to get these clinical systems in place to take advantage of the incentive dollars offered through the Centers for Medicare and Medicaid Services (CMS) Meaningful Use incentive program (ONC, 2013). Adoption has been swift since 2009, yet enhancements to usability have been slow.

The challenges that we face regarding usability in healthcare IT are several. First, there is no standard and accepted definition of usability in the healthcare IT industry. Several are offered that are very good, but none seem to be the gold standard from which we all work. Nielson (1995) defined usability as "a quality attribute that assesses how easy the user interfaces are to use."

Further, Zhang and Walji (2011) noted that usability "...refers to how useful, usable, and satisfying a system is for the intended users to accomplish goals by performing certain sequences of tasks" (p. 1056).

Second, we have the issue of individual perspectives and paradigms. What may make perfect sense on a display screen to one person may not be as clear to another. Reasons for this are several and may be due to the person's level of exposure to technology, their age and education, and perhaps gender.

The bottom line is that healthcare is complex, EHRs are complex, and attempting to visually display the nonlinear work of caring for patients is a huge challenge. However, several core concepts that are evidence-based can help lay a strong foundation for those informaticists working in the area of system design. This chapter will focus on those core concepts and give readers the tools to evaluate and improve their systems.

Assessing Usability

The current state of usability leaves us with much work to do in a complex and fast-paced, ever-changing environment. Middleton et al. (2013, p. 3), in a position paper on behalf of the American Medical Informatics Association (AMIA), stated, "[T]he ability to perform meaningful, reproducible, objective usability metrics for EHR systems is limited by the socio-technical nature of the systems. They are typically highly configurable and different providers will implement them in different ways, with markedly different process."

So, what is the big deal with usability? What are the origins? What are the side effects of poor usability? Why is it important to you and your users?

First, a historical perspective. Studies of usability have a long and distinguished history. In the early twentieth century, during the Industrial Age, pioneer studies were conducted on human interaction with machines to increase productivity and improve worker safety. Usability and human interactions took on a new level of importance in the World War II era, specifically in aviation. During this time, human interaction with the electronic control panel was more complex than ever before.

Quite obviously, technology grew more sophisticated over the decades as did the science of usability. In the 1960s and 1970s, the first homegrown electronic records were introduced, including one of the largest at Veterans Administration (VA) Medical Centers

(Atherton, 2011). In the 1970s, Xerox was one of the first technology companies to incorporate the user experience in design of their systems, hardware, and software. In the 1980s, when the PC became a commonplace device, the industry took the concepts from earlier decades and spun off a number of user interfaces.

This is also when the electronic gaming industry began to take off. The entertainment factor—and therefore usability—has been essential to success in this sector. Some of these same gaming concepts are present today in more recent EHR development. Notably, in the 1980s, Apple launched the Macintosh user interface. Needless to say, its success has been evident in the usability arena (Spillers, 2007).

In the 1990s and early 2000s, usability was recognized as a strategic element to success in system implementation. Tools exist through the Usability Professionals' Association (UPA) to measure usability concepts from acceptance to return on investment (UPA, 2012).

What happens when a system is designed with poor usability? Koppel et al. (2005) published a bold study noting that poorly designed computerized physician order entry (CPOE) systems were the cause of 22 types of medication errors risks. The methods used in the study included direct observation, expert interviews, staff interviews, focus groups, and surveys to garner the most complete information. Of the identified medication error risks, a few of the types included medication discontinuation failure, wrong medication selection, and conflicting or duplicative medication selections. Also noted in this study, "...fifty-five percent of house staff reported difficulty identifying the patient they were ordering for because of fragmented CPOE displays; 23% reported that this happened a few times weekly or more frequently" (p. 1200). While noting the importance of how clinicians' work is organized, independent of the technology, the most significant findings were related to the human interaction with the technology: the usability of the system. The study conclusion was that the use of the CPOE system as it was evaluated actually *facilitated* medication errors rather than reducing them.

Wow! Let that sink in for a minute. We just answered the question about why usability is important to you and your users. Poor usability has the distinct potential to lead to errors, which is the very thing we try to prevent. If we get down to brass tacks, we know that errors are costly from the patient's standpoint and organizationally. It makes sense and "cents" that we give usability due attention.

Applying Usability Evidence

Comprehensive tools for usability evaluation can be found through a number of sources, both internally and externally to the healthcare IT industry. One helpful site that contains numerous links to practical resources on user experience with technology, evaluation tools, and concepts of visual design is an interactive website managed by the Digital Communications Division in the U.S. Department of Health and Human Services (2014) Office of the Assistant Secretary for Public Affairs. This website contains links to valuable information on the "what and why" of usability in addition to access to a wide variety of tools and methods to assess the design and usability in clinical systems (http://www.usability.gov).

Two additional resources stand out as being very usable themselves, and are based on evidence with the guidance of industry experts. In the sections that follow, fundamental and practical examples of usability in a healthcare environment are presented, using these tools as the foundation from which informatics specialists can begin to evaluate and improve the systems they are responsible for designing.

One of these tools is the document, "Defining and Testing EMR Usability: Principles and Proposed Methods of EMR Usability Evaluation and Rating," published by the HIMSS Usability Task Force (Belden et al., 2009). Its usability rating tool includes a five-star rating system and defines the necessity of formative and summative evaluation, the first of which is the responsibility of the vendor and the latter, the responsibility of the customer. These concepts are further defined in an article by Boone (2010), "EMR Usability: Bridging the Gap between Nurse and Computer." These resources identify nine areas where informatics specialists should focus attention not only during the initial design phase of system implementation but at any time during the system's lifecycle. These nine areas of focus are:

- Simplicity
- Naturalness
- Consistency
- Minimizing cognitive load
- Efficient interactions
- Forgiveness and feedback

- Effective use of language
- Effective information presentation
- Preservation of context

Simplicity

The essential message here is *the simpler, the better*. "Simplicity is concise information displayed to the user, including only the functionality and data needed to effectively accomplish tasks and decision making" (Boone, 2010, p. 15).

Designing screens that are clean, clear, and as intuitive as possible is the goal of simplicity. The concept is exemplified by building stackable content within the EHR, giving users only what they need to make the best decisions for the patient and move smoothly to the next step. By *stackable,* we mean segments of content that can be added together, or "stacked," to best paint the care picture for your patient.

Take order sets as one example of stackable content. As healthcare providers, we want to ensure that the latest evidence-based content is reflected in ordering processes and the needs of the patient are addressed. While attempting to accomplish just that, many users find order sets to be cumbersome and time consuming. Order sets are often built as a "laundry list" of every possible order that a patient could need, from admission to discharge for a given diagnosis. The sets might be broken into categories of like orders, diagnostics, imaging, and medications with only a few defaults selected; or perhaps the selections are left entirely to the user to discern. Although the intent of an order set is to ensure that the provider has the needed content and does not miss a critical step, the end result is lots of scrolling and frustration, which could lead to the exact opposite of the intent.

So, how to solve this conundrum? How do we motivate providers to use evidence-based order sets? The takeaway: Do not overthink it. Keep it simple. Make it as easy as possible for the end user to do the right thing, enter what they need to enter for the patient, and move on. Providers need to get to the business of tending to the patient, not tending to the system.

Walk through this scenario. Your patient comes through the Emergency Department and has a diagnosis of sepsis. We know that a sequence of events, if implemented in a timely fashion, increases the chance of survival (Society of Critical Care Medicine, 2012). Rather than complicate the process with extraneous orders, imagine using a quick order set with just the necessary elements needed for this immediate care. We would want most of those necessary elements already entered (default presets) to save time and ensure consistency.

Before we move on, think about a few stumbling blocks on the road to simplicity. Here's an example. What about all of the possible antibiotics that could be used in the initial treatment? Here is an opportunity to use the *80/20 rule*, which states that when looking at a page within the application, the user should be able ascertain the needed information 80% of the time, and the user will need to dig a little deeper 20% of the time. Look at the evidence-based guidelines for the diagnosis and the data for your facility. Are there recommended antibiotics? Which antibiotics do you use most frequently in your facility? Which are most cost effective? So, perhaps in your quick order set, you have a maximum of three choices, with one of those choices defaulted for the provider. Any outlying factors, such as a patient allergy to the three choices, could be covered by a single standalone order.

Back to our scenario. We know there will be a need for admission and ongoing care of this septic patient. Imagine a stack of building blocks that snap together like the tiny plastic bricks kids play with, as shown in Figure 3.1.

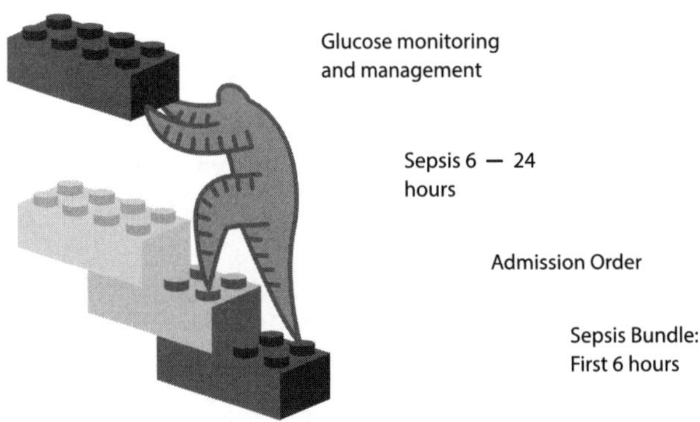

FIGURE 3.1 Stackable content concept.

Our first building block is the bundle of elements for immediate care (sepsis). Our next block is the order for admission, including elements such as the diagnosis and reason for admission, type of bed, and service. The next block might include things critical for the first 24 hours of care, such as continued antibiotics and any other pertinent medications, labs, diet, and nursing orders for frequency of monitoring.

We also know that rarely do patients present with a single problem to be addressed during a hospitalization. Still using the idea of simple, stackable content, imagine that our septic patient is also diabetic. Make it easy for the provider to pull in the block of orders appropriate for glucose management to stack with the sepsis orders. This block might include orders pertaining to glucose-monitoring frequency, appropriate glucose range, and any medications needed for glucose control.

Overall, we would expect the end result to be easy to use, guiding intuitively from one step to the next, capturing the pertinent data needed for care. In their simplest form, the blocks stack together, connecting the care logically for the patient and the EHR user.

Here are some questions to ask when implementing simplicity:

- Is the system easy to navigate from one step to the next? Take into account workflow process here.
- Does the system present information in a way that is simple, easy to read, and easy to understand?

Naturalness

Boone (2010, p. 15) noted, "[N]aturalness means the end user should be immediately comfortable and familiar with the system." What does "immediately comfortable" really mean to the user? How do we remove the subjectivity of individual user perceptions? Well, step outside the healthcare setting for a moment to something more universal. How many times have you heard someone say, "Google it!"? When that phrase is mentioned, there is an immediate familiarity with the concept and the look and feel of "Google-ing." You likely conjured up an image of the rainbow-colored word GOOGLE above a search bar. You have come to expect completion matching on what you are typing in that search bar, and the results page is easy to navigate. You know what to do and what to expect at each step in your search process.

Take that same idea and apply it to the EHR. The user should never have to guess about the next step. She should never be too timid to click a button for fear of where it will take her and worry that she cannot get back to where she started. When searching for a definition of *intuitive,* Google offers, "a) using or based on what one feels to be true even without conscious reasoning; instinctive; b) (chiefly of computer software) easy to use and understand" (2014). That is exactly the point of "immediately comfortable and familiar."

Here are some questions to ask to facilitate naturalness:

- Does each screen in your EHR indicate how to get back to the previous screen?
- Is it clear what the next step is when proceeding through the ordering process?

Consistency

With any software application—but particularly in healthcare when safety is at stake—consistency is crucial. Nielsen noted, "[U]sers should not have to wonder whether different words, situations, or actions mean the same thing" (1995, para. 4). Think of some of the most popular software programs in use today. The *graphical user interface (GUI)*—what the user sees and interacts with on the electronic page—provides consistency. The user may navigate deep into the application, but the consistency with which information is presented, how icons appear, the behavior of the icons, and the overall layout of the screen provides a sense of ease from one task to the next. "The application's structure, interactions, and behaviors match a user's experience with other software applications and are consistently applied throughout the EMR" (Boone, 2010, p. 15).

We know that electronic health records (EHRs) are data-rich, including discrete data, subjective data, report data, and so on. We have data that, after being filed, can be seen in multiple locations within the chart. Often those data can be pulled or auto-populated into reports and notes. The question of consistency is not a question. In order to expect consistent results in human behavior and potentially prevent errors, users should expect consistent software behavior.

A few practical examples of consistency included the following:

- A toolbar across the top of the page that never changes, regardless of location in the chart

- An icon that looks like a house to symbolize returning to the Home screen from anywhere in the application
- An expectation that clicking the Next button, for example, will open a similar user workspace
- Despite differing information in reports, a consistent appearance to reports
- Consistent naming conventions and use of a style guide to provide searchable results for builders and users alike (for example, care plans for behavioral health may contain "Behavioral Health" in the title)

Here are some questions to ask regarding consistency:

- Do all your order entry screens and all your clinical documentation screens have a Submit or Save button in the same location?
- Is there a consistent button for the user to return to the Home screen? Is that button in the same location on each screen?

Minimizing Cognitive Load

Make sure that users are not overwhelmed by what they see and how they interact with the system. "Minimizing cognitive load ensures density, poor end-user feedback, and inadequate data entry field cues don't lead to sensory overload" (Boone, 2010, p. 15). Too much at one time or in one place takes away from the intention of providing needed information.

Take a minute to explore density a little further, because this concept can sometimes be confusing. One of the simplest definitions of density comes from the world of instructional design. First, for those unfamiliar with instructional design, it is "the entire process of analysis of learning needs and goals and the development of a delivery system to meet those needs" (University of Michigan, 1996, para. 1). In the world of instructional design, density is important to the successful result of a learning experience. Likewise, it translates to the world of electronic records. Density can enhance or detract from the EHR user experience. Gibbons and Fairweather (1998, p. 359) defined density as "the amount of new information knotted up at one new information location."

An example of poor density may come in the form of a patient information report within the EHR. In this example, we are referring to a report housed within the EHR, not a printed report. How many times have you heard a user say, "Give me a one-stop shop" with all the pertinent information? This request is often fraught with competing priorities. On the one hand, giving users the information they need with minimal clicks or system movement is a plus. However, the density with which the information is presented can be tricky. Too much text, expecting the user to determine new versus old information, or the text size may lend itself to poor density. Beldon et al. (2009) offered the 80/20 rule in this circumstance as well.

A few strategies for minimizing the cognitive load of this report and achieving a balanced density might include the following:

- Ensure that the text size is easy to read.
- Flag new information with a symbol.
- Allow hovering or hyperlinks to gain more details, if desired.
- Use simple, natural, and consistent concepts in the screen layout.

Here are some questions to ask regarding minimizing cognitive load:

- How old is the information that's displayed? For example, when placing orders for potassium, does the user need to remember the last potassium lab value from the results screens, or is it displayed on the ordering screen?
- Is the text size from screen to screen consistent and readable?

Efficient Interactions

Inefficiencies cost users time. You have likely been to a website filling out information, and you are not able to do something as simple as tab to the next field. The form's flow does not seem logical and clicking in and out of boxes with your mouse and typing takes you extra time. This is an example of inefficient workflow design and interaction. In context of the EHR, imagine the time it takes away from the patient.

Workflow can be optimized by setting logical default tabs, large-enough lists, and text boxes to limit scrolling and prevent frequent switching between keyboard and mouse. In a systematic review, Poissant, Pereira, Tamblyn, and Kawasumi (2005) noted that end-user efficiency is a hallmark goal of successful EHR implementation. The authors' findings include the idea that time savings is most frequently measured by pre- and post-implementation documentation times. They go on to note that time savings is often achieved in the broader sense of patient care through enhanced ability, including simultaneous access to the chart and immediate availability of information. Thus, clinicians are focused on the tangible time with the patient.

Although the documentation of care is a necessary part of what we do and translates a patient's story among colleagues, direct care is equally important. Therefore, an efficient EHR gets clinicians back to the bedside interacting with the patient and family. Efficiency may seem like a grand idea given our complex environments, but incorporating some simple tasks that save clicks—therefore, time—can increase user satisfaction.

Most of us are quite familiar with the head-to-toe assessment. Within the EHR, end users likely document on a flow sheet of sorts. Many design options in this example could be implemented to improve efficiency. One option could order the systems of the body from head to toe (Neuro, EENT, Cardiac, Respiratory, and so on). For each system, the user could select a *Within Normal Limits* option if the assessment warranted such a response. When an assessment requires an exception to normal, capturing the exception should be easy for the user. The user could select *Exception,* causing buttons for the most common exceptions to appear within the workspace, and allowing the user to select more than one button to describe the exception accurately. In this example, the user is consistently clicking; switching the interaction to typing would reduce efficiency. Typing (or free-texting), although generally an option on any assessment field, should be a last resort.

NOTE

A helpful by-product of well-designed efficiency is discrete data that can be used for future evaluation, research, and process improvement within your system.

Here are some questions to ask to ensure efficient interactions:

- On a given screen, is the expected user behavior consistent (typing versus clicking)?
- Are there actions or buttons within the EHR that can be added to make documentation accurate and efficient?

Forgiveness and Feedback

To expect that a user will never need to go back and make a correction is unrealistic. "User forgiveness occurs when errors are made, such as the use of the undo button found in many applications" (Boone, 2010, p. 15). Applying the concepts we have discussed thus far in this chapter will minimize the need for user forgiveness. However, there are different levels of forgiveness to consider within the EHR.

First, how easy is it for a user to correct information prior to finalizing or making it part of the permanent record? This may be as simple as backspacing or clicking an Undo button and then typing in or clicking the correction.

Second, what happens when the data is finalized as part of the chart, but in error? An example of this might be that the user filed erroneous finger stick glucose data by accidentally "fat fingering" the value. Likely, the same simple fixes are applied, but a record or an audit trail of the correction is filed or flagged in the chart. This harkens back to the paper charting days when clinicians would strike through and initial a charting error. Nielson (1995), one of the first to study usability, stated in his concept of allowing user control and freedom to simply support "undo and redo."

"Feedback ensures users that their input has had the desired effect, such as immediately indicating a critically high fever in red when entered" (Boone, 2010, p. 15). Another example of feedback is noting a percentage of change that is clinically relevant. For instance, it is important to know when a newborn has lost 10% of its birth weight. Flagging the percent change is relevant to the clinical care of the newborn. Using concepts previously discussed and based on the appropriate feedback received, suggesting nutritional supplements or a change in feeding schedule may be an appropriate next step guiding the clinician simply and naturally through the clinical process within the EHR.

Forgiveness and feedback work hand in hand in the EHR. Rarely are they mutually exclusive. An example is setting parameters within the EHR to prevent error. Nielson noted design to support correct data entry is better than a good error message. He stated, "...either eliminate error-prone conditions or check for them and present the user with a confirmation option before they commit the action" (1995, para. 5). Using weight and a percent change again as an example, the weight of your patient yesterday was 67 kilograms (kg), but today, the user attempts to enter 76 kg, which is a significant change in a 24-hour span. Prior to signing off on the entry of 76 kg, the system recognizes this is a potential error and gives appropriate feedback to the clinician. Options would include affirming the value as correct and moving forward, or allowing the clinician to easily go back and correct the entry.

Here are some questions to ask regarding forgiveness and feedback:

- Are you asking for the right format in each of the data fields to eliminate potential for error? For example, weight is numerical, so allow the field to accept only a numerical response. Thus, alphabetic characters cannot be entered.
- Is it easy for your users to correct an entry error with proper tracking when necessary?

Effective Use of Language

Language is a big deal—so much so that in 2010, the United States government passed the Plain Writing Act stating the government had to "write all new publications, forms, and publicly distributed documents in a 'clear, concise, well-organized' manner" (Office of Management and Budget [OMB], 2011, p. 1), and government health agencies are no exception to the rule. Furthermore, The Joint Commission (TJC) has long been a proponent of minimizing the use of abbreviations to reduce the risk of harm, and published in 2004 the well-known "Do Not Use" list (TJC, 2010).

Have you ever thought about how we speak in code and in the context of our own sphere of expertise, often without realizing those around us may not understand the message we are attempting to communicate? The user should never have to guess what the EHR is asking for or question what information is presented. "Language used in an EMR is concise, unambiguous, familiar, and meaningful to end users in the context of their work. Abbreviations and acronyms should only be displayed when they're commonly understood and unambiguous. Text in upper case should never be displayed because it takes longer to read and increases perceived density" (Boone, 2010, p. 15). Nielson noted, "The system should speak the users' language, with words, phrases, and concepts familiar to the user…follow real world conventions, making information appear in natural and logical order" (1995, para. 2). The takeaway: Say what you mean, and mean what you say.

Here are some questions to ask regarding the effective use of language:

- Have you asked for information in a clear, concise, and consistent format?
- Is the language appropriate to the discipline and understood across disciplines?

Effective Information Presentation

Effective information presentation "ensures the appropriate density of data, readability, and the meaningful use of color. Comprehensive guidelines on use of color have recently been developed by the Human Factors and Ergonomics Society (HFES):

- Red: stop, hot, danger, error, extreme warning, severe alert, emergency, alarm
- Yellow: caution, potential or mild warning, requires attention, slow, moderate alert
- Green: go, safe, normal, good, proceed
- Blue: cold, advisory" (Boone, 2010, p. 15)

Using color coding in the EHR is meaningful to how a clinician perceives and reacts to the information presented. Belden et al. (2009, p. 9) noted, "[F]or color to convey meaning, there cannot be a larger number of colors used than the user can remember, and they must be used consistently throughout the application." For example, say your patient has an anaphylactic reaction to amoxicillin. The physician places an order in the same medication class. Before completing the order, the system presents the physician with a red stop sign alerting that the patient has a potentially fatal reaction to a medication in this same class. Similarly, if the patient received a critical value lab result, that information may displayed in red or contain red exclamation points to bring the same level of awareness and expected reaction.

As previously discussed in this chapter, data density and readability lend to effective information presentation. This includes the effective use of language, font size, background color versus text color, and simplicity. The user should be able to quickly look at the screen and comprehend the necessary information and intuitively understand the expected level of attention and required reaction.

One tool that you may find useful as you are designing and evaluating your EHR is the Colour Contrast Analyser. This tool evaluates the contrast of text to background color. It also takes into account the accommodations for color blindness. This tool can be accessed for both PC and Mac users at

http://www.paciellogroup.com/resources/contrastAnalyser

Upon downloading and running the tool, the user receives a box like that shown in Figure 3.2, noting whether the contrast is appropriate:

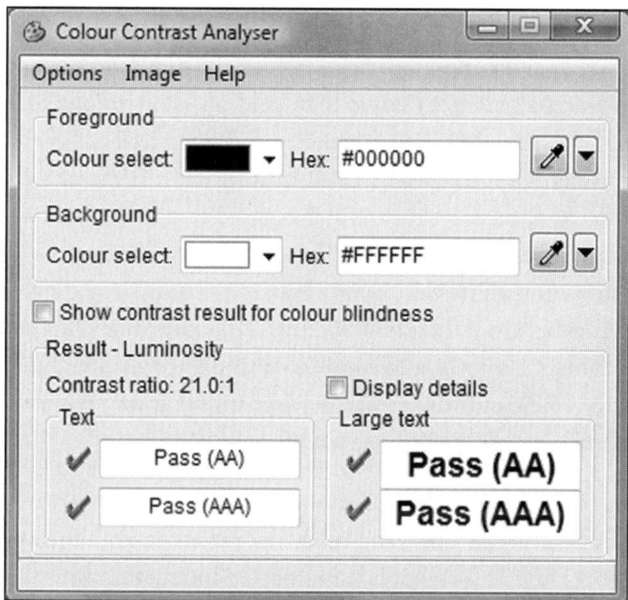

FIGURE 3.2 Paciello Contrast Analyser.

Here are some questions to ask regarding effective information presentation:

- Is the text contrast optimal?
- Is the color coding consistent throughout the record?
- Is the use of color in line with more global concepts of color coding (red = warning)?

Preservation of Context

Work to minimize alerts and interruptions as much as possible. "This ensures screen changes and visual interruptions such as pop-ups, instructions, and screen repaints are kept to a minimum during completion of a particular task. Visual interruptions include anything that forces users to shift visual focus away from the area on the screen where they're currently reading and/or working to address something else and then re-establish focus afterward" (Boone 2010, p. 16). Certainly, there are times when critical information is needed prior to proceeding with a workflow, but be diligent in determining your definition of "critical."

Alarm fatigue is a phenomenon that has a potentially negative effect on efficiency and patient safety. Dolan (2012, para. 1) stated that "...alerts are designed to inform (users) of possible patient safety issues, but their frequency and often lack of necessity make them the electronic equivalent of the boy who cried wolf." The intention of an alert is to protect the patient, but too often, we are not careful and consistent about how we design, deploy, and monitor the alerts. Van der Sijs, Aarts, Vulto, and Berg (2006, p. 147) noted that 49% to 96% of drug interaction alerts were overridden for reasons including design and sensitivity. Dolan (2012, para. 2) went on to note that, "[I]t's clear that the answer is to create systems that take human behavior and supplemental patient data into account when writing rules that decide when and why an alert is fired off. That way, the alerts could have more success in their purpose: protecting patient safety."

When deciding to interrupt a clinician's workflow and take them out of context, be mindful of the why behind the what. Is it really important enough to stop the clinician? Is the gain worth the pain? If so, what is the expected interaction with the alert? Make the interruption as minimal as possible and guide the user to the appropriate action. Nielson (1995, para. 9) encouraged that, "[M]essages should be expressed in plain language, precisely indicate the problem, and constructively suggest a solution." Finally, plan to evaluate the behavior associated with the alert at specified time frames: perhaps 30, 60, and 90 days out from implementation of the alert. Make informed adjustments based on discrete data collection and end-user feedback.

The Agency for Healthcare Research and Quality (AHRQ) (2009) completed a study measuring the percentage of alerts or reminders that resulted in desired action. The overall conclusion indicated that alerts in general—and particularly asynchronous alerts—can "...improve compliance with recommended care and adherence to practice guidelines" (p. 1). Asynchronous alerts occur outside of the standard workflow within the EHR: For example, the order process for a vaccine is complete. However, the system does not allow the discharge paperwork to be completed until documentation occurs on the medication administration record (MAR) regarding the status of the vaccine. Within the same study, the AHRQ offered tools on how to conduct your own study regarding alert effectiveness (www.ahrq.gov).

Here are some questions to ask regarding preservation of context:

- What are the acceptable circumstances in your organization to stop a clinician's workflow with an alert?
- How will the effectiveness of the alert, including the usability, be monitored to ensure the desired result is achieved?

Usability Testing for Your EHR

One of the many challenges that confront the informatics specialist is the development of methods to assess the EHR for the concepts described earlier in this chapter. One method that can assist in the evaluation is user acceptance testing, as described in Chapter 4. As part of any system implementation, upgrade, or enhancement, user acceptance testing should be part of the standard process prior to actual implementation. It is during this testing that system end users are asked to take the system for a test ride.

Figure 3.3 is a simple checklist to consider as you begin your usability journey. Each of these items can certainly be explored in more depth. This is by no means an exhaustive list but a quick tool to give you a sense of where you are good to go and where you may have an opportunity.

	A	B	C	D
1	Quick Usability Checklist: People, Process, Technology	Yes	No	Additional Comments
2	People			
3	Does your organization have human resources dedicated to usability?			
4	Do the people involved in usability testing understand the concepts of system usability?			
5	Will you involve end users in user acceptance testing?			
6	Process:			
7	Do you have a process outlined for testing usability/user acceptance testing?			
8	Is your testing format consistent?			
9	Do you have a plan for incorporating feedback from user acceptance testing into the system?			
10	Technology:			
11	Is the system simple to use and understand?			
12	Is there naturalness in system interaction (i.e., the user does not have to wonder what to do next)?			
13	Are the screens consistent (i.e., buttons in the same location, behavior of buttons makes sense)?			
14	Is the text size appropriate, consistent, and easy to read?			
15	Is the text and screen contrast optimal?			
16	Is the density of information on the screen appropriate (hint: 80% of what the user needs should be presented)?			
17	Is the interaction consistent (typing vs. clicking)?			
18	Does the system allow error correction?			
19	Does the system track error correction?			
20	Does the system ask for information in required formats (alpha, numeric, decimal, etc.)?			
21	Is it clear what information the system is asking for or presenting?			
22	Is the language consistent with the discipline and understood across disciplines?			
23	Are alerts presented at appropriate points in workflow?			
24	Does the alert achieve the desired result?			

FIGURE 3.3 Quick Usability Checklist. Courtesy of C. St. John, 2014.

Future Directions

One would like to assume that by ensuring a usable, useful, and meaningful EHR, attestation for various regulatory programs, such as Meaningful Use and Value-based Purchasing, would become less burdensome. This may or may not prove to be true in our complex, highly regulated environment and offers an opportunity for further study. Also, in light of EHR certification programs, determining a common set of usability criteria for evaluation and rating would offer weight to the concept. As noted in earlier discussion, by nature of the complex interactions and scenarios inherent in healthcare, as well as the subjectivity of the user, this will prove to be a difficult but not insurmountable task. Continued work by the ONC and HIMSS, partnering with informatics organizations, will yield further research on usability and its role in patient safety. Staggers, Weir, and Phansalkar (2008) noted that "studies in sociotechnical and human-computer interaction are needed. This would help us understand the complex processes inherent in technology design and adoption. Interdisciplinary examinations are needed in future research to understand interdependent roles" (p. 125).

Conclusion

We initiated the chapter with a brief overview and definition. To conclude, we will wrap back to the core of the definition. Usability, in addition to usefulness, equates to a usable EHR and meaningful end-user experience. In your vision and strategy to raise the bar as it relates to usability, employ the concepts discussed and include stakeholders in every step of the journey. The study of usability in our complex, technology-saturated world will continue to evolve. Be innovative in your efforts to ensure that users have a seamless experience with the EHR. Be diligent in considering these concepts and using the tools presented as a springboard to ensuring your systems are usable, useful, and effective in promoting safe patient care.

References

Agency for Healthcare Research and Quality (AHRQ). (2009). *Percentage of alerts or reminders that resulted in desired action.* Retrieved from http://www.ahrq.gov/

Atherton, J. (2011). Development of the electronic health record. *American Medical Association Journal of Ethics: Virtual Mentor, 13*(3), 186–189.

Belden, J., Grayson, R., & Barnes, J. (2009). *Defining and testing EMR usability: Principles and proposed methods of EMR usability evaluation and rating.* HIMSS EHR Usability Task Force. Retrieved from http://www.himss.org/files/HIMSSorg/content/files/himss_definingandtestingemrusability.pdf

Boone, E. (2010). EMR usability: Bridging the gap between nurse and computer. *Nursing Management, 41*(3), 14–16.

Dolan, P. (2012). Search is on to cure EHR alert fatigue. Retrieved from http://www.amednews.com/article/20120416/business/304169973/1/

Gibbons, A., & Fairweather, P. (1998). *Computer-based instruction: Design and development.* Englewood Cliffs, NJ: Educational Technology Publications.

Google. (2014). Definition of intuitive. Retrieved from https://www.google.com/webhp?sourceid=chrome-instant&ion=1&espv=2&ie=UTF-8#q=intuitive

Gregg, H. (2014, June 2). Survey: Providers investing heavily in EHRs, but dissatisfied with purchase. *Becker's Hospital Review.* Retrieved from http://www.beckershospitalreview.com/healthcare-information-technology/survey-providers-investing-heavily-in-ehrs-but-dissatisfied-with-purchase.html

The Joint Commission. (2010). *Facts about the official "Do Not Use" list.* Retrieved from http://www.jointcommission.org/assets/1/18/Do_Not_Use_List.pdf

Koppel, R., Metlay, J., Cohen, A., Abaluck, B., Localio, A., Kimmel, S., & Strom, B. (2005). Role of computerized physician order entry systems in facilitating medication errors. *Journal of the American Medical Association, 293*(10), 1197–1203.

Middleton, B., Bloomrosen, M., Dente, M., Hashmat, B., Koppel, R., Overhage, J., . . . Zhang, J. (2013). Enhancing patient safety and quality of care by improving the usability of electronic health record systems: Recommendations from AMIA. *Journal of American Medical Informatics Association, 20*(e1), e2–8.

Nielsen, J. (1995). *10 usability heuristics for user interface design.* Retrieved from http://www.nngroup.com/articles/ten-usability-heuristics/

Office of Management and Budget. (2011). *Final guidance on implementing the Plain Writing Act of 2010.* Retrieved from http://www.whitehouse.gov/sites/default/files/omb/memoranda/2011/m11-15.pdf

Office of the National Coordinator for Health Information Technology (ONC). (2013). *Update on the adoption of health information technology and related efforts to facilitate the electronic use and exchange of health information: A report to Congress.* Retrieved from http://www.healthit.gov/sites/default/files/rtc_adoption_of_healthit_and_relatedefforts.pdf

Poissant, L., Pereira, J., Tamblyn, R., & Kawasumi, Y. (2005). The impact of electronic health records on time efficiency of physicians and nurses: A systematic review. *Journal of the American Medical Informatics Association, 12*(5), 505–516.

Society of Critical Care Medicine, Surviving Sepsis Campaign. (2012). *Sepsis bundle.* Retrieved from http://www.survivingsepsis.org/Bundles/Pages/default.aspx

Spillers, F. (2007). *Usability from WWII to the present: The historical origins of usability testing.* Retrieved from http://www.usabilitytestingcentral.com/2007/02/the_history_of_.html

Staggers, N., Weir, C., & Phansalkar, S. (2008). Patient safety and health information technology: Role of the electronic health record. In R. G. Hughes (Ed.), *Patient safety and quality: An evidence-based handbook for nurses* (chapter 47; pp. 3-91–3-133). Rockville, MD: Agency for Healthcare Research and Quality.

University of Michigan. (1996). *Definitions of instructional design.* Retrieved from http://www.umich.edu/~ed626/define.html

Usability Professionals Association (UPA). (2012). *Usability book of knowledge.* Retrieved from http://www.upassoc.org/upa_projects/body_of_knowledge/bok.html

U.S. Department of Health and Human Services. (2014). *Usability guide.* Retrieved from http://www.usability.gov

van der Sijs H., Aarts J., Vulto A., & Berg, M. (2006). Overriding of drug safety alerts in computerized physician order entry. *Journal of the American Medical Informatics Association 13*(2), 138–147.

Zhang, J., & Walji, M. (2011). TURF: Toward a unified framework of EHR usability. *Journal of Biomedical Informatics, 44*(6), 1056–1067.

"Testing leads to failure, and failure leads to understanding."
–Matthew Gionta (Freedman, 2005)

Testing in the Healthcare Informatics Environment

4

Seth D. Carlson, BS

OBJECTIVES

- List and describe the phases of testing.
- Discuss the importance of test scripts and testing requirements.
- Describe the steps of the testing process.
- Describe electronic tools to support testing.

Software testing is a crucial phase of the Systems Development Life Cycle (SDLC), but without the proper planning and timeline, it may become a casualty from missed deadlines in prior phases of a project. One reason that this may happen is that while most methodologies and organizations recognize its importance, there is also a level of uncertainty built into testing complex clinical systems.

Each type or phase of testing is designed to cover key functionality and use cases given that there are far too many individual logical pathways for testing to be completely certain. Testing is therefore a tool to identify and mitigate risk, and different phases of testing expose different aspects of that risk. These phases will be explained with examples in this chapter. Function testing is more likely to uncover functionality bugs and training issues. Integration testing may identify issues with the process flows built into the application, if certain use cases are not supported.

After each type of issue is identified, it must be triaged by the project's implementation team to determine the severity of the issue and how it should be addressed. Some issues uncovered are severe enough that testing must halt until the problem is addressed. Others may be deemed "working as designed" or as issues which should be covered in user training.

The goals of testing, particularly in a healthcare environment, are to:

- Evaluate whether a given system is built according to its specifications and design.
- Reduce the risk of critical problems being present when the system begins to be used.

Testing in Clinical Systems

A clinical system is used to support clinical care, and one that is operating without meeting all its specifications may at best be costing the clinician time and attention—and at worst may present a severe risk to the patient's health. With those sorts of potential consequences, establishing a robust testing process is key to the development of sound clinical systems both in the initial project implementation and in the ongoing operations and maintenance phase.

Given that clinical systems and their use cases are highly complex, the challenge for an implementation team is to prioritize where testing can have an impact. What are the areas of the system that carry the highest risk? What can be fixed if problems are found? As an implementation evolves, there may be fixed deadlines that necessitate "going live" if there is not strong evidence that going live would lead to poor outcomes. There is a need for both establishing a functional baseline through testing (each phase of testing builds on the previous phase) and running through enough use cases that the significant problems of the system are found before the go-live date. The challenge in this scenario is that the prior phases of the SDLC (Planning and Analysis, and Design and Usability) will often encroach upon the testing phase if deadlines are not met. The training period that follows testing is also required in order for users to know the processes around the system. Testing must therefore be well planned but also efficient and well understood so that prioritization decisions can be made if the allocated time period for testing shrinks during the implementation.

For those working in the informatics field, the concept and practice of testing can be daunting. The informatics curriculum in many educational programs merely brushes the surface of testing, yet the consequences of inadequate testing can be disastrous. Informatics specialists may serve in many roles related to the healthcare information technology (IT) testing process, including: consultant, developer, analyst, or even the person conducting the actual testing. This chapter will provide informaticists with enhanced knowledge regarding the testing phases and the process to conduct quality testing to provide a clinical system that meets and exceeds user expectations.

The Phases of Testing

Testing of clinical systems is performed in multiple phases. Not all phases are required, but usually some combination of function testing, integration testing, and user acceptance testing is performed. The following sections provide a brief overview of each testing phase.

Unit Testing

Unit testing is performed while a component is being developed and before it is turned over to the test team. It is typically performed by the developer who is creating the component. Because the developer understands the underlying design and coding of the component, this testing should be fairly low level and include testing of the logical pathways that the code follows. For example, if there are two sections of code that are run depending on a logical condition, unit testing should be performed on both conditions so that all of the code is logically tested. After this testing is completed, the component can be turned over to the test team for function testing.

There are no testing predecessors to unit testing other than that the component needs to have completed development so that it can be properly tested.

Unit Testing

1. Developer configures order set "Diagnostic Tests" including CBC, Chem 20 Panel, Chest X-Ray, Acetaminophen, and Vital Signs.
2. Developer includes defaults for days to perform different orders in order set.
3. Developer logs into Hospital Information System.
4. Developer opens order set "Diagnostic Tests."
5. Developer verifies that all orders are included and that default dates are present for order set.
6. Developer enters order set on test patient.
7. Developer validates orders appear correct on test patient Orders tab.

Function Testing

After different functional components of the system have been developed, they can be provided to the test team for function testing. This phase requires that the functional requirements of the system have been defined and documented. Test scripts are written to evaluate whether the system meets the functional requirements, and each requirement is mapped to a test script. This testing phase assumes that unit testing has already occurred on the components being tested.

A test script is a series of steps that can be taken to execute a test of a system. Test scripts are run by the group designated to perform the phase of testing (testers, users, or developers) and are usually designed to test specific requirements or business scenarios.

Examples of Function Testing Requirements

- The system shall send Lab orders to the Lab system on the day they are scheduled, 6 hours in advance.
- The system shall set any order that has been Active for 365 days to a status of Auto Complete.

Some of the concepts of clinical systems testing involve an understanding of some more technical concepts, such as Health Level Seven (HL7) and Structured Query Language (SQL). Tables 4.1 and 4.2, adapted from Henderson 2007, contain definitions of these terms.

Table 4.1 Health Level 7 Interface Definitions

Clinical System Term	*Definition*
Health Level Seven (HL7)	A standard series of predefined logical formats for packaging healthcare data in the form of messages to be transmitted among computer systems
HL7 Message	A collection of data that sends information about an event in the healthcare enterprise
Interface	The data connection between two computer systems

Unless the system is *self-contained* (an integrated hospital information system containing additional components, such as pharmacy, lab, and radiology), there will be a need to integrate multiple applications together and keep their data consistent. An interface engine that communicates with the HL7 standard is a methodology for creating a consistent set of clinical data across systems.

Function testing of HL7 interfaces consists of entering data into one system and validating that it is appearing properly in another system. This can be in the form of patient demographic data, where a patient can be registered and admitted using a registration system; or with orders that are entered in a hospital information system and sent by interface to another more specialized system used by a department: for example, a lab system. The lab system would then be used to document the results of lab testing, and those results would be sent back via an HL7 interface to the hospital information system. A test script might consist of a test order being entered in one system, and validated to have crossed the interface to the lab system. Then results would be entered in the lab system and validated in the hospital information system.

Another component of a system that may require function testing is the database. Although clinical applications are built upon databases that maintain the patient and application data and help render it to the user, some systems also include a data warehouse or other downstream databases that are used to provide reporting or querying capabilities to the user. Function testing can include validation that the correct data are being written to the database. This type of testing requires the tester to have a more technical background in order to find their way around the database and put together SQL queries. Table 4.2 contains definitions related to SQL and databases.

What are SQL queries?

SQL queries are a method to display data that are contained within a database. The query identifies the different data elements that are to be displayed, and can identify a single or multiple tables which contain the data. The methodology is a powerful way of combining data and searching for specific elements in the database. An example would be a query that is to identify a patient's orders.

```
SELECT order.name, order.enteredwhen, patient.name
FROM Patient_Table patient
INNER JOIN Order_Table order ON order.PatientID = patient.ID
WHERE Patient_Name = 'Sam Smith'
ORDER BY order.enteredwhen
```

In this example, there are two tables in the database: Patient_Table and Order_Table. The Patient_Table contains data about different patients, and the Order_Table contains data related to the orders placed on patients. The common identifier between the two tables is the patient's ID. Each record in the Order_Table contains a reference called PatientID that can then reference the Patient_Table ID field. In this way, all of a patient's orders can be retrieved by the query. In this example, a single patient (Sam Smith) is being specified, so that only this patient's orders are retrieved.

Table 4.2 Standard Query Language Definitions

Database Term	***Definition***
SQL	A query language used in conjunction with databases for the purposes of defining tables and relationships between tables; adding, modifying, retrieving, and deleting data; along with administrative purposes
Query	A structured request to the database in SQL to retrieve data from existing tables

Adapted from Gallardo, 2003

A key feature of any clinical system is how data can be rendered on printed media, in the form of paper, labels, or patient identifiers. Although clinical systems are evolving to a model that is less dependent upon paper, some processes still involve printing in most clinical settings, and printing takes on an important role, at times supporting regular processes, but also in the event of a system downtime.

Testing printing can be complex and detailed. It can include printing locally or printing via a broader network (for example, Citrix). It can involve printing-on-demand or on a scheduled basis. It can involve testing each custom report that has been developed for the system, which can number in the hundreds. Additionally, each report may have different conditions, which exercise different logic, so this testing can be a daunting task! Because of the sheer volume of testing that needs to happen with reports, collaboration between developers and testers can often be the best way of executing enough testing to minimize the risk of critical error.

User security and roles are another area that should be thoroughly vetted in function testing. The assignment of security rights to different user roles—to grant them sufficient access and permissions for the duties that their job entails, but not to provide inappropriate access which may lead to problems—is the basis of a functional security model. Testing of this model will involve the creation of multiple user accounts, each of which can assume a role, and exercising the functionality of that role to make sure that security permits the approved actions. Additional testing can be performed to ensure that the roles do not have permissions to perform unapproved actions.

Testing medical devices, such as bedside monitors interfaced into a hospital information system, can be challenging to function-test. These devices often require a real-time data feed, and simulating that feed without an actual patient may not be possible. Still, with any clinical system, there should be a way to execute testing before the setup is promoted to the live or production environment. In the case of devices, sometimes using either a pre-production feed or a development setup including a tester can be effective. The pre-production feed would be set up so that actual device data would be sent to both a development and a production clinical system, allowing for testing in the development system with information from the devices. The development setup using a tester would require devices dedicated to testing as well as a subject to try the devices so that data would be fed into a development system. In either case, the functionality and areas where the data are stored (result or flowsheet data) can be evaluated as it would be in production, with a supply of production data values, to verify the system functionality.

Integration Testing

Integration or *scenario testing* involves the development of common scenarios that will exercise the integrated components of the clinical system. The goal of this type of testing is to ensure that the individual components work together as a fully developed application to support the intended business processes (Garton & McCulloch, 2012).

In this sort of testing, it is important to have a consistent test patient who will receive the activity, and to make sure that the users who are executing actions on the test patient are assigned appropriate security rights for their roles. This will help to ensure that the system is properly configured to allow users to take expected actions and that the application will deliver the expected results without running into any consistency issues.

The first step to developing testing scenarios is for the business process of the application to be properly defined. An analyst, working in conjunction with a tester, can then work with the subject matter experts to identify what typical scenarios would look like when using the clinical system. Different users who will be interacting with the clinical system should be defined, and separate logins created for these users with appropriate security rights attached. The number of patients who would be seen in the scenario will also be identified so that they could be made available for testing. Any other components that would be necessary to execute the scenario could then be identified and made available, including printing and interfaces to other systems.

The testing scenario could then be broken down into steps taken by each of the users, with a test script created for each of the steps. The test scripts would contain, in smaller increments, the exact steps necessary to perform for testing, along with identifying the user executing the steps and the test patient that the steps will be performed on in the clinical system.

It is important that the scenarios covered during this phase of testing represent some of the more common or important scenarios that may be performed by the user population with the system, and also that function testing has been completed before this phase of testing begins. This will help to ensure that the problems that might have existed in the system during the function testing period have already been addressed and are known to the testers, and new problems that are found relate more to the intended business process of the system and how well the system can meet those business needs.

Clinical Integration Testing

The testing of a barcode system involves multiple components and setup, and can lead to a high volume of testable clinical scenarios. Patient identification, specimen collection, transfusion verification, and medication administration are some of the applications for barcode clinical workflows. Each clinical workflow involves multiple functional components, including the barcode application, printing capabilities, scanning capabilities, and often a mobile computer platform to run the clinical application, attached to a scanner, and enabling the generation of barcoded media. Additionally, there is the infrastructure of the hospital information system to allow order entry as well as an ancillary system (depending on the function: pharmacy, lab, or blood bank) to assist in the management of orders, medications, specimens, and blood units. Here is a sample testing scenario:

1. Physician logs into the hospital information system.
2. Physician selects the test patient.
3. Physician enters a lab order to collect a CBC + Diff.
4. Nurse logs into the barcode specimen collection application.
5. Nurse scans the patient ID.
6. Nurse verifies that CBC + Diff order is present in specimen collection application.

7. Nurse prints a label for CBC + Diff order and affixes to tube.
8. Nurse draws a sample in tube.
9. Nurse scans a label barcode to indicate that specimen was collected.
10. Physician validates in the hospital information system that the order is updated to "specimen collected" status, and that date/time associated with order is date/time of specimen collection.
11. Nurse sends tube to the lab.
12. Lab scans label barcode to indicate that the specimen was received.
13. Lab performs tests with analyzer on the specimen. Results are documented in the lab system.
14. Prescriber validates in hospital information system that the order is updated to "resulted," and that all results documented in lab system are visible under results view for patient.

Performance Testing

A more technical type of testing is *performance testing*, which generally involves the concept of creating user load to validate that the components of the system are robust enough to support the anticipated volume of usage at different times. This type of testing usually involves the application itself, the underlying database, and any other system components that are used in common scenarios, and also how they perform together as a whole (Garton & McCulloch, 2012).

You may (or may not) appreciate the analogy of the performance testing that a new football stadium performs prior to opening, where they flush all the toilets at once to ensure that halftime will not result in a major plumbing issue!

In performance testing, the tester creates scripts that are executed by a performance testing program. Sometimes if the tester does not have a sufficient technical background, this scripting may be developed by both a member of the test team and a member of the technical team. The performance testing program will generate multiple instances of the script, which simulate the volume of users performing the tasks multiple times on the system. These instances will all run against the system resources concurrently, which can test how the system setup and components stand up to the demands of multiple users.

Monitoring software should also be in place at this time to help validate that system memory, processor allocation, and response time still fall within the acceptable levels defined in the technical requirements of the system. The database server can also be validated in this approach to help ensure that the database can also support multiple read and write requests at an acceptable level as defined in the requirements.

After the testing has been performed, the monitoring results can be reviewed, and any issues addressed. This testing can help identify whether the server random access memory (RAM) or central processing unit (CPU) need to be enhanced to support the system function. Before investing in performance testing software, an organization should identify whether it is willing to correct any performance issues found, as well as what additional cost may be required.

If there are limitations on improving performance, sometimes it is not a cost-effective approach to run performance testing. Still, performance testing can reveal any bottlenecks and risks that might otherwise be found in the production phase, and may factor in to when a site can go live with their application.

Clinical Performance Testing

A new clinical system to support surgical functions is being installed in a hospital, and the installation team is interested in determining if the technical resources in place to support the surgical system are adequate. A tester creates a performance test script that simulates common user actions within the surgical system. As peak user volume is anticipated to be 25 concurrent users, the performance testing software is configured to run 25 concurrent sessions using the performance test script. Monitoring software is in place to observe how many system resources are utilized during the performance test. The test is run, and the results of the system resource monitoring are reviewed to determine if the system components need to be augmented to support the anticipated usage of the system.

User Acceptance Testing

After function and integration testing have been completed, a final testing phase is *user acceptance testing*, where the final software product is used as it will be used after deployment (Garton & McCulloch, 2012). During this phase, the system users will interact with the system and identify any problems or issues that they perceive with the functional aspects of the system, or with the process flow. Because this phase can be the first exposure of the users to the system, the system should be functioning reliably to provide a positive impression.

User acceptance testing may involve the users alone as testers, or it may involve others—from the test team or from another team, as someone who is present at the time of testing with the user—to record the user's observations and also help provide guidance about the system if there are questions. Choosing one strategy or the other is dependent upon what outcome the team wants to achieve through user acceptance. If the team wants to determine whether the system is intuitive enough for a new user to understand without assistance, then having them run through scenarios alone may be more appropriate. Otherwise, it may help facilitate the user getting familiar with the system to have someone else from the team partnered in this phase of testing.

Regression Testing

After the clinical application has gone live and is in use, the system moves to the operations and maintenance phase. Change needs to be introduced on a periodic basis, either based on improvements to the systems (upgrades, new releases) or configuration updates (new configuration or build). Along with testing that the specific defects have been corrected, a standardized set of regression test scripts should be developed and maintained to verify that no functionality that was previously working is now failing as a result of the change that was introduced (Garton & McCulloch, 2012).

Regression testing is a testing methodology that provides coverage of basic system capabilities to validate that any change to the system has not caused an issue with that basic functionality.

Additionally, other types of change, such as operating system *hot-fixes* (which are software updates to the operating system) or database changes, may have an impact on the clinical application. Often the specific change will not be known to the test team, so the best that can be done is to run the set of regression test scripts to help reduce the risk of a major impact to system functionality.

Common Components to Regression Test

- Order entry
- Clinical documentation
- Order HL7 interface
- Preview of reports
- One or two custom Medical Logic Modules (MLM) functions: for example, drug-allergy interaction
- Patient Admit-Discharge-Transfer (ADT)/demographic change

When change is promoted to the production environment, there is usually a limited window of time to run testing before releasing the system back to users. It is often regression testing that is performed rather than testing every new function and feature that has been deployed. Through the configuration management process, the same changes that were thoroughly vetted in development have been moved to production, and so a lesser extent of testing is performed in production.

What Helps Testing Run Efficiently?

With the focus on efficiency and planning for testing, what can help testing run smoothly? Before a test case can be run, planning tasks must occur to help define the testing schedule, process, and the scope of testing. After scope is defined, including what phases of testing will be included, test scripts are written to capture the different requirements and use cases. This task can be straightforward when firm decisions have been made, and requirements have been documented in the analysis phase of implementation. However, if decisions and requirements are still changing, preparing for (and executing) testing becomes much more challenging.

There will always be a few changes to process as the product becomes sufficiently well developed, and things emerge that must be addressed. That being said, there should always be an emphasis on freezing new development and processes to give the testing phase a better chance at success. Changes that come after testing begins place the testing methodology at risk, because the assumption is that what has already passed testing will continue to function. Strategies, including regression testing, can help if changes are introduced after testing begins, but there will also be testing resource costs in executing regression testing, and problems with system development may go undiscovered if not enough ground is covered.

The testing process includes the execution of test scripts by testers who may not be experts at the clinical system or clinical process. While they are running through their test scripts, they may have questions about the intended functionality or process, which could be either problems or just gaps in understanding. The availability of subject matter experts—usually in the role of analyst, informaticist, developer, or clinical user—will help expedite testing and quickly help identify if a problem has been found. If these resources are mostly unavailable, the testing process will be slowed down, especially with integration/scenario testing where testing scenarios can run for multiple days, and delays can be more costly.

What is the purpose of the different phases of testing? Testing phases tend to build on each other, and establishing a firm foundation before running more complex testing will help simplify the process of troubleshooting and redevelopment. The simplest parts of testing are run first: *unit* and *function* testing, which test individual areas of functionality, or requirements. After these have passed testing, *integration* or *system* testing is possible, where use-cases and scenarios are tested. If problems are found in this phase, it can often be a result of putting the individual functions together in a sequence, rather than an inherent issue with functionality, given that the functionality has already passed testing. *Performance* testing will often be run after function testing as well, because this is a process that involves testing the execution capacity of different system components. *User acceptance* testing is run after the other phases because this will be the user's first exposure to the system, and all the obvious errors should have been discovered and corrected at this time.

The Testing Process

When assessing any system from a testing perspective, you must develop a plan for how to develop an understanding of how the system operates, how to create the necessary scenarios and test scripts, and how to execute those test scripts using a testing methodology must be developed. Here are the beginning steps for how such a process can be assembled.

Identify the requirements to be tested, the key stakeholders, and the business processes involved.

Ideally, the requirements will have been identified and documented in a previous phase of the project, so the translation of requirements to test script is simplified. The tester must get familiar with the clinical application to be tested so that they understand how the requirements can be represented in terms of actions in the system, and then those actions documented into a test script. Similarly, scenarios and business processes will need to be translated into actions in the system so that they can be tested.

Identify the relevant types of testing to be performed.

Of all the different testing phases, some testing will be appropriate and considered in the testing scope, and other phases may not be necessary. Unit, function, integration, and user scceptance testing are usually necessary with any new implementation. Performance testing may be required with some implementations with a high anticipated user volume.

Engage your clinical users in the process.

An experienced tester may understand a lot about how systems work as well as the common issues involved, but clinical users can be extremely helpful. They can help with the use cases and scenarios that will be supported by the system but also in determining the severity and nature of issues found with the system. They are the ones who will tell the testers, "That will never work!"

Identify key requirements (both functional and technical) to be tested.

If time and resources are limited, there may be more requirements (both functional and technical) than can be tested within the allocated timeframe. Only some requirements can be tested, and an assessment should be performed of the testable requirements, along with a prioritization of requirements.

Identify key business processes/scenarios to be tested.

Common scenarios should be incorporated into integration testing, along with capturing the different types of user who will be interacting with the system in these scenarios.

Define criteria on whether a test script passes or fails.

Work out the rules for the testers so that they know how to proceed with a test script when they find an issue. Should they keep executing the script? Should they stop and report the issue to someone? The decision points should also be defined around a test script passing or failing, to identify whether every test step must pass. Usually, each step of the script must pass for the test script itself to pass. Later, after an issue has been triaged, it may be found that the system was working as designed, which may allow the script to pass.

Define how issues/bugs are identified, prioritized, and followed up on with the developer and determine whether software will be used to document each issue.

For any testing phase, a process needs to be developed on how issues are identified, triaged, and followed up. Ideally, testing issues are reviewed once per day during a system implementation, and any critical items are reviewed immediately. This timeliness will help ensure that the testing progresses on its anticipated timeline, and any items that place the system at risk can be quickly analyzed to determine an appropriate resolution plan. Often, a database or a tracker tool can be useful for documenting testing issues and assigning them to analysts or developers to further review and determine a resolution plan. Someone with an overall knowledge of the system and its processes should also be involved to prioritize issue resolution, or make the determination to proceed and accept the issue and train users on how to handle it.

Define when you will know that testing is completed for a given phase.

Along with creating a testing plan and a scope to the testing phases, it is important to know when testing for a certain phase is complete. This will often include a group of test scripts that must be executed and cover the system functionality to be tested. It may also include follow-up on any testing issues that were identified. Ultimately, there will be a decision-maker on the project team who can decide when to conclude testing for a given phase, and that the remaining issues are acceptable for the application, if any have not been resolved.

Create a testing timeline.

The testing tasks should be mapped into a timeline and calendar so that each day has a planned activity and a schedule can be developed, including the days that are required for putting together test scripts, along with executing those test scripts. Time should be given after test script execution for the correction and retesting of any incidents found. This helps guide the assessment if testing is ahead or behind schedule for planning and status-reporting purposes.

Define reporting metrics.

As testing progresses, the team will need to determine how to best report testing status and give an estimate of how much work remains. Status can usually be rolled into the number of test scripts or testing scenarios that have been run (with the results as a pass or fail) and the total number that will be run per phase. From a testing incident perspective, the number of incidents found at each level of severity can also be reported, along with the number open and the total number remaining.

How much testing is enough?

As testing is being planned, it may become clear that there is more out there to test than there are resources. In those cases, a nontraditional approach may need to be considered. The goal in testing is to minimize the risk of a critical issue being present in the system when the system becomes live, along with ensuring that the system has the desired capabilities which were defined when it was being built. Depending on the type of testing being performed, sometimes it can be more efficient to author an SQL query to help compare what has been built with the desired result. For instance, a system may have 200 types of orderable items configured in it, each with a separate message. If the messages are defined in a database table, and what has been built in the system is also defined, then using an SQL query can help compare the two and identify any deviations.

Perhaps a combination of this SQL query approach along with a spot-check of the application's front end may provide the most assurance that things are working as they should. Checking the database table may not guarantee that what is stored is actually what is displayed to the user. Checking the application side will help provide more of a guarantee of continuity between the content in the database and what the user sees.

Other times, despite efforts to keep to a schedule, testing tasks may take longer than planned and there may not be time to execute all of the planned testing. In those cases, decisions will need to be made about what the highest priority items are that need to be tested. Those decisions may depend on the critical nature of the functions or components that are being tested, and what the level of risk is if one of them has issues. Other ways to prioritize would include how frequently the use case or function may be employed in the system: An issue that the user runs into every day will be more frustrating than one that may be encountered to a lesser extent. Finally, testing the key functionality of a system can be the highest priority; if the system is advertised as assisting research and graphing key clinical indicators, the graphing functionality of the system should be tested so that it can meet those requirements and perform as desired for the user.

Applying the Technology

The previous section describes some aspects of broad testing methodology. There are some differences found within the composition of a clinical application as to where testing should be focused, how detailed the requirements will be that are provided to test, and the ability of the developer/vendor to change items within the application if they do not match the requirements/workflow. This section addresses some specifics when testing is required for vendor products, "home-grown" products, and web-based applications.

Testing Commercial Off-the-Shelf Applications

Many commercial off-the-shelf (COTS) clinical systems are available for purchase, and an organization will encounter some tradeoffs when purchasing them. The main tradeoff is that the vendor supplies resources to enhance the product, but there can be a lack of control over the direction that the product will take, because the vendor will be developing changes and upgrades for all of their clients rather than for one specific site.

The roadmap to testing these applications may be somewhat different than a custom-built application. Requirements may be defined at a higher level, and the focus of testing could be on the sections of the application that can be customized (for example, order forms, clinical documentation) and on interfaces (if they exist) to other systems. Performance testing can be conducted, but the question should always be asked whether there are appropriate methods to resolve issues if they are found.

Sometimes the project team may retain some control in resolving issues: for example, increasing the capabilities of the application servers or the capacity of concurrent users on virtual client servers (if such servers are part of the architecture). Other times, the problems will lie in the application software itself, and it may be costly to present compelling evidence to the vendor that their software is the root cause of the issue. Even if this can be done, if the contract that was signed does not include clear language around performance requirements, the vendor may not be required to correct the performance issues.

Albeit potentially frustrating, these limitations should be understood when planning where testing will be focused so that testing resources can be used strategically, where the issues that they identify add value and reduce risk.

As upgrades are released for a COTS product, the implementation team will want to analyze what new features and functionality they wish to use from the upgrade and then develop test cases to validate that the new functionality works as expected. This phase will also be where regression testing is important, given that an upgrade should be installed only in the live production environment after determining that major use cases and functionality still work without issue in the new release.

Testing Custom Applications

Custom applications are generally "home grown" by the developers in a company or organization. They will generally be more flexible when it comes to functionality and use cases, but they may also be impacted by a lack of resources if the developer team is not staffed to a capacity where they can maintain their existing applications and develop new ones.

Assuming that the analysis phase has been completed and requirements documented, the functional requirements and scenarios should be documented at a detailed level, allowing the test team to draw on those requirements for developing their function test scripts. Testing can be run to the approved specifications because there should be flexibility in the design and implementation to account for the system functionality. Any deviations from the design should be documented, and the requirements updated to reflect the current state of the system as well as any subsequent decisions. Integration testing and user acceptance testing are key. If a high volume of users is anticipated on the system, performance testing would add value because of flexibility in terms of updating the application code itself if performance issues are identified.

Upgrades and new versions of the application would be handled in similar fashion to a COTS product. New functionality would be tested with new function test scripts, and regression testing would be used to ensure that the existing functionality was maintained in the new version.

Testing Web-Based Applications

Web-based applications have additional requirements, mostly concerning browser compatibility and security (depending on what information is available within them). They can either be COTS or custom-developed, but additionally, they do not operate based on a client-server model but rather a web-based model where the system may be more broadly available (unless restricted by a firewall). In this case, additional technical requirements around security and authentication may come in to play.

Much of the testing that would occur would likely be unit testing or testing performed by the security team. However, the test team can assist with testing browser compatibility, validating authentication into the application, and verifying that it is available from appropriate locations—for example, if the application should be available while the user is on the company network but not available from a public network. Users may be accessing the application from a PC or a Mac, along with different browsers offered from these operating systems.

If mobile devices are being used to access the web application, those devices and browsers should also be included in testing. If the application is compatible with only certain web browsers and certain versions, both (acceptable and not acceptable) those should be published into the application so that users know that they are using an incompatible browser or version. If the application is assumed to function on many browsers, then testing should be performed on those browsers to validate that there are not significant deviations in display or functionality. Similarly, if multiple types of mobile devices will be used in accessing the web application, each type of mobile device should be tested when accessing the application. Additionally, test the combinations of web browsers for the mobile device that may be invoked in accessing the application. Testing can get complicated quickly, which is why some developers limit their support to specific devices and browsers.

What Software Tools Can Assist with Testing?

Software tools are available that can assist with making testing more efficient as well as keeping testing better organized so that reports can be generated quickly, tasks can be assigned, and status can easily be visualized.

- **Tools to assist with defining requirements and mapping to test cases:** Software tools are available that can be used to document the requirements for a software application, and then make sure that they are mapped to test scripts. During the testing phase, the test script status can then be updated to Pass/Fail, allowing an overall status to be conveyed around which requirements are met within the system. An example of a requirements management tool is Borland Caliber:

  http://www.borland.com/products/caliber/

- **Tools to assist with tracking and reporting issues/incidents:** Issue-tracking software will help document issues found in testing. Many contain custom abilities to define a state flow—what states an issue will take on: for example, Open, Assigned to Development, Ready for Retest, Retest Passed, Closed—along with characteristics of the issue, such as which test phase and script it was identified in, and whom the issue is currently assigned to. Capabilities of these systems include customization of the state flow and issue form, email notification to assignees, and the generation of reports in different formats. Some examples are Atlassian Jira and Serena Business Manager:

  https://www.atlassian.com/software/jira

  http://www.serena.com/index.php/en/products/featured-products/sbm/

- **Tools to assist with performance testing:** Performance testing tools are available as both proprietary software and open source, and can assist with the generation of simulated user load on a software application. These tools require some customization before they can run so as to define the user workflows in the application that will be simulated, but can then evaluate the performance of a clinical application in its environment. Examples include HP LoadRunner and Borland Silk Performer:

  http://www8.hp.com/us/en/software-solutions/loadrunner-load-testing/

  http://www.borland.com/products/silkperformer/read/

- **Tools to assist with the automation of testing:** If testing is to be repeated on a clinical application, as may be the case for regression testing scripts, it may be worth creating automated test scripts, which can run automatically rather than having a tester manually execute each step. There is an initial setup cost, along with the cost of the automated testing tool (if an open source tool is not identified), but the time spent in recurring testing will then be lessened through the automated tool. An example is HP Unified Functional Testing:

  http://www8.hp.com/us/en/software-solutions/unified-functional-testing-automation/

Future Directions

As new frameworks for understanding emerge in the realm of healthcare informatics, some of these can be leveraged to enhance testing practice and help identify areas for a testing focus to reduce the risk for implementations.

Proprietary and Open Source Software

Proprietary software is commercial software which is sold and maintained by a vendor and tends to have configurable settings, but also limits to how much the user can customize the software. *Open source* software is publically available with "no software costs or licensing fees" (Sanzeri, 2008), with the expectation that it will be downloaded and instantiated by different users.

Both proprietary and open source software have initial setup costs, and require skilled developers to install and prepare for use (Sanzeri, 2008). Over time, there are tradeoffs about how the software can be modified and maintained. Proprietary software can be modified by the software vendor, and modifications usually require a new release or a change to the software application. Open source software can be customized and modified at any time, but requires the developer resources to do so. An important point is that with proprietary software, the vendor must evaluate change to a software application across all of its users, and some changes may not be approved. This can come into contention with business process workflows that an organization may have, and may require the modification of business processes to conform to the application (Sanzeri, 2008).

Including the Underlying Architecture/Authentication Mechanisms in Testing

A more technical form of testing—but important in terms of ensuring the security and data flows within a clinical application—involves testing that includes the architecture and authentication mechanisms. Such testing is important with web-based applications, applications with multiple components, or applications that share data with other applications. As part of the design for the system, a plan related to disaster recovery and system component unavailability should be generated; and in that plan, recovery procedures should be documented. The testing of those recovery procedures would be part of this testing, addressing items such as failover server clustering to provide high availability of the system, restoration of databases from backup, and the resending of HL7 messages to recover a system to an appropriate point in time. After these processes have been performed, regression testing and validation would be important in helping to ensure that the system has been put into a workable state for future use before being released to users.

Testing in the Cloud

Cloud computing has become a more popular method of virtualizing aspects of a computerized network. Applications, platforms, and servers can be virtualized and service can be provided by a group that sells that aspect of the network "as a service" (Kuo, 2011), thus creating a different infrastructure that can be more adaptable and increase flexibility of allocation of system resources to multiple clients. The idea of putting part of a system "in the cloud" means to outsource the maintenance of those parts of the computer network to another group that will provide those services.

The three layers of Cloud services are outlined below, per Kuo (2011).

- *Software as a service (SaaS):* The clinical applications are hosted by a cloud service provider and made available to users over a network, such as the Internet.
- *Platform as a service (PaaS):* The operating systems are hosted in the cloud and accessed through a browser. With PaaS, developers can build clinical Web applications without installing any special tools on their computer, and then deploy those applications for use.
- *Infrastructure as a service (IaaS):* The cloud user outsources the equipment used to support operations, including storage, hardware, servers, and networking components, upon which the clinical applications are run and accessed. The cloud provider owns the equipment and is responsible for housing, running, and maintaining it.

To a functional tester, if the application is being provided through SaaS, then the access mechanism to the application may relate to this relationship. The authentication mechanism can then be tested, and functional requirement testing would proceed as with any other implementation technique. Many of the other aspects of cloud computing are abstracted from the functional testing methodology. Performance testing could still be performed to ensure that the PaaS and IaaS layers are sufficiently robust to support the anticipated user load on the system, if those layers are being outsourced.

Testing for Mobile Devices

Mobile devices are becoming a more common access mechanism both for systems tied to monitoring and barcoded workflow, along with systems that are integrated into the clinician's documentation or order entry process. The availability of the application on a mobile platform brings into play the wireless network (which allows the device to connect to remote resources) but creates additional security concerns, such as how to protect data that flows along those wireless pathways, along with how to protect the physical devices themselves. Some security concerns can be alleviated through enforcing effective password policies and ensuring a way to remotely erase the memory of any stolen devices (Carr, 2011).

Along with testing some of these capabilities, testing of mobile devices can also include testing of availability along the wireless network (performing testing in the different areas where the mobile device is expected to function) and function testing of different expected functions. For example, if a device will allow printing to a wireless printer, then execute that printing function in various locations and validate that both the device and the printer behave as expected in conjunction with the clinical application.

The Importance of Understanding Enterprise Architecture for Testing

Enterprise Architecture encompasses an understanding of business, application, data, and technology architecture, and drills down from the business needs and capabilities into a specific implementation at the server and database level (The Open Group Architecture Forum, 2011). As part of the definition of the architecture, business process requirements, technical requirements, and business scenarios are developed and documented, which can be incorporated into the development of testing scripts. The mapping of higher-level capabilities into testing scenarios can also help to ensure that the application has met the business needs that drove its creation.

Conclusion

Although the testing process can be quite technical, it requires informatics expertise in all phases. Whether to determine and prioritize testing requirements, develop testing scripts, or actually conduct testing, informatics knowledge and expertise will help ensure that quality testing processes are carried out. Many of us have lived the experience of inadequate testing in our organizations and know the unpleasant and potentially unsafe consequences that result. This chapter, while providing a broad, fairly high level of understanding of testing in a healthcare environment, builds a foundation to continue to develop expertise in this important phase of our clinical systems.

References

Carr, D. F. (2011, May 19). Healthcare puts tablets to the test. *InformationWeek.* Retrieved from http://www.informationweek.com/mobile/healthcare-puts-tablets-to-the-test/d/d-id/1097846?

Freedman, D. H. (2005, January 1). Entrepreneur of the year. *Inc. Magazine.* Retrieved from http://www.inc.com/magazine/20050101/eoty-rutan.html

Gallardo, D. (2003, May 30). SQL essentials. *InformIt.* Retrieved from http://www.informit.com/articles/article.aspx?p=31829

Garton, C., & McCulloch, E. (2012). *Fundamentals of technology project management* (2nd ed.). (pp. 397–400). Boise, ID: MC Press Online, LLC.

Henderson, M. (2007). *HL7 messaging* (2nd ed.). (pp. 11–12). Aubrey, TX: OTech, Inc.

Kuo, A. M-H. (2011). Opportunities and challenges of cloud computing to improve health care services. *Journal of Medical Internet Research, 13*(3) e67. doi: 10.2196/jmir.1867. Retrieved from http://www.ncbi.nlm.nih.gov/pmc/articles/PMC3222190/

The Open Group Architecture Forum. (2011). Part I: Introduction > Core concepts. TOGAF 9.1. Retrieved from http://www.togaf.org/togaf9/chap02.html

Sanzeri, S. (2008, November 20). Proprietary software vs. open source – The hidden costs [Web log post]. *Trellon.* Retrieved from http://www.trellon.com/content/blog/proprietary-software-vs-open-source-hidden-costs

"Ignorance of all things is an evil neither terrible nor excessive, nor yet the greatest of all; but great cleverness and much learning, if they be accompanied by a bad training, are a much greater misfortune."

–Plato

Delivering Healthcare Informatics Training

5

Brenda Kulhanek, PhD, MSN, MS, RN-BC, CPHIMS

OBJECTIVES

- Describe the purpose of health information technology training.
- Arrange training tasks within a training development framework.
- Explain the purpose of learning theory.
- List the five types of learning evaluation.

The introduction of healthcare information technology (IT) into the already complex healthcare environment has triggered the need for a new approach to training. In this chapter, you will learn how to use well-established training frameworks and models to implement effective training in the rapidly changing world of healthcare. Implementation of healthcare IT has been associated with the introduction of new leadership structures, disciplines, and patient care practices (Shea et al., 2014), and may be correlated to a decrease in patient safety during and after the initial implementation period (Meeks, Takian, Sittig, Singh, & Barber, 2014). Managing change through effective training becomes extremely important in light of the potential for unplanned consequences and organizational turbulence.

Assessing Training

The *Nursing Informatics Scope and Standards* (American Nurses Association, 2008, p. 25) stated that "[E]ducation is a critical component of many NI functions and may directly affect the success or failure of any new or modified IT solution." Despite the inclusion of education as a functional area for nursing informatics, little is found in healthcare-related literature about the process of developing and delivering effective training for users of healthcare IT (Alpay & Russell, 2002; Bredfelt, Awad, Joseph, & Mark, 2013; Page, 2011). Most concerning is that the results of poor training can produce decreased efficiency, staff turnover, patient care errors, and poor quality documentation followed by decreased billing revenue. Training is the final opportunity to positively influence performance and attitude toward change.

Business, education, and the military spend billions of dollars annually on training (Morrison, Ross, Kalman, & Kemp, 2011), based on effective training models developed over decades and based on the science of human performance improvement (HPI). The good news is that these models can be used to successfully address the challenges of healthcare IT training in our current fast-moving and unique healthcare environments. Grounded in psychology, organizational behavior, performance improvement, quality, and other disciplines (Pershing, 2006), training is different from education (Morrison et al., 2011, p. 4):

> "Specific job training has precise, immediate requirements with identifiable and often measurable outcomes. …Formal education, on the other hand, often has broad purposes and more generalized objectives. Application of the knowledge and skills taught may not become important until sometime in the future."

Implementing an effective and accountable training model in healthcare requires a different approach along with new models and frameworks to guide the process.

Informatics in Action

This true story, possibly repeated many times in many organizations, demonstrates the role that training plays in patient safety. The surgeon, new to use of healthcare IT, ordered antibiotics to be given 30 minutes before surgery and every 6 hours post-surgery. A dose of the antibiotic was given in the operating room with the expectation that the next dose would be given in 6 hours.

When the patient arrived in the recovery room, the recovery nurse, also new to the healthcare IT system, viewed the order for an antibiotic, along with the many other post-operative orders that were in the system. The nurse proceeded to hang another dose of the IV antibiotic, just 45 minutes after the first dose was given.

When the patient was transferred to the inpatient unit after leaving the recovery unit, the admitting nurse, also new to the healthcare IT system, reviewed the list of post-operative orders, noted the antibiotic order, and administered another dose of the medication just 1.5 hours after the last dose. At the same time, the pharmacist, also new to the system, reviewed the antibiotic order and sent the next dose to the patient care unit so that it would be ready for the next dose in six hours.

At the change of shift, the oncoming nurse reviewed the patient care orders, noted that an antibiotic was due, and administered another dose of the medication, 6 hours after the operative dose has been given. In total, it was discovered that the patient received four doses of the ordered antibiotic within a 6-hour period.

A root-cause analysis was performed and concluded that each person that administered the medication improperly during the 6 hours under review had failed to read the patient chart and the medication administration record completely. The involved staff were coached, and the incident was filed away into the quality and risk records. There was no attempt to review the training that each of the staff received prior to using the healthcare IT system to determine whether the training was effective or if the staff had even attended training. Even more concerning, there had been no post-training evaluation designed to assess whether the staff were competent to perform their jobs after the conclusion of training.

Because training was not considered as a causative factor in this medication error incident, the training program was not examined or adjusted in any way. Because the training program was not examined, there was no assurance that future trainees would not replicate this same error. Could this type of incident occur again?

Applying the Technology: Tools and Evidence

Why do we need to train in the first place? Why can't members of the patient care team intuitively figure out how to use a new healthcare IT system? Unlike many computer applications that can be used almost immediately with little effort, a healthcare IT system is a very complex application that introduces new equipment, unfamiliar physical skills, changed processes, and altered workflows into the patient care setting (Runy, 2005).

Many nurses lack basic computer skills. According to a 2008 Health Resources and Services Administration (HRSA) survey, the median age for registered nurses in the United States is 46 years old (HHS, 2010). Nurses and other healthcare workers may need to become comfortable with computer functionality before they can begin to learn and apply a new system for patient care (Alpay & Russell, 2002; Jacques, 2002; Runy, 2005).

Prior to the implementation of healthcare IT, new healthcare and medical information was delivered using educational models that included lecture and demonstration, often led by an expert clinician. This method of education provided a reliable way to deliver clinical and medical training. However, existing educational models and frameworks familiar to healthcare are now challenged to produce successful and cost-effective training, especially when faced with the complexities and unique issues associated with healthcare IT.

Benefits of using the evidence-based HPI models in our healthcare IT environment are numerous. The models can provide a consistent framework of established models and methods that are used to analyze, design, develop, implement, and evaluate training. By using the established framework, training can:

- Focus on those elements that are critical for the learners to understand.
- Produce more cost-effective training.
- Continually improve the training process through evaluation.
- Deliver the right content to the right learners at the right time using the right method.
- Use learning theory to increase relevance and applicability to learners.
- Leverage design theory to facilitate learner engagement.
- Relate results to performance improvement.

HPI training models provide a flexible framework that can be used successfully for training healthcare providers to use healthcare IT.

In order to understand the framework, it is important to learn about the foundations upon which the framework is based. HPI theory views the stimulus for training as a gap in performance (Morrison et al., 2011). Approaching a training project from this perspective allows for the measurement of current knowledge or skills against post-training knowledge and application. Human performance technology seeks to identify the root cause of performance gaps and apply the best and most effective intervention to address and measure the gaps. Training as an intervention is just one of the tools used by the human performance improvement specialist.

Multiple learning theories drive the design of training and include behaviorist theory, cognitive theory, constructivist theory, social learning theory, adult learning theory, learning styles, and more (Morrison et al., 2011). Theories help performance improvement specialists to understand how the brain learns, how to best structure instruction, and what motivates learners. Of these many theories, adult learning theory takes into consideration the unique needs and perspectives of the adult learner. Failure to understand and use these foundational principles can result in increased learner resistance and reduced training effectiveness.

Adult learning theory is one of the major frameworks used for developing successful healthcare IT training, and includes the following six principles (Knowles, Holton & Swanson, 2005):

1. The learner wants to know why learning is necessary before investing the time and energy into pursuing learning.
2. Adults have life experiences and are accustomed to being responsible for their own decisions. Adults tend to resist learning that they perceive is forced upon them.
3. Adults have a great volume of life experience and appreciate learning experiences that acknowledge the value of their past experiences.
4. Adults seek to learn those things that will prepare them for situations or tasks that are imminent and seek learning that will help them progress in life or accomplish tasks more readily.
5. Adults learn best when information is presented or aligned with the context of life or life situations.
6. The greatest motivator for adult learning is intrinsic rather than extrinsic.

NOTE

Incorporating adult learning theory into training will ensure that your training plan does not run into common roadblocks that will disengage your learners. Roadblocks can include covering information that the audience already knows, failing to link new information to upcoming job tasks, or delivering training before the learners have developed an understanding of the need for training.

Teaching to learning styles has been popular in healthcare for many years. The theory of learning styles states that each individual has specific ways in which they prefer to learn, and these preferences may influence the success of training. Learning preferences can include visual, auditory, verbal, kinesthetic, logical, social, solitary, and experiential; subdivided into converger, diverger, assimilator, and accommodator (Brady, 2013). The effort to accommodate diverse learning styles in the development of training materials can add a significant amount of work and time to the training design and development process, and the effectiveness of instructing to learning styles has not been demonstrated (Choi, Lee, & Kang, 2009).

A Training Development Model

The use of a training development model will help to develop solid training design, which ultimately results in effective training. The five steps to the training development process are analysis, design, development, implementation, and evaluation, often referred to as "ADDIE." Although other training development models are in use, ADDIE provides a straightforward, iterative process that provides a methodical model for training design.

Analysis

Training should always be approached as an intervention that is delivered in response to a gap in performance. Why is it important to start the training design process with analysis? Even though you may very clearly understand what your audience needs to learn, analysis can help you understand the characteristics of your learner audience to prevent redundant or unnecessary training and allow you to meet the learner at their current level of function. Analysis helps you to understand the technology environment needed to support the delivery of training and the amount of current support from the organization and your leaders. Analysis will also uncover other organizational initiatives that may affect resources for your project.

The analysis portion of the design framework can be quite lengthy; however, the information gathered during this phase of the project is critical and will be used to make decisions through the remaining steps of the design framework. The types of analysis that you choose to perform will vary, depending on the type of learning project and the amount of information previously collected. A robust analysis can prevent wasted work and effort during the entire course of the project by uncovering barriers and identifying sources of support. Types of analysis are listed in Table 5.1, grouped by general category. Information gathered through analysis can be very enlightening, and sometimes changes the direction of the training project.

Table 5.1 Categories of Analysis

Organizational Analysis	
Needs Assessment	A broad view of organizational needs. What are current initiatives, drivers, and barriers?
Gap Analysis	What is the gap in performance? What is the expected performance?
Cause Analysis	What contributed to the gap in performance?
Root Cause Analysis	What is the root cause of the gap in performance?
Technology	What is the status of the current technology environment?
Stakeholders	Who are the stakeholders? What is the level of awareness? What is the level of support?

continues

Table 5.1 Categories of Analysis *(continued)*

Learner Analysis	
Worker	Who are the workers?
Environment	Where do the workers perform their work?
Motivation	What motivates the worker?
Knowledge	What is the base of knowledge of the worker?
Attitude	What is the attitude of the worker toward change?
Skills	What skills do the workers possess?
Roles	What are the different worker roles?
Task Analysis	
Task Inventory	What are all the steps in the new process?
Job performance requirements	What is the expected performance? What are the objectives of each task?
Content	Is there any previous content that can be utilized?
Workflow	What is the specific workflow for each learner role?

© B. Kulhanek (2011)

As you can see, the initial analysis is fairly comprehensive, gathering information that may help or hinder your training project, identifying areas of resistance and communication needs, and defining the value of the training and the expected benefits, helping you design training that is concise and matched to the learner's needs. Although the initial training analysis is labor-intensive, information can often be re-used for similar training projects in the future, allowing for updates as learning audiences and stakeholders change.

One of the most critical portions of the analysis phase is the task analysis, which builds the backbone of the training content. A *task analysis* divides the processes to be trained into pieces so that the most important training elements can be identified and prioritized for efficient end-user training. Although the term "task" is used in many settings, "task" is used in a different context in the instructional design process. Simply put, a *task* is a single technical procedure within a healthcare IT application that has a start and an end point. An example of a task would be the process of logging into a computer application, which has a start and an end point. Grouped together, tasks form complete processes, such as order entry or clinical documentation, typically found in a healthcare IT application. A task analysis is very similar to a workflow but includes the specific actions to be taken at each point in the process.

A task analysis is conducted by using experts in the new processes (subject matter experts) and members of the training team. Subject matter experts play a key role in the design process by outlining processes and clearly identifying tasks. You will refer to the subject matter experts frequently during the design process; their role will include validating key information to be included in training, reviewing training content, and possibly piloting training materials. Although entire books have been written about working with subject matter experts, it is important to remember that subject matter experts typically have full-time jobs, and their time must be used judiciously and efficiently. Because subject matter experts are very familiar with processes, they may skip key steps during task analysis in a process that has become automatic to them. Make sure that you ask detailed questions and map out every single step in a process. Sometimes it is helpful to have both a subject matter expert and a naïve user in the same room during the task analysis.

When processes have been completely mapped out, stakeholder support has been identified, and you have a good understanding of the needs of your learner audience and the nature of the performance gap, you are ready to begin design of the training program. As mentioned earlier, the ADDIE model can be an iterative process, meaning that you may have to conduct more analysis during the design phase as you encounter design issues that were not answered through the initial analysis.

Design

During the design process, the training delivery method is selected, which will guide the design of the instruction. Training may be delivered through web-based training, just-in-time training, paper-based training, instructor-led training, or a mix of these methods. The addition of multiple training delivery methods can add flexibility and efficiency to the training process. However, each training delivery method has pros and cons and is most appropriate for certain learning needs. Regardless of the training delivery method, the design and development process remain the same.

Each healthcare discipline and care setting may have different training delivery preferences. Many physicians prefer on-the-job training and resist extended hours of classroom training (Fisher, Creusat, & McNamara, 2008). Nurses will attend classroom training but must be replaced by another nurse to provide patient care during the classroom training time, resulting in high costs for this training delivery method. Frequently, due to the training delivery method selected, there is no opportunity for care providers to practice in a real-life setting, thus reducing the chances of successful transfer of learning to the care setting. When determining the delivery method for a training program, it is important to refer to learner needs obtained during the analysis phase of development as well as to consider the specific needs of adult learners.

Learning objectives identify what you would like the learner to be able to do at the end of the training session and are developed during the design phase of the project. Learning objectives satisfy two key needs (Morrison et al., 2011):

- Learning objectives guide the designer during development of learning activities.
- Learning objectives provide the foundation for learning evaluation.

Learning objective statements should contain a verb and a noun: Here is an example:

> "At the conclusion of this session, the learner will be able to demonstrate [verb] how to log on to the computer [noun]."

This statement can guide both the content that is delivered during training (the steps needed to log on to the computer) and the plan for evaluation (at the conclusion of training, demonstrate how to log on to the computer). When developing objectives, some designers find it easier to identify what the learner should understand or demonstrate at the end of training, write the evaluation questions, and then create the learning outcomes. Either way, learning objectives and outcomes should be evaluated and approved by your subject matter experts to ensure that your training plan addresses and evaluates the most critical learning elements.

When developing learning objectives, remember that use of healthcare IT involves physical actions, emotion, and knowledge; therefore, learning objectives should be focused on more than knowledge. In fact, attaining knowledge is not an indicator that learners will apply what they have learned on the job (Phillips & Phillips, 2008). However, without knowledge there would be no application of learning. The ability to recite facts after training is not correlated with application of training on the job. Successive levels within each of the learning domains of knowledge (cognitive domain), feelings (affective domain), and actions (psychomotor domain) allow for learning objectives to range from simply knowing to being able to synthesize or evaluate learning (Bloom, 1956). Similar levels of learning are associated with the affective and psychomotor domains.

During the design phase, communicate with project stakeholders to finalize training logistics including the training schedule, equipment, facilities, and budget. Nursing unit managers typically appreciate knowing training dates months in advance so that schedules can be adjusted. When the training has been conceptually mapped out and learning objectives have been created, it is time to begin developing the training materials.

Development

During the development phase, training content is created based on the learning objectives. Outlines developed during the task analysis are tailored to address key training concepts and to follow the flow of the training program. Although it is tempting to create a comprehensive training manual for each learner, these resources represent a vast amount of work and expense and are seldom accessed after the training class has been completed. Rather than printing a training manual, it may be better to develop an accessible online "e-manual" or to focus on creating *job aids* (short documents that help the learner to remember how to complete complex or rarely used processes).

During the development process, you will rely on subject matter experts again to validate the training content as it is being developed. Often the healthcare IT system is under development at the same time that the training is being designed, resulting in many changes and revisions during the development period. When you are nearing completion of the development process, the training materials can be pilot tested and revised based on learner reaction, feedback, and system functionality, using an iterative process.

Important to address during the development phase are any technical links and processes; spelling; and appearance of materials on various-sized computer screens and devices, such as an iPhone or iPad. If technology has not yet been tested, this is the time to ensure that materials can be delivered to the learners without problem. Make sure that learners can access materials on network locations or websites, using several different computers, browsers, operating systems, and connections to test. If possible, schedule your delivery date for a week prior to the training implementation date so that any issues can be resolved prior to training.

When all training materials have been developed, schedule a final review session with subject matter experts and other stakeholders. Review the materials as well as the learning objectives and plans for evaluation. The development phase typically concludes with sign-off of all training materials by the subject matter experts or project leaders and stakeholders.

NOTE

If you will be delivering training through instructor-led classes, your instructors will need to be trained to effectively present the content. Learners will quickly lose faith in an instructor who does not know the materials and processes and cannot answer questions. Many books have been written about skills needed for delivering instructor-led training. One quick tip is to teach your instructors to use a "parking lot" for questions that cannot or should not be answered during the teaching session.

Implementation

The implementation phase involves delivering training materials to the learners through the distribution methods that were determined during the analysis and design phases of the project. Although implementation may seem like a time when you can heave a sigh of relief and relax after the hard work, there is work to be done. Implementation, especially in the first few days, offers the opportunity to gather information that can be used to make necessary changes or improvements to the training plan. It is important to monitor not only that the learners are successfully gaining new knowledge, but that the training materials themselves are effective.

Formative evaluation is typically conducted during the development phase of the training process, but can also be used during a training pilot to evaluate the success of the learning materials. Effectiveness of the training materials can be seen through post-training evaluations and through observation of the learners. If there are areas of the training instructions or content that seems to cause problems, adjustments can be made so that the final implementation of the materials is as effective as possible. If you find that (as seen through evaluation questions) a large percentage of pilot learners are struggling with portions of the content, there may be unclear areas that need to be updated. The goal is to implement your training program with materials as close to perfect as possible. Even small errors in spelling can detract from learner attention.

Summative evaluation refers to evaluation of the training materials and program after the materials have been developed and implemented. Plan for a routine, daily review of the learning evaluation data, especially during the first few days of the training implementation, in order to quickly catch and resolve any problems. If training materials need to be corrected at this point, you may have more of a challenge to update printed materials that are already distributed, or re-publish links to Internet sites or network locations.

If your training program is being delivered through instructor-led training, remember to establish rules of the classroom, including *silencing technology* such as cell phones or smartphones. Allow for frequent changes in activity to relieve the monotony of training. If access to personal communication devices is banned in the classroom, allow for regular email breaks. To assist instructors, plan to collect commonly asked questions or frequently occurring issues so that all are prepared for future classes. You may also need to maintain a roster of training attendees and report back to leaders about attendees and no-shows. In a clinical environment, attendees may be pulled away from training for clinical emergencies. Try to avoid this as much as possible by ensuring that attendees are not in clinical rotation during training. If you do not maintain some control over the class schedule and the classroom environment, you may find that very few people attend the first classes or very little learning occurs, resulting in overflowing final classes with new and repeat learners.

Evaluation

Post-training evaluation is conducted to determine the success of the training program in addressing the previously identified performance gap (Morrison et al., 2011). There are five levels of evaluation, each serving a different purpose within an organization. Table 5.2 contains an overview of evaluation types along with recommended tools for data collection. Each level of evaluation lays the foundation for the next level of evaluation, but does not guarantee the success of the next level of evaluation.

Table 5.2 The Five Levels of Evaluation

Level	*Definition*	*Purpose*	*Examples*	*Question Types*
1. Reaction	Measuring the perception that the training experience did or did not meet the needs of the learner	Immediate feedback on the training experience (Positive feedback on the training experience does not necessarily correlate with learning success.)	• The content will be useful in my job. (Likert) • The visual aids were effective. (Likert) • The training was a good use of my time. (Likert) • What barriers that will prevent you from applying what you have learned? (multiple choice)	• Likert scale • Multiple choice • Open-ended questions • Focus groups • Yes/No

Level	*Definition*	*Purpose*	*Examples*	*Question Types*
2. Learning	Measuring the learning that took place as a result of the training	This measure does not assess what the learner does with the knowledge, but just that there was a change	• Demonstration of correct sequence of steps in a process • Matching or ranking questions • Observation with performance checklist (classroom) • Problem-solving questions	• Multiple choice • Open-ended questions • Observation • Likert scale • Pre- and post-test
3. Application	Measuring the degree of use of the new knowledge and skills on the job	To identify how much of learning is used on the job by an individual or group of individuals	• Measures of efficiency • Measures of error/success • Self-reporting measures • Observation with performance checklist (job setting)	• Observation • Metrics • Likert scale • Open-ended questions • Interviews/focus groups
4. Business Results	Measuring any change in business metrics resulting from the application of new knowledge and skills gained from training	To analyze specific pre and post business metrics to identify changes	• Error rates • Patient satisfaction • Turnover rate • Productivity rate • Outcomes/quality measures	• Customer surveys • Business metrics • Individual metrics

continues

Table 5.2 The Five Levels of Evaluation *(continued)*

Level	*Definition*	*Purpose*	*Examples*	*Question Types*
5. Return on Investment	Measuring the benefits of the training outcomes against the cost of the training	Determining the value of a training program in order to support informed decisions	• Time and cost of training development • Time and cost of delivering training to learners • Value of changes in business metrics	• Typically related to gathering data for business metrics, training costs, and resources used for training

© B. Kulhanek (2011)

Evaluation measurements are taken at different times during and after the implementation period, dependent on the type of evaluation.

Please indicate your reaction to the class.	**Strongly Agree**	**Agree**	**Disagree**	**Strongly Disagree**
The training session was a good use of my time.	4	3	2	1

Reaction evaluation: A Level 1 evaluation, also known as evaluation of reaction, occurs immediately after the training has been delivered. The reaction evaluation collects learner impressions and responses to trainers, training materials, delivery methods, the training environment, and other factors that influence attitude toward training. A reaction evaluation can tell you whether learners liked or disliked a course. Enjoyment or dissatisfaction of a course can influence the attitudes of future attendees.

Although a reaction evaluation can provide useful information, it is not a reliable indicator of whether learning occurred. Many times training is evaluated only at the reaction level, which stops short of providing information about success in closing the performance gap.

Learning evaluation: Learning, or knowledge, is the Level 2 evaluation. A knowledge evaluation determines how well the learners have assimilated facts and figures into short-term and long-term memory. Typically administered during and immediately after training, the knowledge evaluation can assess understanding of terms, workflow processes, and recall of facts or actions.

Again, a successful learning evaluation does not ensure that the learners will apply what they have learned on the job, although understanding key terms and processes is important for successful learning application. The true value of training as a means to resolve a performance gap begins to be seen in evaluation levels 3–5.

Application evaluation: Level 3 evaluation measures the learner's ability to apply the content and processes learned during training. The culmination of a long training development process is to see that learners efficiently and effectively use the information that they have learned after they have attended training. Measurement of the application of training is a more labor-intensive process and cannot be conducted during or immediately after training. Learning objectives related to application of learning will typically contain an action statement such as, *Completes an admission assessment by addressing all interview questions for all assigned patients within 60 minutes of admission.*

Please indicate your level of confidence.	**Extremely Confident and Can Help Others**	**Confident and Need No Help**	**Moderately Confident, May Need Some Help**	**Unsure and Need Some Help**	**Extremely Unsure and Need Large Amount of Help**
Upon completion of training, I can enter orders into the EHR.	5	4	3	2	1

Methods of application evaluation can include observation, audits, reports, surveys, and focus groups. Because evaluation of learning application is more time consuming than the first two levels of evaluation, the evaluation of application is reserved for high-value training programs or key concepts delivered within a training program.

Business results evaluation: The entire training development process is time consuming and costly; therefore, it can be important to demonstrate a positive impact to the business that occurred as a result of training. The Level 4 evaluation is designed to measure business results.

Imagine that a hospital has experienced a high level of urinary tract infections related to urinary catheters. A new system has been designed to alert patient care staff about catheter days and catheter care. Assuming that each urinary tract infection costs the organization $1,000 per incidence, and the organization experiences 100 infections per month, the cost of the performance gap related to urinary catheters is $100,000 per month. If the rate of catheter-related urinary tract infections drops by 75% after training, the business result of this training program is $75,000 per month. If the rate remains constant, the yearly total would be almost one million dollars. Although obtaining and quantifying the business results of training can be difficult, providing training evaluation results in terms of dollars saved or earned can generate quite a bit of attention from leaders and stakeholders.

Return on investment evaluation: The final and most infrequently used level of training evaluation concludes with a calculation of the return on investment (ROI) of the training program. Using a formula that looks at program benefits and program costs, an amount is calculated that shows the return for each dollar that is spent on training. The ROI process uses tangible and intangible benefits to calculate value. Due to the complexities found in the healthcare environment and the difficulty of establishing clear cause-and-effect relationships, ROI training evaluation has rarely been used in the healthcare field.

Future Directions

To develop and deliver maximally efficient and effective training in a health information technology environment, focus on the following areas.

Critical Training Elements

In a healthcare environment where detail is important—and even critical—including a large volume of detail into the electronic health record (EHR) training is tempting. This can quickly lead to overly detailed training that cannot be delivered within a reasonable time frame. Highly detailed training can overwhelm the learner with volumes of details that cannot be placed into a meaningful context.

Instructional design is built on a theoretical model that allows for a concise evaluation and prioritization of design elements during the design phase of the instructional design project. Task analyses and other methods can be used to determine which elements of training should be included and which should be excluded from the training project.

Cost-Effectiveness

Training can be unnecessarily expensive when training is designed and delivered indiscriminately to all types of learners. Failure to analyze the needs and workflow processes for each type of learner can create irrelevant and lengthy training that will waste learner time and create unnecessary antagonism toward the healthcare IT changes that are about to occur.

Relevant Evaluation

Training consumes a large volume of resources in order to both develop and to deliver training. A failure to evaluate the effectiveness of the training program can result in lost opportunities to improve the training or the training process. Determine when it is important to evaluate business results versus application of learning versus knowledge or reaction.

Learner Characteristics

Health unit secretaries, physicians, nurses, and social workers all perform different tasks within a healthcare organization, and all have different learning needs and learning availability. Learning content delivered in a training manual for one group of learners may not be the best training delivery method for learners of another discipline.

For example, medical residents and medical students may rotate quickly in and out of an organization and use healthcare IT less intensively during their time at an organization than a newly hired nurse may use the system. Therefore, the medical student or resident may need short training courses that deliver only the essential content necessary so that they can being to perform their job duties. Nurses, as the primary caregiver for their patients, may need more intensive training that enables them to understand the processes and workflow of other disciplines and how they relate and interact with the nursing processes and workflow.

Using Learning Theory to Improve Acceptance

The principles of adult learning theory help to guide training by providing an understanding of how adults learn. Many of us are only familiar with how we were educated as young students and tend to craft our training according to what is familiar to us.

Design to Increase Engagement

Volumes of research have been conducted to determine what types of design help promote learning and what design elements detract from learning. It is important to understand the basics of these elements in order to produce training that is visually appealing and stimulating to the learner without being distracting, annoying, or overwhelming to the students. Even the best training content can be derailed by introducing it using a hot pink background or by having multiple, distracting pictures, movements, or designs within the training. On the other hand, using page after page of solid single-spaced text will also lose the attention of the learner.

Improving the Performance Gap

The purpose of training is to improve the performance of the learners. Many times we fail to measure the current performance of the learners, and then we fail again to measure performance after the training has been delivered to see if the training produced positive results. The theories of performance improvement can be used to guide the analysis, measurement, selection of interventions, and evaluation of training projects as well as other efforts designed to improve gaps in performance within a healthcare organization.

Conclusion

Training differs from education and focuses on equipping learners to perform tasks that have an immediate and measurable outcome. The need for training is determined by identifying a measurable gap in performance or knowledge. Decades of research and practice in business, education, and the military have produced evidence-based training models and a training development framework that can be used within healthcare organizations to produce efficient and effective training programs. After implementation, training can be evaluated at five levels of impact, ranging from learner reaction to the return on investment for each dollar spent on training. Finally, the goal of training is for each learner to safely and effectively apply what has been learned to their practice setting in order to efficiently and effectively improve patient safety and outcomes.

References

Alpay, L., & Russell, A. (2002). Information technology training in primary care: The nurses' voice. *CIN: Computers, Informatics, Nursing, 20*(4), 136–142

American Nurses Association. (2008). *Nursing informatics Scope and standards of practice.* Silver Springs, MD: American Nurses Association.

Bloom, P. S. (Ed.). (1956). *Taxonomy of educational objectives: The classification of educational goals, by a committee of college and university examiners.* New York, NY: D. McKay.

Brady, C. (2013). Understanding learning styles: Providing the optimal learning experience. *International Journal of Childbirth Education, 28*(2), 16–19.

Bredfeldt, C., Awad, E., Joseph, K., & Mark H. (2013). Training providers: Beyond the basics of electronic health records. *BMC Health Services Research, 13*(1), 1–14.

Choi, I., Lee, S., & Kang, J. (2009). Implementing a case-based eLearning environment in a lecture-oriented anesthesiology class: Do learning styles matter in complex problem solving over time? *British Journal of Educational Technology, 40*(5), 933–947.

Fisher, S., Creusat, J., & McNamara, D. (2008). *Improving physician adoption of CPOE systems.* Retrieved from http://www.strategiestoperform.com/volume3_issue2/docs/Improving PhysicianAdoption.pdf

Jacques, E. (2002). *The impact of selected factors in nurses' attitudes toward bedside computers.* (Doctoral dissertation). Available from ProQuest Dissertations and Theses database. (UMI No. 3049803)

Knowles, M., Holton, E. III., Swanson, R. (2005). *Adult learner: The definitive classic in adult education and human resource development* (6th ed.). Burlington, MA: Butterworth-Heinemann.

Meeks, D., Takian, A., Sittig, D., Singh, H., & Barber, N. (2014). Exploring the sociotechnical intersection of patient safety and electronic health record implementation. *Journal of the American Medical Informatics Association, 21*(e1), e28-e34.

Morrison, G., Ross, S., Kalman, H., & Kemp, J. (2011). *Designing effective instruction* (6th ed.). Hoboken, NJ: John Wiley & Sons, Inc.

Page, D. (2011). Turning nurses into health IT superusers. *Hospitals & Health Networks, 85*(4), 27–28.

Pershing, J. (2006). Human performance technology fundamentals. In James A. Pershing (Ed.), *Handbook of human performance technology* (3rd ed.), (pp. 5–34). San Francisco, CA: John Wiley & Sons, Inc.

Phillips, P., & Phillips, J. (2008). *ROI fundamentals: Why and when to measure return on investment.* San Francisco, CA: John Wiley & Sons, Inc.

Runy, L. (2005). Physician and nurse training: Involving clinicians in planning, teaching eases skepticism. *Hospitals and Health Networks, 4*(2), 30–33.

Shea, C., Malone, R., Weinberger, M., Reiter, K., Thornhill, J., Lord, … Weiner, B. (2014). Assessing organizational capacity for achieving meaningful use of electronic health records. *Health Care Management Review, 39*(2), 124–133.

U.S. Department of Health and Human Services. (2010). *The registered nurse population: Findings from the 2008 national sample of registered nurses.* Retrieved from http://bhpr.hrsa.gov/healthworkforce/rnsurveys/rnsurveyfinal.pdf

"There are no secrets to success. It is the result of preparation, hard work, and learning from failure."

–Colin Powell

Healthcare System Implementation

6

Susan M. Houston, MBA, RN-BC, PMP, CPHIMS, FHIMSS

OBJECTIVES

- Review the importance of planning early for the implementation and activation of a project.
- Develop an activation plan from the initial brainstorming activity to the final version that can help mitigate the risks associated with system activation.
- Describe a variety of plans and tools that can assist with planning for system implementation.
- Articulate the use of a communication plan to document who, what, when, and how activation communication should be conducted.

The activities surrounding the implementation of a new system will vary depending on what is being implemented. Most activities will need to occur, but the specifics may vary. There are very few references on the best practices for implementation planning, but this chapter will provide some guidelines and tools that will assist with implementation, activation, or going live, as well as when variations will occur and why.

The type of project will influence the amount of planning required, when you should start, and what activities will be needed. These activities include determining what needs to be done before, during, and after activation or going live, and who will be doing those activities. When will people need to be onsite, and where will they be located? Communication is always required, along with just-in-time training and support.

One example is the implementation of a new application where the processes are moving from manual or paper to electronic. Everything is all set, and it just needs to be turned on—right? It is never that easy. After the application has been designed, developed, and tested, there are still some details to work out and tasks to be done. For example, will information or data need to be loaded into the new system? If this is an electronic health record (EHR), will all active orders need to be added? When will that occur, and by whom?

> **TIP**
>
> Activation planning should occur early in the project to allow enough time for decisions to be made and details to be worked out.
>
> Small project – start planning 2 months out
>
> Larger, more complex projects – start planning 4 to 6 months out

Another example would be an upgrade to an application that is already in use. Typically, the application needs to be turned off for the upgrade to occur, which results is a period of downtime where the end users cannot access the system. Planning needs to include how patient care will continue without the application as well as how information will be entered after the application is back up and running. Control of the upgrade tasks is essential to ensuring the shortest possible downtime. Adding new functionality or a new interface between two applications may require a different set of tasks and may or may not require downtime.

Activation Planning

Planning for the activation begins at the project's inception, although it does not always happen that way. So much attention is given to the system design, building, testing, and training that thorough activation planning is sometimes an afterthought. The type of project, as mentioned earlier, will help guide the planning, along with the implementation plan.

A *pilot launch* allows for the implementation in a single location with limited users. This allows for the validation of the functionality and impact to workflow. The users are asked to provide feedback to allow the project team to improve the application prior to the implementation for other areas or users. Although the small number of users requires fewer support staff, often they are very involved and visible during the duration of the pilot and ensure good documentation of the feedback and necessary improvements.

A *phased approach* can be accomplished in two ways. One, the functionality is rolled out to all users but in small amounts, such as barcode functionality for specimen collection and then for medication administration. The support for this implementation plan would need to cover the entire user population but would be limited to specific functionality. The upside is that the impact of the change on the users is lessened.

In the second way to accomplish a phased approach, you implement all functionality at one time but roll it out by area or group of users. The support for this implementation would require fewer support staff who would move along with each phase. However, the downside is that the impact of the change is much larger.

And you can use hybrids of both approaches: A *Pop-Bang approach* is a pilot launch followed by full implementation to the rest of the users. A *Big Bang approach* is the implementation of all functionality to all users at one time. This is required when you are upgrading an application or moving from one electronic system to another.

After you choose the implementation strategy, the size of the project will help determine when to actually start the detailed planning. For smaller projects, two to three months prior to the scheduled go-live date would be best. For larger projects, planning should begin up to six months prior. There is no set standard, but obviously, the larger or more complex the project, the earlier the planning should begin. Danaher, Felt, and Sirois (2011) noted that most pre-activation planning should begin no less than four months prior to going live.

It is also important to include the right people at the very beginning of the planning process. The implementation team will vary across different projects and may include staff from the interface, database administration, system administration, configuration or build, communication, project management, training, and testing teams. It is also important to include representatives from the end-user base as well. And although you need to include the right people, it is also essential to keep the team to a minimum. Everyone will want to be involved, and you may need everyone involved, but the planning team should be a smaller group—maybe just a representative of each required team. If your organization has staff in silos, bringing these people together early will help with the collaboration that is needed for a successful activation.

TIP

Involve the right people.

Get the right people in the room – from the beginning!

Take down the silos.

Include system users.

Some elements that all activation plans should include are related to decision-making, communication, risk management, contingency planning, lessons learned process, end-user support, and listing tasks for the actual activation. How you document and track decisions throughout the project should be continued for any activation-specific decisions. Even though there may be a communication plan for the project, an activation-specific plan may be useful because this is when the majority of the communication happens related to the organization and user community.

As the planning team identifies the tasks that are necessary in preparation of the activation day and during the actual activation, discussions should include the identification of any risks. Contingency planning will help prepare for the negative impact of any risks identified. For example, how will an upgrade be backed out if it is unsuccessful? Regroup after each step of the implementation process to evaluate any lessons learned that could be applied to help ensure success at the end of the project. This can occur after a pilot, after each phase of the implementation, or after a rehearsal of the actual activation activity.

Some items to remember during the planning would relate to how long staff will be at work during the actual activation and post-live support. For the best collaboration and communication during the actual activation, it is best if all participating staff is in the same location, such as a large conference room. Space for a call center or help desk is also important if one is not already available. After the location is determined, ensure that there is enough network and power access for all the workstations and also make sure that phones are available. Planning for food and drink will go a long way, especially if these activities will occur when a cafeteria is not available or if the staff will not have time to leave. If staff is expected to be onsite overnight or over an extended period of time, having the option to sleep or take a shower might be necessary or at least a welcomed option.

Communication

Anyone who touches the application, or will be affected by the system being unavailable, needs to receive communication. During earlier phases of the project, the main focus of the communication was with the project team and key stakeholders. The communication during implementation needs to be extended to all end users and also anyone who will be affected by the change being implemented.

TIP

Remember to communicate early and often, and make sure that your communications are clear and concise.

Language choice is also important. Use language that the audience will understand; strive to limit technical jargon. Oftentimes, your target audience may not actually read emails from you or even follow any included directions. For this reason, the communication plan needs to include multiple communication methods. Some options for communication include attending staff meetings, posters, flyers, and making the rounds to the units or departments. Involving the organization's communications and marketing department will help with having clear and consistent messaging. Remember to include communication to patients and visitors if they will be affected by the change being implemented.

TIP

Do not rely on email as the sole source of communication with system users.

Communication must also occur in a timely manner. Managers need to plan different staffing patterns for when the system is unavailable as well as when it becomes available again, and they may need to enter information about care that occurred when it was unavailable. Communication should continue after the system is back up and running, because typically there is information users will need to know as issues are worked through or workarounds are put into place. Having support staff make the rounds during the activation event as well as after will help with any just-in-time training and the quick identification of issues.

The communication plan does not need to be a lengthy document. Rather, it could be a simple table, as long as it includes the key information about who, what, when, and how. See Tables 6.1 and 6.2.

Table 6.1 Communication Plan

Who	*What*	*When*	*How*	*Responsible*
Project Team				
Administration				
Dept./Unit Managers				
End Users				
Marketing & Communications				
Support Staff				
Help Desk				
Vendors				
Other Project Teams				
Governance Committee				
Public				
Other				

Table 6.2 Communication Options

What to Communicate	*When to Communicate*	*How to Communicate*
• Status • Schedule milestones • Issues and resolution • Workarounds • Changes • Action Items • Assignments • Deliverables	• Quarterly, weekly, monthly, and so on • During planning meeting • When milestone achieved • During scheduled meeting • Specific number of weeks/days prior to a milestone	• Newsletter • Internet/intranet • Email • Storyboards • Patient handouts • Marketing materials • Meeting minutes • Posters or flyers

Plans and Lists

Many plans should be documented for clarification or reference during the activation and after. One such plan is a *downtime plan*, which defines how work will continue during anytime the application is unavailable. For example:

- If the electronic medical record is unavailable, how will medication administration be documented?
- What forms will be used for patient documentation or ordering stat lab tests and how will the results be communicated back to the care providers?
- If the nutrition system is unavailable, how will correct meals be prepared and delivered?

These are just some of the details that may be included in a downtime plan. If the organization already has a downtime plan, and the implementation is related to an upgrade, the plan should be reviewed and updated as necessary if any new functionality is being added. The plan should also provide guidance in the event of a single system interruption as well as multiple system interruption. This will be important as more systems are implemented and integrated with the EHR.

During decision-making, many different options are reviewed to ensure the correct decision is made based on the information provided. How this information is provided can help or hinder the decision-making process. If the decision-maker needs to read a lengthy document where details are spread over many pages, it might be difficult to compare them. Using a table to display the different options side by side could make this more efficient. The content of the options document may vary depending on the decision. A decision related to the type of workstation to be deployed may include details concerning the hardware configuration, price, ease of use, or even the physical size. A decision related to the date and time of the activation may include impact to patient care; required staffing; availability of vendor resources; and patient activity, such as quantity of admissions or discharges. Each options document should include a description of the situation, or decision to be made and a recommended option. The table should include rows for the description, advantages, disadvantages, constraints, assumptions, and barriers. As a general rule, these documents should be as simple as possible while providing the information needed for an informed decision to be made. See Table 6.3.

At various times during the planning, the sponsors should review the readiness state for the activation. These are often called "go/no-go meetings" where the decision is made to continue as planned, go live, or modify the plan, or not go live (no-go). If a plan needs to be modified, typically something has caused a delay in the schedule, such as a major issue or that work cannot be completed on time.

A tool to assist with these meetings and decisions is an Operational Readiness Review document. This document lists the major activities and milestones that need to be completed prior to the activation date. They can be sorted by specific categories and include the scheduled due date, actual completion date, and a status comment. They may also include the percent complete and scheduled start date, given that some activities may not start right away. Such a tracking document provides a quick look at the status of the key activities to provide good data on whether the planned activation date is feasible. See Table 6.4.

Table 6.3 Options Document: Description of Situation and Recommended Option with Rationale

	Option 1	*Option 2*	*Option 3*	*Option 4*
Description				
Advantages				
Disadvantages				
Resource Impact				
Workflow Impact				
Budget Impact				
Technical Impact				
Patient Care Impact				
Risks				
Assumptions				
Constraints				
Barriers				

Table 6.4 Sample Operational Readiness Review Document

#	*Readiness Criteria*	*Scheduled Completion Date*	*Actual Completion Date*	*Responsible Person*	*Status*
Management					
1	All go-live related staff identified and available	8/15/14	8/15/14	John Smith	
2	All go-live related space requirements identified and finalized	8/1/14	7/29/14	Kathy Jones	
3	Hospital ancillary support staff identified and available	8/15/14		John Smith	
4	Contingency plan developed and verified	8/15/14		John Smith	
Reports					
5	Order Requisitions built and verified	8/23/14	8/30/14	Dave Johnson	

#	*Readiness Criteria*	*Scheduled Completion Date*	*Actual Completion Date*	*Responsible Person*	*Status*
6	Go-live EHRs built and verified	8/15/14		Dave Johnson	
Hardware					
7	Deployment of user workstations complete	8/1/14	8/3/14	Tom Hark	
8	Deployment of report and label printers is complete	8/23/14		Tom Hark	
Testing					
9	Parallel Testing complete	8/6/14	8/6/14	Susan Hamilton	
10	User Acceptance Testing complete	8/15/14	8/15/14	Susan Hamilton	
11	All test incidents identified as Go-Live Critical resolved	8/29/14		Susan Hamilton	

continues

Table 6.4 Sample Operational Readiness Review Document *(continued)*

#	*Readiness Criteria*	*Scheduled Completion Date*	*Actual Completion Date*	*Responsible Person*	*Status*
Training					
12	All super users have attended training	9/6/14		Harvey Walton	
13	All key prescribers have attended training	8/29/14		Harvey Walton	
14	All nursing staff have completed training	8/29/14		Harvey Walton	
Help Desk					
15	Help Desk staff are available and have been trained	9/6/14		Kathy Jones	

#	*Readiness Criteria*	*Scheduled Completion Date*	*Actual Completion Date*	*Responsible Person*	*Status*
16	Scripts are prepared to support anticipated questions	9/11/14		Kathy Jones	
Operations and Maintenance					
17	System monitoring plan created and verified	9/6/14		Tom Hark	
18	Backup/recovery procedures and schedules in place	9/1/14	8/2/14	Tom Hark	
User Community Readiness					
19	Manual downtime procedures finalized and communicated	8/1/14	8/1/14	Susan Hamilton	

Activation Checklist and Rehearsals

One tool that is critical to a smooth implementation is the activation checklist. This list is similar to a project work plan, which includes the details surrounding the tasks that need to occur during the activation. The difference is that the activation checklist has tasks with duration to at least 5 minutes, and the project work plan rarely gets to this level of detail.

One method of identifying the tasks that will go on this checklist is to use sticky notes. This is a brainstorming activity that includes all the staff working during the activation. Each person has a pad of sticky notes, and then writes down one task per sticky note and turns them in to the facilitator. Tasks might include making a backup copy of the database, turning off interfaces, or even announcing the downtime to the end users.

After it appears that most tasks are documented, the facilitator goes through each note to organize it with input from the group. For example, the tasks might be organized by when they would occur, such as 2 weeks prior to the day of the activation or the day after. The tasks are then organized by when they should occur in relation to the others listed, or in the order they need to be completed. This step helps to determine predecessors and identify whether any tasks can occur concurrently. When possible, the person who will complete the task will also be documented along with an estimated duration. After the meeting, the information is added to the checklist template and lays the foundation for the main control document for the activation. See Table 6.5.

After the checklist is developed, it is good practice to review it with the team until everyone is confident that it is accurate. This step should be completed in meetings to ensure that the checklist is actually reviewed and to encourage dialogue among the team. With a large project, the checklist may have 75 to 80 tasks listed and will take multiple meetings to just get through the checklist once.

Table 6.5 Activation Checklist

Done	*#*	*Task*	*Estimated Duration*	*Estimated Start*	*Estimated Finish*	*Predecessor*	*Resource*	*Comment*
X Weeks Before Go-Live								
	1	Prep task	X days				Name	
	2	Prep task	X days				Name	
	3	Communication	X days			1,2	Name	
Week of Go-Live – MM/DD/YYYY								
	4	Prep task	X days				Name	
	5	Prep task	X days			4	Name	
Activation – MM/DD/YYYY								
	6	Communication	X min				Name	
	7	Task	X min			6	Name	
		System Down						
	8	Task	X min			7	Name	
	9	Task	X min			8	Name	
	10	Task	X min			9	Name	
		System Up						
	11	Communication	X min			10	Name	
		Activation Complete						
	12	Issue Management	X min			11	Name	
Post Go-Live Support – MM/DD/YYYY								
	13	Task	X min				Name	
	14	Task	X min			13	Name	
	15	Task	X min			13	Name	

During the review meetings, each task should be reviewed to make sure the task name is correct and that the person completing the task knows what this means and what he will need to do. The duration is reviewed along with when the task can occur. Do as many tasks ahead of time as possible to limit the work effort on the actual activation date. This also allows for any issue or unexpected delays without impacting the actual event. Understanding the predecessors will help to determine whether any tasks can occur at the same time for efficiency. It may seem obvious, but remember that tasks that require the same resource cannot be done concurrently, so predecessors and resources must be reviewed when the timing is being set for each task.

TIP

The checklist development is an iterative process and will change frequently during the reviews. This checklist also becomes historical information that can be used as a starting point for similar activations in the future.

After the checklist is to a point where the team believes it is as accurate as possible, it is ready to add the estimated start and end times, which are derived from the durations and predecessors. The first time through, setting the start time as midnight will easily show how far into the event each tasks occurs and what the total estimated duration would be. If the validation task occurs at 4:00 a.m., for example, it will be easy to determine that it occurs four hours into the event. Knowing the total estimated duration provides input to the decision on when to begin the work, given that the best time to start something lasting 2 hours is vastly different then the best time to begin when the duration is 12 hours.

When the checklist is in a final state, a schedule can be created for when resources are needed. The tasks, times, and resources are known, so the resource schedule can be prepared. For lengthy events, all staff will not need to be onsite working for the entire event. For example, the test team that will do validation prior to the system being considered "live" for end users will not be required until the end of the event.

When developing the resource schedule, schedule people to arrive early so there is time for them to set up their computer, log on, and get prepared. This extra lead time also allows for some variation in the timing of the tasks and their arrivals. Having contact information for each person allows for the possibility of needing to contact him or her if the event is ahead or behind schedule.

Support staff should be included in the resource schedule even if they do not have an official task. Curtis (2013) noted that the go-live support plan should be confirmed for each location with specific roles, responsibilities, and a defined schedule. This will help to avoid any confusion or gaps in the required support, such as vendor staff who are available for issues or department staff who are providing support to their users. This schedule will need to be updated whenever the activation checklist is modified—which is why it should be completed later in the review process.

During the checklist development, the identification of tasks will help to determine where contingency plans are needed. Where are there high-risk tasks that may not go as planned or changes that might need to be backed out? Detailed contingency planning is the best form of risk mitigation for this event. Remember that after data has been changed, there is no going back. If you turn on interfaces and the messages populate data into the database, the system has changed, and you are committed.

Here are potential questions to help with contingency planning:

- What happens if you need to back out the change you just made?
- What if you need to uninstall what you just installed?
- What if the database is corrupted?
- What is the upgrade is interrupted or does not complete?

If there will be tasks that require configuration or multiple settings, these can be documented separately from the checklist. This will allow for the contingency of someone not being available for the activation and the need for a replacement. Also, it is much easier to make the configuration changes when it is being read rather than relying on memory, and documentation also ensures that the settings are what was actually tested and planned.

If this activity is complex or has not been done before, it is good practice to rehearse. Go through the entire checklist in as real of a situation as possible prior to the actual activation date. If this is an upgrade, use a copy of the production system to simulate the actual event. This is the time to make mistakes. If the rehearsal does not go well, review, learn, and repeat. During the rehearsal, the checklist is validated. Are the right tasks listed, and are they in the right order? Do tasks have the right duration, and are there any tasks missing? The intended outcome of the rehearsal is to have staff who are much more comfortable with the tasks they will be doing as well as a more refined checklist and estimate for the total duration. As the tasks are completed, the actual start and end times should be documented and the checklist updated if tasks are changed. Having a single person who manages the checklist will free up the rest of the team to focus on their tasks. The project manager is available to communicate and manage risks and issues that might arise.

TIP

Rehearse your activation.

Conduct all tasks scheduled during downtime in a practice database.

Validate that you have the:

- Right tasks
- Right order
- Right duration

After the rehearsal is completed, a "lessons learned" meeting should be held. Reviewing the checklist and the specific tasks provides input into the next version with more realistic durations and sequencing of tasks. It is important to understand that some tasks might not be completed during the rehearsal: For example, end users will not need to have their access turned off, and end-user communication is not necessary. Any issues or problems that were encountered during the rehearsal will provide input into additional contingency planning that might be needed. During this meeting, it can be discussed whether a second rehearsal is required or desired to ensure a successful activation. Reviewing what went well and what could be improved will help to better the activity. A revised activation checklist will provide better clarity to each task and task detail.

A lessons learned meeting should occur after each rehearsal and after the actual activation. The outcomes will help to improve the process for the next step or for the next project of this type.

Activation

Well, all the planning is done, and the big day is here. As you move through the checklist, remember to document the actual start and end times as well as editing any task information. To provide good documentation and assist with learning for next time, all changes can be documented in a different font style or color. Even during the actual activation, there are still lessons that can be learned for future projects.

Final checklists are invaluable historical information. Tasks that typically have most variability in the durations include any data loads (due to variations in the network speed) and regression testing (due to unexpected issues that require resolution). Having clear lines of communication for all interested and involved stakeholders is important, especially for lengthy activations.

When possible, it is beneficial to isolate those with assigned tasks from administration or sponsors that want an update. This prevents interruptions and allows the staff to stay focused on their tasks. This can be accomplished by the project manager sending out regular updates by email or by having questions go directly to her or him (not having people come in and out of the conference room).

> Regression testing during activation validates that the changes made did not introduce unexpected consequences.

Support

Support actually starts during the activation event. Support staff, which might include "super users," can assist with communication by making rounds on the units or in the departments. They can share how the activation is going, make sure everyone is ready for when the application is live, and answer any last-minute training questions. Danaher et al. (2011) stated that experience shows large implementations should plan for a 3:1 or a 4:1 ratio of additional support staff to internal support staff. Having a clear and consistent way to report issues, whether they come from the end users directly or through support staff, will make sure each one is properly documented and assigned to the right person for analysis and resolution.

The use of a central support or help center will facilitate this process. End users can be directed to contact the support center for all issues or questions. Anything identified while the support staff is making rounds can be documented and delivered to the support center for data entry and assignment. Any "how-to" questions can be routed to the training team so they can evaluate the need for additional training or communication. Technical support should be available for any issues requiring additional expertise beyond the support desk. Jaén (2011) identified readily available technical resources as a common pathway for success.

Having regular post-live meetings to review issues will ensure proper assignment and escalation as well as communication. Categorizing the issues can help to determine which are critical to be resolved quickly and which can be a lower priority. Typically, the project manager stays involved for a period of time after the activation to facilitate the issue resolution and ensure proper transition of activities to the support manager. This keeps a single point of contact for communication, questions, and issue resolution.

The number of support staff will depend on the quantity of users to be supported and how widespread they are. Super users provide support on various shifts and for an extended period of time because they often work in the same areas as their normal assignment. The duration of the support will depend on the amount of change being introduced with the project. A new EHR system that includes the first time users have entered orders or completed their documentation online will require much longer support than an upgrade with limited new functionality. It is wise to schedule support staff for longer than expected, because it is easier to cancel shifts than to fill a schedule at the last minute.

Conclusion

Planning for the implementation activities should start early and follow an iterative process as more details are identified. Using tools and templates will assist with communicating the plans across the project team and beyond to extended stakeholders. Learning from previous implementations can give the team a head start and eliminate the need to start from scratch. Ensuring that the right people are involved in the development of the plans will ensure they cover all the necessary activities and details. Comprehensive communication and contingency plans will cover most risks that may occur during this period. A comprehensive checklist is a very valuable tool, but does take time to create, review, and validate. Mistakes are learning opportunities, but it is best to make them during rehearsals; and if necessary, repeat the rehearsal event until the team is comfortable with what is expected of them and the outcome is successful. The most important aspect is to learn. Learn from the reviews of the plans, checklists, and rehearsals. Review and update as you learn, and make sure everyone is ready for the big day when the application goes live. And when it is all done, remember to celebrate all of the hard work and the success.

References

Curtis, S. (2013, April 30). Driving EHR adoption: Activation plan 10 considerations. Electronic Health Record (EHR) expert blog. Retrieved from http://blog.projectnavigation.com/blog/bid/272700/Driving-EHR-Adoption-Activation-Plan-10-Considerations

Danaher, S., Felt, P., & Sirois, M. L. (2011, May). Lessons learned: Avoiding some of the common pitfalls of EHR activation. *Divurgent, 1*(8). Retrieved from http://divurgent.com/wp-content/uploads/2013/12/Newsletter-May-2011.pdf

Jaén, C. R. (2011). Successful health information technology implementation requires practice and health care system transformation. *Annals of Family Medicine, 9*(5), 388–389.

"...that it will ever come into general use, notwithstanding its value, is extremely doubtful; because its beneficial application requires much time and gives a good bit of trouble to both the patient and the practitioner; and because its hue and character are foreign and opposed to all our habits and associations. It is just not going to get used."

–The Times (London), 1834; regarding the stethoscope, invented by René-Théophile-Hyacinthe Laënnec in 1816

7 Maintaining and Optimizing a Healthcare Information System

Theresa (Tess) J. Settergren, MHA, MA, RN-BC

OBJECTIVES

- Describe the maintenance phase in relation to the system life cycle.
- Discuss the importance of robust change management, downtime, and business continuity processes and tools.
- Examine optimization in the context of the system life cycle, user adoption, and resource allocation.

After the implementation phase is complete and the "switch is flipped" on a clinical information system, many think that the most difficult work is behind them. However, this next phase of a system's life cycle can be just as challenging as the preceding phases. The system life cycle definition of post-implementation activities comprises support, maintenance, and project evaluation (Dennis, Wixom, & Roth, 2012; Saba & McCormick, 2011). Phrases used to describe this phase include "winding down," "turning over to support staff," "moving on to the next project," and other terms that denote significant reduction in the quality and quantity of dedicated resources.

Traditionally, this approach is well established, particularly from a fiscal perspective. Accounting principles distinguish capital versus operating expenses. New information system implementations are capital projects that have budgetary and temporal limits. Funding for a capital project ends when the project is deemed closed, typically soon after go-live. In the world of the Chief Financial Officer (CFO), a completed system installation signals the end of the capital project and a subsequent dramatic decrease in the human and monetary resources dedicated to that information system.

Ongoing system maintenance and support is resourced from the operations budget. Operations budgets in hospitals and other healthcare provider organizations undergo perpetual scrutiny for opportunities to reduce costs. Because information technology (IT) and informatics experts are expensive resources and are not revenue generators, naturally, budget trimming after a system installation will include proposals for reduction in staff. The net effect is that experts who are essential to optimize—not simply maintain—the electronic health record (EHR) are at-risk resources in operating budgets. Why is this important to explore?

In the former IT world of financial and departmental management systems, the philosophy of "install, stabilize, and redeploy resources" was appropriate for new information systems. End users of these systems were accustomed to using information technology; and typically, a new system meant enhanced departmental workflows and functionality for a relatively small user population.

EHRs created a new and unexpected level of complexity to system implementations in terms of the integration of multiple upstream and downstream systems, medical devices, and clinical analytics, as well as factors such as human change readiness and the introduction of complex integrated interdisciplinary workflows. Physicians, nurses, and other clinical staff were generally not adept IT users.

Interdisciplinary team members could no longer remain in their departmental silos: Workflow changes became ubiquitous, creating new expectations of collaborative work processes and thus system design decision-making. The focus of clinical information systems was centered on patient care needs and cross-functional workflows, rather than on department management. Decisions made in departmental isolation in the past now had to be socialized across multiple stakeholder groups before system changes could be implemented. Data entry requirements changed for departments that had never collected those data elements in the past—such as race and ethnicity collection—by registration staff to support clinical research objectives and meaningful use. Stakeholder expectations around clinical analytics and point-of-care clinical decision support rose exponentially. This unprecedented magnitude of change for all care team members and the expectations for care delivery transformation was almost impossible to achieve at the initial go-live. The mantra of "perfection is the enemy of good enough" was coined to help manage stakeholder expectations.

Care transformation is not achieved at go-live. It is not achieved by traditional maintenance and support alone. Sustained significant effort is required to achieve the efficient, effective workflows and system tools that enable care transformation. "Go-live is a critical step in EHR implementation. However, rather than marking the end of your work, it marks the beginning of the next phase—several years of enhancing the EHR system and the skills of your users" (Henry, 2005, p. 124).

Optimization is the key to making the EHR (and the clinical intelligence that it enables) the "stethoscope" of this century. Optimization is ordinarily subsumed under maintenance, and thus is underrepresented and underfunded. Maintenance implies *stagnation*—that is, continuing the status quo—and is not ordinarily associated with major EHR enhancements. In contrast, optimization is dedicated to making a clinical information system work better to support users, patients, operations, quality, research, and other goals. Optimization involves continual evolution and progressive improvements that may be incremental or comprehensive.

Just as the stethoscope evolved from Laënnec's single wooden tube to the later binaural flexible tube versions, the EHR can and must be improved as a bedside tool for caregivers. This chapter will explore the benefits of optimization, as distinct from maintenance, and will offer ideas for securing resources to enable ongoing optimization. First, the maintenance phase of the system life cycle is important—and deserves attention.

System Maintenance Components

Maintenance is usually described as the final phase in the system life cycle, and includes minor system and workflow adjustments intended to correct errors, update metadata, accommodate regulatory changes, and similar activities. Hunt, Sproat, and Kitzmiller (2004) defined system maintenance as day-to-day management, including preventing downtime, ensuring user access and data integrity, routine system upgrades, and constant reevaluation for needed enhancements. Ensuring business continuity, providing support to users, and hardwiring a robust change control process (Dennis et al., 2012) should be added to this list of post-live activities. Senft and Gallegos (2009) broadly categorize system maintenance as adaptive, corrective, perfective, and predictive.

- *Adaptive maintenance* occurs when improvements to the system are necessary to adapt to changing working procedures or legislation (see Table 7.1).

Documentation improvements that support core measures, other quality measures, meaningful use requirements, and other externally driven requirements are included in adaptive maintenance.

- *Corrective maintenance* refers to ongoing system functionality improvements that are made (*bug fixing*) to ensure the system still meets the original user requirements: in essence, fixing functions that were working and are now broken. System issues categorized under corrective maintenance are frequently the result of planned or unplanned changes in system configuration. Both adaptive and corrective maintenance can be characterized as passively reactive to a changing environment.
- *Perfective maintenance* denotes improving the system so that it becomes more refined and more efficient at processing. This type of maintenance is more proactive than adaptive or corrective maintenance, but it does not represent optimization because the focus is technical throughput, and database administrators and programmers are more likely to perform perfective maintenance than are system or informatics analysts.
- *Predictive maintenance*, defined as strategic changes made in anticipation of likely changes to technology or working practices in the future, begins to describe a concept closer to optimization.

Change and configuration management, downtime and business continuity management, and handling requests for enhancement are key processes in the maintenance phase.

Change and Configuration Management

The IT Infrastructure Library (ITIL) service management framework defines the roles, functions, and services that collectively balance system stability with adaptability (Farenden, 2012). Change management—often labeled "change control" to differentiate it from human change and transition facilitation—and configuration management are two intricately linked ITIL processes. *Configuration management* pertains to all the assets, as well as the relationships between assets, required to deliver an IT service, whether at a macro or micro level. A robust configuration management process allows the creation of a logical model that enables the following activities:

- **Predicting change impacts:** What intended and unintended consequences could occur as a result of the change?

- **Root cause analysis:** What are the possible underlying causes for a change-related problem?

Table 7.1 Maintenance Types

Type	*Driver(s)*	*Example*
Adaptive	New requirements: Regulatory bodies, accreditation agencies, other	• ICD-9-CM to ICD-10-CM • Annual CPT code updates • Core Measures/Meaningful Use
Corrective	Bug fix for nonworking functionality to meet original user requirements	Role-based EHR tools suddenly unavailable to clinicians: unintended consequence of a code change
Perfective	Changes to improve data processing efficiency	Code changes to application or database management system that improve system throughput and response time
Predictive	Preparation for upcoming technology or practice changes	• Addition of field to capture ethnicity • New visit navigator (documentation, orders, patient/family education, care plan elements, billing codes) for post-discharge home visits by advanced practice nurses

Although the term “configuration management” is frequently used in reference to technical infrastructure, the same principles apply to clinical information systems and are especially relevant to electronic health systems, which typically have complex interrelationships with upstream and downstream systems and processes. For example, a change in a charge capture configuration may cause unintended effects in clinical ordering and documentation tools and vice versa. Or, a small modification in one component of a role-based security template may result in a physician suddenly losing access to personalized orders pick-lists. Blueprints of clinical system configuration decisions and logical interrelationships can accelerate identification and resolution of change-induced issues. Configuration management is also instrumental to proactively evaluate the impact of a proposed change.

The ITIL framework defines a *change* as an addition, a modification, or a removal of anything that could have an effect on IT services, including architecture, process, tool, metrics, and documentation changes, as well as configuration changes (Farenden, 2012). If you contemplate EHR availability to an end user as a single IT service, it is easy to imagine potential impacts from hardware and network configuration changes, changes in interfaces, or changes in application functionality. *Change management* in the ITIL framework describes the methods and tools used to maximize system stability while supporting adaptability to customer needs. Strategies for successful system change management include the following characteristics (McCormick & Gugerty, 2013):

- **Transparency:** As evidenced by well-informed stakeholders
- **Tracking:** Includes both request management and request-related communications
- **Organization:** Bundling requests in various ways, such as by requestor and/or by impact
- **Prioritization:** Through thoughtful governance and decision-making processes

The change management process's overall goal is to, through the use of standard processes and procedures, reduce risk and ensure that changes are scheduled, implemented on time, meet the specified requirements, and not break anything. Changes are commonly initiated through a request process. Figure 7.1 describes a simplified example of a request management process.

Change management procedures indicate how the requested change will be appraised—and, if approved to move forward, how the requested change will be prioritized, planned, tested, trained, implemented, and evaluated. Kulhanek (2011) described effective electronic medical record change management processes to include the following key elements:

- Linking requests to organizational priorities
- A single change request method
- User-based ranking of the change priority

- Standard tracking mechanisms
- Interdisciplinary review of requested changes
- Regularly scheduled change batching
- Communication mechanisms to ensure all users are informed

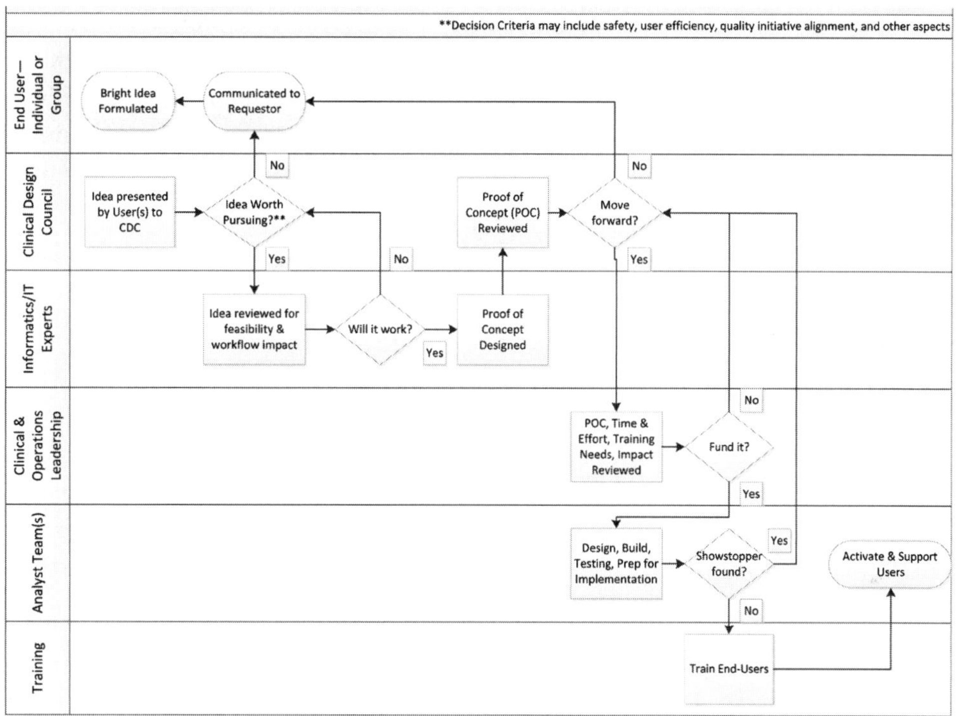

FIGURE 7.1 Request management process example.

The scope and magnitude of the requested change will determine the degree to which the change must follow an exhaustive change control process. Small daily changes that have limited impact are defined as "business as usual" (BAU) and thus require minimal review, unit testing, no end-user training; these changes are migrated into production the same day as the change request. An example of a BAU change is the addition of a retail pharmacy that can be selected as the patient's preferred pharmacy during e-prescribing.

On the other end of the spectrum is the major version upgrade or implementation of a new module that has broad impact and requires a tight change control process, multiple testing cycles, and classroom training for end users: that is, the full system life cycle process.

Between the two extremes lie innumerable shades of gray, with no uniformly accepted definition of the demarcation between post-live enhancement and a project. Figure 7.2 illustrates a simplified technical change control process. Figures 7.3 and 7.4 are examples of the first few steps of a major EHR module implementation, including a subset of the multiple subtasks and timing required for a successful cutover. Informatics nurses are well positioned to interpret and communicate end-user impact of changes, and also to advocate for proper levels of change control to reduce unintended consequences of said changes.

Downtime and Business Continuity

System downtime is inevitable. Changes to application functionality, the technical infrastructure, or other system components may require scheduled system downtime. Scheduled downtimes will vary in frequency and duration, but timing nearly always occurs in the wee hours of a Saturday or Sunday morning, when user impact is minimal. Changes that require the system to be unavailable to users are typically bundled—hardware, middleware, software, upgrades to interfaced systems, and so on—unless the risk is deemed to be lower by not bundling the downtimes.

Risk criteria include complexity and replicability of the system change or changes. For example, a routine server upgrade that has been well tested and has been successfully completed on the organization's fail-over servers can be bundled with software configuration changes that likewise have been successful in the past. The risk is low in this example, given that unintended consequences are not common, and the changes are not likely to require reversal.

On the other hand, an extensive upgrade of the EHR database that cannot be fully tested prior or requires a new technical approach, and does not have a successful track record in other organizations using the same software, probably will not be bundled with any other changes. This is important because the risk of unintended ripple effects or system errors is higher, and root cause analysis is facilitated by limiting the number of concurrent changes.

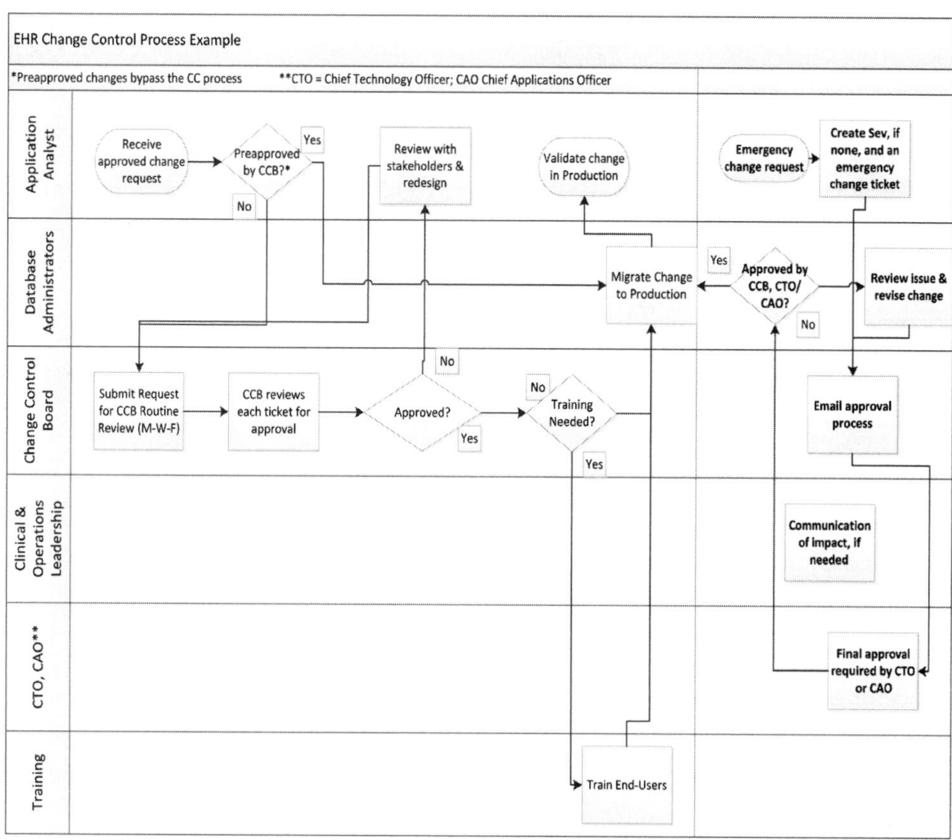

FIGURE 7.2 Change control process example.

Status	Date	Start Time	Duration	PGL Start Date/ Time	PGL Duration	PGL End Time	ITG #	Depend-encies	Task	Team	Resource	Validation Resource	Notes
Completed - Cutover Preparation Steps													
Complete - Cutover Pre-Steps: Week Of													
Cutover Pre-Steps: Friday 11/8													
Begin Downtime Steps: Friday 11/8 at 9:00PM													
Bring Down Interfaces and PRD: Saturday 11/9 at 1:00AM													
RA/SU Bundle Validation and Optime and Anesthesia Migrations: Saturday 11/9 Approx 2:30 AM													
Restart and Validate Device, ADT and 3M Interfaces: Saturday 11/9 Approx 3:00 AM													
Replay BCA and ADT and RX Recovery: Saturday 11/9 Approx 3:00 AM													
Enable Epic Interfaces: Saturday 11/9 Approx 3:30 AM													
Validation and Down-Stream Testing: Saturday 11/9 Approx 3:30 AM													
End Downtime - Disable SRO and Resume PRD Access: Saturday 11/9 Approx 4:50 AM													
Users back in PRD: Saturday 11/9 Approx 5:00 AM													
Post Cutover Steps													
Next Week Follow Up Tasks													

FIGURE 7.3 Implementation cutover major steps.

Status	Date	Start Time	Durati	Dependencies	Task	Team	Resource	Validation Resource	Notes
Completed - Cutover Preparation Steps									
Complete - Cutover Pre-Steps: Week Of									
Cutover Pre-Steps: Friday 11/8									
					Citrix and DME Pre-Steps				
Complete	11/08/13	7:00 AM			Apply CWS screensaver notification on clinical workstations (post Saturday AM shift)	DME Team	(Name/Names)		
Complete	11/08/13	9:00 AM		Complete RA list	Install RA Update and Onbase update on servers 1-5	Citrix Team			
Complete	11/08/13				Reboot servers 1-5	Citrix Team			
					BCA Pre-Steps				
Complete	11/08/13	9:00 AM			Confirm if BCA ADT is being populated with data from PRD.	ADT Team			
					Reschedule Batch Jobs				
Complete	11/08/13	9:00 AM	All Day		Grant access to App Teams members to reschedule batches	Change Team			Nothing to run between 0:30AM and 5AM
	11/08/13				Unschedule Cancer Center Batch	Bridges Team			
Complete	11/08/13				Delay Clarity extract and jobs that normally run daily and schedule for a later time	DBA Team			
					DBA Pre-Steps				
Complete	11/08/13				Preload SU's into Production	DBA Team			
Complete	11/08/13				Sync \\cshsnfsblobp\epicshare with \\cshsepicblobp\epicshare	DBA			Sync before the downtime
Complete	11/08/13				Write a global on Production and confirm it is shadowed over to the RSHD	DBA Team			
Complete	11/08/13				Verify directory for access logging daemons exists on the RPTSHD d ^E -> E1M Utilities Event Management	DBA Team			
Complete	11/08/13				Verify directory for audit trail logs exists on the RPTSHD (setting is in HDF)	DBA Team			
Complete	11/08/13				Publish MOTD on Production and Shadow	DBA Team	(Name/Names)		
Begin Downtime Steps: Friday 11/8 at 9:00PM									
Open	11/08/13	9:00PM			**Pre-Steps Wintel Maintenance**				
Complete	11/08/13	9:00PM			Remove All Pre-Down servers from BigIP (verify connections on target node have terminated on BIGIP) cshsmychart01 eswepicintcnt1p esxwepicsoap1p cshsepicwrprp1 eswepiccslblob1p eswcesf01p	Network Ops	(Name/Names)		
Complete	11/08/13				Begin Pre-Downtime Maintenance	Wintel Team			
Complete	11/08/13				Patch/TSM Upgrade cshsmychart01	Wintel Team	(Name/Names)		Notify (name) when complete
Complete	11/08/13				Patch/TSM Upgrade eswepicintcnt1p	Wintel Team	(Name/Names)		Notify (name) when complete
Complete	11/08/13				Patch/TSM Upgrade eswepiccslblob1p	Wintel Team	(Name/Names)		Notify (name) when complete
Complete	11/08/13				Patch/TSM Upgrade cshscslvpsx3-1	Wintel Team	(Name/Names)		
Complete	11/08/13				Patch/TSM Upgrade eswepicpls2p	Wintel Team	(Name/Names)		
Complete	11/08/13				Patch/TSM Upgrade esxwepicsoap1p	Wintel Team	(Name/Names)		
Complete	11/08/13				Patch/TSM Upgrade cshsepicwrprp1	Wintel Team	(Name/Names)		
Complete	11/08/13				Patch/TSM Upgrade cshscslepsp02	Wintel Team	(Name/Names)		
Complete					Patch/TSM Upgrade eswcesf01p	Wintel Team	(Name/Names)		
Complete	11/08/13				Turn Over above listed servers to DBA team as soon as ready	Wintel Team	(Name/Names)		
Open	11/08/13	11:00PM			**Pre-Steps DBA Maintenance**				
Complete	11/08/13	11:00PM	10 mins		Stage and pre-load RA's into Production script lister	DBA Team	(Name/Names)		
Complete	11/08/13	11:10PM	10 mins		Stage RA's to be loaded into the Reporting Shadows	DBA Team	(Name/Names)		
Complete	11/08/13	11:00PM	10 mins		Stage new cpf on Production and all shadow servers and PSUP	DBA Team	(Name/Names)		
Complete	11/08/13	11:10PM	10 mins		Stage new jmadmin on Production server and DR shadows and PSUP	DBA Team	(Name/Names)		
Complete	11/08/13	11:20PM	30mins		Create directories for new datasets on Production and shadows, verify permissions	DBA Team	(Name/Names)		
Complete	11/08/13	11:50PM	30mins		Create CACHE.DATs for new datasets on Production and shadows, verify permissions	DBA Team	(Name/Names)		
Complete	11/08/13	11:00PM	10 mins		Apply (EHR) client packs to cshscslvpsx3-2	DBA Team	(Name/Names)		
Complete	11/08/13	11:00PM			Apply VPSx Upgrade to cshscslvpsx3-2	DBA Team	(Name/Names)		
Complete	11/08/13	11:10PM	10 mins		Apply (EHR) client packs to cshscslvpsx3-2	DBA Team	(Name/Names)		
Complete	11/08/13	11:00PM	30 mins		Apply (EHR) client packs to cshscslvpsx3-2	DBA Team	(Name/Names)		
Complete	11/08/13	11:30PM	30 mins		Apply (EHR) client packs to cshscslvpsx3-2	DBA Team	(Name/Names)		

FIGURE 7.4 Implementation cutover detail example.

Scheduled downtime is usually preceded by a testing phase congruent with the magnitude of the change. The process is orderly, following specific and well-orchestrated steps. Communications to end users should focus on what to expect and what to do.

Unscheduled downtime is anything but orderly. Sources of unscheduled downtime can include loss of power, network outages, natural disasters, equipment failures (software or hardware), and deliberate actions. A substandard change control process may cause 50% or more of an organization's EHR corrective maintenance issues and outages.

CAUTION

Failure to follow a robust change control process as it relates to any key component of the EHR is likely to impact users and patients negatively.

Informatics nurses need to be the advocates for meticulous change processes because they are often best suited to understand and communicate the impacts to their information technologist colleagues. A weekly scorecard of information technology issues, with process (not people) failures as the focus is a powerful tool to raise awareness of change control importance and impacts of process failure.

Clinical system failure risk can also be mitigated through infrastructure redundancy planning. Hospitals have back-up systems to maintain power for critical equipment. It is important to plan uninterrupted power supply (UPS) availability for critical workstations and associated devices, in addition to medical devices and other patient care equipment.

TIP

Network components and EHR infrastructure components should be redundant wherever possible to enable rapid failover in a system outage. Redundancy is a key success factor in system disaster recovery.

Examples of system redundancy include:

- **Data center:** Replication of infrastructure for all mission-critical systems in a second data center, which should ideally be remotely located
- **Network:** Two or more sources of and paths for connectivity for all mission-critical buildings, including the data centers
- **Replication of all key EHR support systems:** The application database, file servers, application delivery servers, print servers, user authentication servers, and so on, with regularly tested fail-over processes

Even the most superlative technical disaster recovery planning will not prevent unscheduled downtime. Excellent business continuity processes are, however, critical to maintaining patient safety during scheduled and unscheduled downtimes. Hospitals are required to have business continuity plans that cover mission-critical systems and services, within the broader context of an emergency operations plan.

Business continuity comprises the procedures undertaken to "keep the business running" and to protect information assets during planned or unplanned system unavailability. The business continuity plan (BCP) also includes the operational activities required at resumption of system availability. Business continuity toolkits are widely available online, and include impact assessment tools and planning tools. One good example with links to resources can be found at the California Hospital Association website:

http://www.calhospitalprepare.org/sites/main/files/file-attachments/hcp_checklist_0.doc

TIP

Informatics nurses bring practical knowledge of clinical workflows and systems, as well as the downtime impact, to include in business continuity plans.

Although there are technical safeguards that support business continuity, the plan belongs to the operational and clinical areas responsible to deliver and support care. As end users become more highly dependent on EHR systems, it is vital to have standardized processes for nurses and other members of the care team to follow during a system outage. Because scheduled downtimes invariably occur during the night on a weekend, the majority of nurses and other staff members may not know what to do during a daytime outage. Best practices for downtime planning include the following (Vaughn, 2011):

- A clear, readable, up-to-date *downtime policy and procedure* that is reviewed, updated, and communicated with every new implementation, new interface, and upgrade.
- A *standard procedure* that everyone follows during system downtime, and covers the transition process to paper and back: which downtime forms to use, which data have to be entered into the system when it is available, and what to do with the forms afterward.
- A *downtime toolbox* on every unit that contains a copy of the downtime procedure, downtime forms that are to be used (may be customized for the unit's population), who maintains the toolbox for that unit (assign an owner!), quick references and samples to guide end users, and flowcharts that depict the major workflows.
- *Downtime access* to patient data that may include access to a shadow copy of the database for view-only, and locally stored clinical summaries and medication administration records that are updated at regular intervals and can be printed locally in the event of network outages.

- *Education* for nurses, physicians, and other members of the care team. Examples of education include poster boards, flyers, newsletter articles, computer-based training modules, refresher classes, and downtime drills or mock downtimes. When a prolonged scheduled downtime is anticipated, a downtime drill for day shift staff is excellent preparation.

In addition to education, policy, and tools for downtime, it may be advisable to incorporate a staffing plan for response to downtime. Unscheduled downtime could be extended and could put patient safety at significant risk. Emergency preparedness plans should include the components of downtime procedures and an emergency staffing plan. Additional staff can ensure a higher level of safety for patients during the downtime, when clinical decision support, patient medication profile, and barcoding mechanisms are not available.

After the downtime, the additional staff can ensure that key patient data are backloaded into the EHR promptly and accurately, without decreasing staff availability for direct patient care. Informatics nurses can advocate for the right level of support for these activities.

Enhancement Request Management

EHRs are never perfect at go-live. There are invariably functionality and workflow glitches that despite extensive user input and testing, manifest themselves only at go-live. The first few weeks post-live typically focus on prioritizing and resolving as many of these issues as possible. Simultaneously, end users are building skills proficiency and learning how the system really works.

As the go-live issues list dwindles down to unresolvable and low-priority issues, great enhancement ideas begin to pour in from users. Remember that this is around the same time that the project is deemed "completed," and resource reductions are anticipated. Often, those resources are redeployed to new strategic projects, resulting in a request backlog—an abundant demand of worthy enhancement ideas, but a modest supply of resources to implement them along with the adaptive and corrective maintenance that is now required in a live system. A well-defined and governed request-management process is needed at this point.

Structure and process for request management will depend on the organization's culture, but in general, there is a process for end users to ask for enhancements; a tracking system for the requests that usually also captures corrective maintenance; and a process for requests to be reviewed, approved or denied, prioritized, and scheduled. Ideally, a configuration database is updated when the change is implemented. Figure 7.5 is an example of a request governance structure.

Requests come in from multiple sources. The appropriate clinical, operational, or interdisciplinary group discusses the merits and impacts of the proposed change. If supported, the request is sent to a group of clinical and technical EHR experts for a feasibility discussion. If the request is technically workable, it is presented to the decision-making group, along with expected work effort and anticipated workflow and end-user training impacts. The decision group approves or denies, then prioritizes the approved work so that the teams responsible to build and test the enhancement can schedule the work.

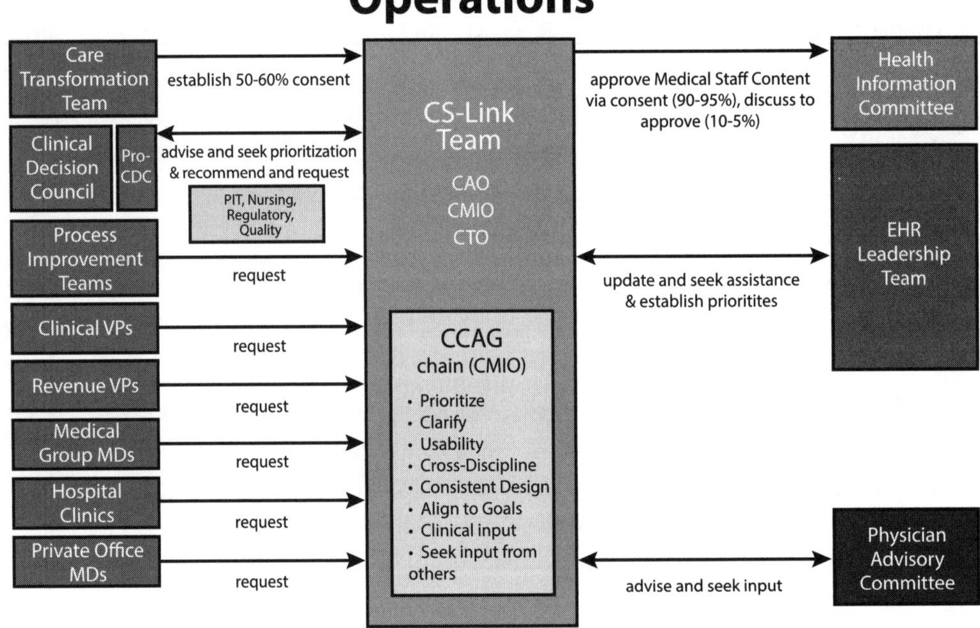

FIGURE 7.5 Request governance structure example.

Optimization

Definitions of EHR optimization vary, but common themes include strategies to improve processes, maximize effective use, reduce errors, reduce costs, eliminate workflow inefficiencies, improve clinical decision support, and improve end-user skills and satisfaction with the system. Optimization is all too often lumped into post-live maintenance and support, but it should be treated separately from maintenance: Optimization is more akin to innovation than to maintenance.

Henry (2005) talked about optimization starting long before system installation and then continuing during implementation and maintenance phases of the system life cycle. Anticipatory optimization of workflows and basic computer skills, prior to any training on the new clinical system, better prepares end users for go-live. Workflow optimization prior to go-live is preparatory to the changes expected with go-live. Superfluous pre-live process steps should be eliminated, and the end users should be engaged in the expected workflow changes.

System optimization can similarly occur prior to go-live. Simulation is an extremely effective tool for optimizing user tools and workflows, especially when the simulations are interdisciplinary. Organizations are beginning to invest in simulation labs for various training purposes; Ideally, EHR installation and significant changes should be tested in a simulated scenario. End-user involvement with testing cycles and early training phases may provide invaluable feedback on workflows and functionality for pre-live optimization. A great example is the discovery of a medication-related nurse/pharmacist clinical messaging gap, enabling just-in-time optimization of the messaging workflows to improve user experience and medication safety.

Post-live optimization is similarly composed of three primary and perhaps inseparable aspects: workflow, system functionality, and training.

NOTE

Remember that no clinical information system is perfect at go-live. No user is perfect at go-live. Most end users undergo a massive learning curve during the first several months of using a new EHR system.

Frequent reinforcement of key workflows is vital. No matter how good the training strategy and delivery, users will not remember everything they learned, and will tend to fall back to previous workflows. This is the opportunity to learn how well workflows have been designed as well as how well the functionality supports the workflows.

Frequent observation, monitoring, and re-training are essential during those first critical months. Some organizations deliberately budget for post-live classroom training to occur three to four months post-live. Reinforcement of key workflows and functionality, as well as significant changes to the system as a result of post-live discoveries, are included in post-live training. Complex workflows that were deliberately not implemented in the initial system activation may also be introduced at post-live training. As users become more proficient and gain understanding of how the system works, they generate ideas for improvements. The volume of these often innovative ideas tends to greatly exceed available resources.

Given that implementing multiple enhancements in rapid succession would unduly burden users' capacity for change, using a goal-based decision process is important. Table 7.2 demonstrates an optimization checklist used at two to three months post-live in an ambulatory clinic, with a strong focus on making everyday tools more efficient and effective.

Table 7.2 Ambulatory EHR Optimization Check List

Task	*Status/Date Completed*
1. Schedule in-clinic optimization kick-off meeting:	
a. Meeting date/time	
b. Request users' top ten wish list for optimization	
2. Review wish list items:	
a. Build out in-scope items from wish list in proof of concept (POC) environment.	
b. Review data on current use of tools.	

Task	*Status/Date Completed*
3. Kick-off meeting agenda:	
a. Review purpose of optimization process, including scope, expectations, timeline. (Note: Standardization of tools/content is an expectation: one set of tools per specialty. MD leader for specialty to gain consensus on tools/content).	
b. Review process for approval of out-of-scope requests.	
c. Gather potential build items:	
i. Wish list items (minor content changes can be prebuilt and demonstrated).	
ii. Preference lists (additions, deletions, synonyms/mnemonics).	
iii. Review in-office procedure workflow and documentation.	
iv. Review specialty-specific text documentation tools.	
v. Review flowsheets (additions, deletions)	
vi. Review specialty-specific radio button documentation tools	
vii. Check whether more Smart Sets are needed.	
viii. Check whether changes are needed to unused Smart Sets.	
ix. Review history tools (additions, deletions).	
x. Patient education content: Check whether all key education needs covered by content vendor, or whether additions are needed.	
xi. Coding/billing issues or improvements.	
d. Review reporting needs (data warehouse, application-level reports).	
e. Other requests not submitted on top ten wish list. (Discuss whether formal approval process will be required for these.)	
4. Schedule site visits (group "like" specialties as much as possible):	
a. Dates	
i. Clinic A:	
ii. Clinic B:	
iii. Clinic C: (and so on)	
b. Attendee list	
i. Clinic manager	
ii. Physician department lead	
iii. End users representing front office, back office, billing providers, ancillary areas, and coding	

continues

Table 7.2 Ambulatory EHR Optimization Check List *(continued)*

Task	*Status/Date Completed*
5. Site visit items:	
a. Review and evaluate items discussed in kick-off meeting.	
i. Decide whether to strive for consensus on new build items that impact a single specialty.	
ii. Organize requests that have broad impact and/or require significant resources (40+ hours), because these will need to go through an approval and prioritization process. (Remind the site visit group what the process looks like and the likely timeline.)	
b. Observation of workflows:	
i. Look for retraining needs.	
ii. Look for opportunities to streamline.	
iii. Look for secret paper processes.	
iv. Look for poorly designed workflows or tools.	
v. Check whether the hardware is working.	
vi. Check whether clinicians are ready to offer patient portal. If not, what is needed to get them ready?	
vii. Check whether clinicians are ready for additional "intrusive" clinical decision support tools.	
viii. Check whether super users are actively assisting co-workers.	
ix. Check whether the clinic manager and MD leader are engaged and actively managing to the EHR world. Do they need additional tools or training?	
c. Review findings with clinic leaders:	
i. Training needs assessments:	
1. Targeted or full retraining?	
2. Training delivery options	
3. At-the-elbow support options	
4. Recommendations for clinic-wide and individual training, including leadership and super users	

Task	*Status/Date Completed*

- ii. Workflow changes needed for efficiency/effectiveness/safety
- iii. Change management needs (user non-adherence or workarounds):
  1. Recommend change management strategies to clinic leadership.
- iv. System build needs:
  1. Anticipated time and effort for the department-specific and low-effort items
  2. Anticipated time and effort for the items requiring approval process
- v. Hardware issues, if any
- vi. Billing issues, if any

6. Validation preparation:
   - a. After consensus within specialty is attained, rebuild old and build new tools, content in POC environment.
   - b. If approved, build system-wide and high-effort requests into POC.
   - c. Schedule validation meetings (same attendees as site visit).
   - d. Build the scenarios in POC (right patients, demographic clinical data, appointments, and so on for end-to-end demo).
7. Validation meeting items:
   - a. Demonstrate enhancements built into POC (scenario-based).
     - i. Elicit feedback. Approved? Unapproved? If unapproved, what fixes are needed?
   - b. Discuss communications plan for requests that are in the approval process by governance groups.
   - c. Discuss any requests that governance declined and will be approved. Communicate appeals process if needed.
   - d. See whether new needs have arisen that are higher priority (usually happens).
   - e. Follow up on other needs: Has training been completed? Hardware issues resolved? Reports more usable? Other?

continues

Table 7.2 Ambulatory EHR Optimization Check List *(continued)*

Task	*Status/Date Completed*
8. Submit approved items through change control process to production: a. Job aids to clinic leadership for distribution prior to migration.	
9. Revise unapproved items, demo by webinar, and move through change control process when approved.	
10. Communicate migration to production to clinic leaders, super users, and so on.	
11. Follow-up visit in 30–60 days: a. Observation of workflows: Are gaps closed? b. Hold a brief meeting with leaders and staff for feedback on optimization completed and outstanding requests. c. Discuss timelines for approved governance items and communication of any additional denied requests. d. Discuss user satisfaction survey to elicit additional feedback and items for future optimization rounds.	

Goals of Optimization

Optimization goals may vary within organizations, but are commonly focused on usability and patient/population care improvements. Usability centers around specified users achieving specified goals with effectiveness, efficiency, and satisfaction in a specific use context, based on the 1998 International Organization for Standards 9241-11 definition (Usability Net, 2006). Patient-centered goals include quality, safety, evidence-based care, and patient/family engagement. Both of these general categories of optimization goals should include innovation.

Optimization is not maintenance. Adaptive maintenance does not, by definition, include innovation. Quality improvement related to external entity requirements is appropriately included in adaptive maintenance—enhanced documentation to support core measure data collection, for example.

Enhancement of documentation tools to enable measurement of nursing intervention impacts on a given population's clinical outcomes may represent an innovation. An example of innovation is creating clinical documentation tools with coded interventions, using standardized terminologies, to enable evaluation of independent and interdependent nursing interventions related to 30-day readmission rates of patients with heart failure.

Usability issues can instigate the development of workarounds. Nurses are intelligent and creative process-improvers. If the clinical system design is suboptimal, nurses will modify the way they use the system. Stoots and Manzi (2013) termed deviation between work-as-designed and work-in-practice as *drift*, which is a potential source of risk to patient safety and quality goals, and recommended using an "accountability for workarounds" scorecard to educate various stakeholders to their responsibilities; provide tools for assessment, planning, and evaluation; and report on metrics.

One tool to consider is usability evaluation, performed at intervals during the system life cycle. Several standard instruments for measuring usability are outlined in Table 7.3. Yen and Bakken (2012) found in their review of usability study methodologies that the most frequently used instruments were the questionnaire for user interaction satisfaction, the modified Technology Acceptance Model (TAM) questionnaire, and the IBM usability questionnaires (see Table 7.3). Usability efforts may be under-resourced in healthcare organizations, despite the value that usability principles and practices can bring to patient safety and clinical efficacy. Staggers and Rodney (2012) presented a new health usability maturity model that informaticists can use to assess their organization's level of usability, from a Phase 1 level (in which usability is largely unrecognized) to Phase 5 (in which usability is mandated, resources, budgeted, and measured).

Table 7.3 Selected Standard Usability Questionnaires

Instrument Name	*Type*	*Typical Use*	*Cost*
System Usability Scale (SUS)	10 items; Likert 1–5 scale	Assess overall user satisfaction in learning, consistency, training, integration, and complexity aspects for software, mobile apps, and hardware. http://www.measuringusability.com/sus.php	Free*

continues

Table 7.3 Selected Standard Usability Questionnaires *(continued)*

Instrument Name	*Type*	*Typical Use*	*Cost*
After Scenario Questionnaire (ASQ) IBM	3 items; 1–7 scale	Intended for use immediately after completing a task http://oldwww.acm.org/perlman/question.cgi?form=ASQ	Free*
Post Study System Usability Questionnaire (PSSUQ) IBM	19 items; 1–7 scale	Usability evaluation in a scenario-based laboratory setting; most useful in competitive analyses or iterative design/development. Measures overall usability, system use, information quality, and interface quality. http://www.interaction-design.org/	Free*
Computer System Usability Questionnaire (CSUQ) IBM	19 items; 1–7 scale	Variant of PSSUQ intended for field studies and surveys (rather than in the lab) http://oldwww.acm.org/perlman/question.cgi?form=CSUQ	Free*
Questionnaire for User Interaction Satisfaction (QUIS)	9-point scale; items per focus area	Overall satisfaction along several scales: screen factors, terminology and system feedback, learning factors, system capabilities, technical manuals, online tutorials, multimedia, teleconferencing, and software installation http://lap.umd.edu/QUIS/	$50–1,000
Software Usability Measurement Inventory (SUMI)	1–3 scale; item pool (150 items)	User satisfaction with affect, efficiency, helpfulness, control and learnability aspects of the computer system: prototype or the live product. Subscale and global scores are provided.	$1,200

Instrument Name	*Type*	*Typical Use*	*Cost*
		Reliability and validity information: http://www.ucc.ie/hfrg/questionnaires/sumi/sumipapp.html#sumidev Pricing: http://www.ucc.ie/hfrg/questionnaires/sumi/pricing.html	
Perceived Usefulness and Ease of Use (PUEU)	12 items; 1–7 scale	Instrument based on the modified Technology Acceptance Model. The first six items measure perceived usefulness; the second six items measure perceived ease of use. http://hcibib.org/perlman/question.cgi?form=PUEU	*Free
Website Analysis and Measurement Inventory (WAMMI)	1–8 scale and free text items	Get early feedback on a prototype, monitor ongoing reaction to a website, and compare with competing websites. Measures attractiveness, controllability, efficiency, helpfulness, and learnability aspects. http://www.wammi.com	$350+

**Free as long as source is acknowledged by investigator. (Wilson, 2013; Yen & Bakken, 2012)*

In addition to usability testing, safety evaluations should be routinely employed as part of the system life cycle. Health information technology impacts on patient safety can be positive or negative. An example is barcoded medication administration. When the workflow and technology configuration are right, and the end user knows how to safely use the technology, medication administration safety is significantly increased, as measured by reduced medication errors and the discovery of medication administration near-misses. A poorly designed workflow, misconfigured barcoded medication administration technologies, or deficient integration of the technologies have the potential to increase medication errors, particularly if users feel compelled to devise workarounds. Collins, Fred, Wilcox, and Vawdrey (2012) found that nurses employed inefficient documentation workarounds when EHR flowsheet design did not support communication of clinically significant relationships.

The ECRI Institute regularly publishes reports on the top patient safety hazards and the top health technology hazards. In the 2014 patient safety concern and health technology hazard reports, clinical system/EHR data integrity failure were number one and number four, respectively (ECRI Institute, 2013, 2014). This topic is covered in Chapter 3, but it bears repeating that safety evaluation should be part of optimization efforts. Specific areas for concentration include clinical workflows, data collection and displays, system and interface testing, user training and support, and an incident reporting system.

Optimization of nursing clinical decision support to drive evidence-based practice and innovation is crucial to improving efficient and effective safe care. Clinical decision support takes multiple forms, from displaying the right data and information in the right way to the right person at the right time in the workflow, to intrusive *hard stops* that do not allow the nurse to continue.

Clinical decision support (CDS) is fully covered Chapter 11, but one important purpose of optimization is to enhance existing and devise new clinical decision support. Optimization efforts take into account the growing user proficiency with the EHR (change readiness), the priorities for evidence-based workflow changes, and resource requirements. In addition, there is no single source of truth for how to implement. Nursing does not have a recipe for CDS in EHRs.

Informatics in Action

Anecdotally, seasoned informatics nurse leaders speculate that nursing CDS maturity is still a future goal for the profession. Predictive modeling is a worthy optimization goal that combines process redesign, redesign of EHR design, and perhaps integration of enabling technologies and analytics to improve a selected population's outcomes. This approach could be employed for any at-risk population. One example from the author's organization is innovation in clinical services for heart failure patients. The new program included redesign of evidence-based interdisciplinary care planning and delivery within the acute care episode (starting with identification of the patient) and following through post-discharge: all transitions of care, all disciplines. The process changes necessitated innovation in documentation, patient/family education, and decision support as well as analytics.

Resource Considerations

Making the business case for optimization resources can be challenging. In healthcare organizations, there is fierce competition for scarce resources, both human and monetary, and there tends to be a backlog of IT projects. As operating budgets continue to shrink in the face of dwindling reimbursement for services and rising costs, allocation of resources for clinical system optimization will require additional justification. Options for gaining the critical resources include the following:

- Include optimization as one component of maintenance, but prioritize partial resources for optimization.
- Build in a Phase 2 to the original implementation project that is focused on optimization activities. This is ideally done as part of the original project planning. Phase 2 should be a capital project.
- Treat optimization as a completely new capital project with a well-delineated set of deliverables.

The first option in the preceding list is the least effective and produces the lowest gains, but the organization might not be able to afford more resources. Many organizations do not plan a second phase project for EHR implementations. There is often a perception that a big bang go-live of all modules and functionality is more efficient ("cheaper"), and it is in some cases. However, the trade-off may be lower user satisfaction, higher patient safety risk, and less-effective system use, which may translate into lower-than-expected return on investment (ROI) and failure to meet care quality goals.

Advocating for a Phase 2 optimization should focus on gains expected from higher user adoption and attaining the highest possible return on investment, as well as quality goals. Whether optimization is treated as Phase 2 of the EHR project or as a new standalone project, informatics nurses are well prepared to secure optimization resources by identifying the impacts of optimization and project deliverables aligned to organizational priorities: It is important to connect the dots between optimization goals and organizational goals to influence prioritization of resources.

Another consideration is workforce retention. Highly skilled informatics professionals need opportunities for growth, and are not satisfied if relegated to maintenance work. Optimization is an opportunity for innovative system design that improves usability and helps the organization to attain higher-level goals while preventing talent leak.

Innovation may include integration of additional systems to improve nursing efficiency. For example, streamlining physiological data acquisition and validation into the EHR may save time that allows staff to focus more time on patient/family education; and simultaneously, the real-time documentation of vital signs is used to drive rules that alert nurses to early sepsis or other complications. Nurses and other caregivers can focus time on value-added activities that may prevent readmissions while reducing patient morbidity and mortality. Informatics nurses translate the value of optimization to gain the resources, and then apply those translation skills to ensure that the functionality, workflows, training, and metrics are executed in the most effective way to meet identified goals.

Conclusion

The system life cycle maintenance and support phase should not be perceived as an opportunity to dramatically cut resources. In addition to the vital activities required to provide a stable, reliable clinical information system that receives prompt attention to adaptive and corrective maintenance, minimizes unintended consequences of system change, and ensures business continuity, a case can be made for significant, ongoing optimization of the workflows, functionality, and user informatics competencies. There is never a shortage of organizational goals that can be supported or enabled by clinical systems. Ongoing optimization of those systems can be the key to goal attainment.

References

Collins, S. A., Fred, M., Wilcox, L., & Vawdrey, D. K. (2012, June). Workarounds used by nurses to overcome design constraints of electronic health records. Presented at *11th International Congress on Nursing Informatics.* Montreal, Canada.

Dennis, A., Wixom, B. H., & Roth, R. M. (2012). *Systems analysis and design* (5th ed.). Skillsoft Books24x7 version. Retrieved from http://common.books24x7.com/toc.aspx?bookid=45140

ECRI Institute. (2014a). *Top 10 health technology hazards for 2014: Executive summary report.* Retrieved from http://www.ecri.org/2014hazards

ECRI Institute. (2014b). *Top 10 patient safety concerns for healthcare organizations for 2014.* Retrieved from https://www.ecri.org/PatientSafetyTop10

Farenden, P. (2012). *ITIL for dummies.* John Wiley & Sons: Skillsoft Books24x7 version. Retrieved from http://viewer.books24x7.com/Toc.aspx?bookid=46158

Henry, E. E. (2005). Optimizing primary-care practices. In J. M. Walker, E. J. Bieber, & F. Richards (Eds.), *Implementing an electronic health record system* (pp. 120–127). New York, NY: Springer.

Hunt, E. C., Sproat, S. B., & Kitzmiller, R. R. (2004). *The nursing informatics implementation guide.* New York, NY: Springer.

Kulhanek, B. J. (2011). Creating effective electronic medical record change management processes. *CIN Nursing Magazine, 29*(8), 431–435.

McCormick, K. A., & Gugerty, B. (2013). *Healthcare information technology exam guide for CompTIA, healthcare IT technician, and HIT Pro certifications.* New York, NY: McGraw Hill.

Saba, V. A., & McCormick, K. A. (Eds.). (2011). *Essentials of nursing informatics* (5th ed.). (Kindle edition).

Senft, S., & Gallegos, F. (2009). *Information technology control and audit* (3rd ed.). Skillsoft Books24x7 version. Retrieved from http://common.books24x7.com/toc.aspx?bookid=26441

Staggers, N., & Rodney, M. (2012, June). Promoting usability in organizations with a new health usability model: Implication for nursing informatics. Presented at *11th International Congress on Nursing Informatics.* Montreal, Canada.

Stoots, M., & Manzi, A. (2013, May). Got workarounds? Strategies and tools to get the most from your EHR. Presented at *American Nursing Informatics Association 2013 annual symposium.* San Antonio, TX.

Usability Net. (2006). Usability definitions: International Standards Organization (ISO) 9241-11: Guidance on usability 1998. Retrieved from http://usabilitynet.org/tools/r_international.htm#9241-11

Vaughn, S. (2011). Planning for system downtimes. *CIN Nursing Magazine, 29*(4), 201–203.

Wilson, C. (2013). *Credible checklists and quality questionnaires: A user-centered design method.* Skillsoft Books24x7 version. Retrieved from http://common.books24x7.com/toc.aspx?bookid=54049

Yen, P., & Bakken, S. (2012). Review of health information technology usability study methodologies. *Journal of the American Informatics Association, 19*(3), 413–422.

"True genius resides in the capacity for evaluation of uncertain, hazardous, and conflicting information."

–Winston Churchill

Conducting Quality Healthcare IT Outcome Evaluations: Guidelines and Resources

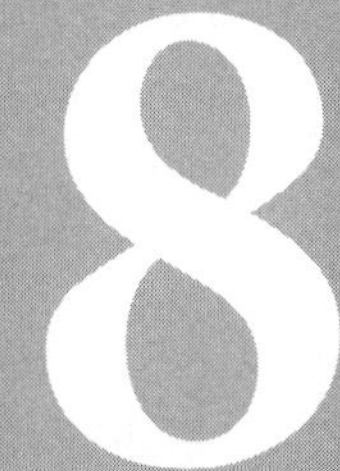

Patricia P. Sengstack, DNP, RN-BC, CPHIMS

OBJECTIVES

- Discuss challenges in conducting outcome evaluations for health-care IT.
- Describe methods to prioritize evaluation projects.
- Discuss the importance of developing a research question.
- Identify appropriate data types for various types of evaluation studies.
- Understand components of a quality publication for an outcome evaluation study.

Clinical information systems are a major investment for healthcare organizations, not just in terms of dollars but human resources as well. Millions of dollars are being spent on electronic health records (EHRs), and the U.S. federal government is contributing billions to advance the adoption of healthcare technology. With more than 80% of U.S. hospitals and 72% of U.S. office-based physicians now using at least a basic EHR, the need to address some fundamental questions becomes essential (ONC, 2013):

- Are EHRs improving patient care and reducing healthcare costs?
- Are EHRs reducing duplication of services?
- Are EHRs reducing time spent documenting patient care?
- Are EHRs reducing medication errors and improving the safety of care delivery?

These questions and others are becoming more and more important to answer. Many organizations are looking to their informatics specialists to help lead the way and provide the expertise in determining the outcomes of their major investment. One might think that organizations have invested significant time and resources to answer these questions throughout their EHR implementation journey, yet that is not currently the case. Relatively few healthcare organizations have developed formal health information technology (IT) outcome evaluation programs.

Although the literature is growing and evolving in the area of healthcare IT outcomes research, these studies are typically conducted in academic medical centers with ample resources, money, and the right skill sets. With EHRs representing a significant portion of an organization's bottom line, it is surprising that formal evaluation programs are not more prominent. This chapter will provide guidelines and the steps that your organization can use to develop and carry out healthcare IT outcome evaluations. It includes examples, ideas, and tools for informatics specialists to use to determine whether their EHR is truly helping.

The Healthcare IT Climate

The adoption rate for clinical information systems is on the rise, with the primary driver being the Centers for Medicare and Medicaid Services (CMS) Meaningful Use incentive program through the Health Information Technology for Economic and Clinical Health (HITECH) Act of 2009. The pace has been fast and furious to implement these systems and capture the incentive dollars. Now that they are in place, it is time to determine their effectiveness.

For an explanation of Meaningful Use, see Chapter 1.

Taking on the task of improving how healthcare IT systems are evaluated is the next phase of technology adoption in healthcare. Between 2000 and 2010, hospitals and ambulatory settings have focused on just getting these systems in place and understanding how best to get the data into them. We are now reaching a point where clinical systems have been in use long enough to develop the expertise and knowledge to get the data out—data that can answer the outcomes questions that will drive improvements in both the system itself as well as the care we deliver.

Starting the journey of healthcare IT evaluation should be fun and informative. If the objective is to evaluate, learn from the evaluation, and make continuous improvements to our systems, then we will need methods that we can all understand and use. The ultimate goal is to be able to answer an evidence-based and confident "yes" to the questions asked earlier, including whether clinical information systems are improving patient care and reducing costs. To use an IT term, we need "usability" in the methodology to evaluate outcomes. It needs to be elegant in its simplicity and optimally become a standardized approach in order to allow for meaningful comparisons, benchmarking, and even (in our wildest dreams) a true meta-analysis of studies.

Assessing Healthcare IT Outcomes

Review of the current healthcare IT outcomes literature finds a lack of standard methods used to evaluate systems, less-than-ideal rigor surrounding the methodology used in the evaluation process, and conflicting results as to whether or not clinical systems are truly helping (Nykanen et al., 2011, Poon, Cusak, & McGowan, 2009; Talmon et al., 2009). Rationale for much of this is the fact that each system is configured uniquely, and the heterogeneity makes it difficult to use similar methods, metrics, and data collection strategies during the evaluative process. Poon et al. (2009) mentioned that in most cases, evaluation is left as an afterthought, and also found many projects without any plans to evaluate the healthcare IT they were tasked with implementing. Additionally, the 2012 report from the Institute of Medicine (IOM), "Healthcare IT and Patient Safety: Building Safer Systems for Better Care," documents the many research gaps in their investigation of the evidence to determine how to most effectively and safely adopt healthcare IT (IOM, 2012).

The Agency for Healthcare Research and Quality (AHRQ) recognized the need for guidance to organizations as they attempt to evaluate the outcomes of their clinical systems. The agency published the Health Information Technology Evaluation Toolkit in 2007 with an updated version in 2009. This resource provides a "fill in the blanks" guide to develop an organization's plan to evaluate healthcare IT. There is an emphasis on the selection of measures or metrics, along with several tools to help project owners determine the best and most accessible measures to select for study. The appendix contains multiple examples of measures that may be used to evaluate a project, including clinical outcome measures; clinical process measures; provider adoption and attitudes measures; patient adoption, knowledge, and attitudes measures; workflow impact measures; and financial impact measures. Additionally, there are examples of outcome evaluations that provide scenarios where the following questions are answered as part of the planning for a study (Cusak et al., 2009):

- Describe the expected impact of the intervention and briefly describe how you think your project will exert this impact.
- What questions do you want to ask to evaluate this impact? These will likely reflect the expected impact (either positive or negative) of your intervention.
- What will you measure in order to answer your questions?
- How will you make your measurements?
- How will you design your study? What comparison group will you use?
- For quantitative measurements only: What types of statistical analysis will you perform on your measurements?

Although this toolkit is helpful, it stops at the step to "write your evaluation plan." The importance of reviewing the literature for any current evidence is not mentioned nor is the importance of the analysis and dissemination of results. Commitment of resources to conduct an outcomes evaluation can be significant, and any quality study should be submitted for publication so that all can learn.

One of the largest healthcare IT industry leaders, the Healthcare Information and Management Systems Society (HIMSS) assembled the *Health IT Value Suite* in 2014, which is a comprehensive knowledge repository that classifies, quantifies, and articulates the clinical, financial, and business impact of healthcare IT investments. HIMSS recognizes that the value of healthcare IT is being questioned through news articles, high-profile EHR implementations, clinicians, buyers, patients, and congressional committees. HIMSS has developed a consistent way to understand, evaluate, and communicate the real-world impact of healthcare IT.

HIMSS has also collected examples from around the world in a library of value-focused, evidence-based examples of healthcare IT evaluations using a common vocabulary, referred to as the *HIMSS Health IT Value STEPS,* as shown in Figure 8.1. The intent is to provide a standard way to categorize healthcare IT evaluative efforts in five areas. As of 2013, HIMSS have demonstrated 56 different documented benefits of healthcare IT across the five categories. Organizations are encouraged to submit their outcomes work to the website, which can be accessed at

http://www.himss.org/valuesuite

	Value Category (STEPS™) and Subtype	Documented Examples
S	Satisfaction: Patient; Provider; Staff; Other	Improved communication with patients; improved patient satisfaction scores; improved internal communication
T	Treatment / Clinical: Safety; Quality of Care; Efficiency	Improved patient safety; reduction in medic errors; reduced readmissions; improved scheduling
E	Electronic information / Data: Evidence Based Medicine; Data Sharing and Reporting	Increased use of evidence-based guidelines increased population health reporting; improved quality measures reporting
P	Prevention and Patient Education: Prevention; Patient Education	Improved disease surveillance; increased immunizations; longitudinal patient analysis; improved patient compliance
S	Savings: Financial / Business; Efficiency Savings; Operational Savings	Increased volume; reduction in days in accounts receivable; reduced patient wait times; improved inventory control

FIGURE 8.1 HIMSS Health IT Value STEPS.
© 2013 Healthcare Information and Management Systems Society (HIMSS). Reprinted with permission.

It is a well-known saying, "If you can't measure it, you can't improve it." This is clearly the case with the evaluation of clinical information systems. They play a vital role in patient care and in an organization's daily operations. It seems common sense that the evaluation of these systems would be an integral part of ongoing activities, yet overall this is the exception and not the rule. One reason perhaps is the fact that there is no industry standard or common method that organizations can use to evaluate the performance of systems to determine if they are achieving desired outcomes. And again, due to the significant heterogeneity among clinical information systems, the standardization of evaluative measures becomes challenging. On the positive side, however, a literature review reveals several methodologies, many of which include evaluative frameworks described herein that can be implemented regardless of the configuration specifics of the system.

Steps, Tools, and Resources to Evaluate Healthcare IT Outcomes

The following steps provide a starting point for developing and conducting healthcare IT evaluation and outcome studies. They are intended to be easy to use for both novice and expert informatics specialists. Start-to-finish steps are provided that can guide organizations through the process while ensuring key components of quality research are not overlooked. The steps describe different types of evaluation studies that can be conducted along with examples of metrics that can be used to represent the issue under study. The focus is on outcomes specific to clinical system implementations or enhancements that are felt to be directly attributable to a system change, and it all starts with getting the right stakeholders around the table. Any outcome evaluation project needs the support and resources that only a multidisciplinary team can provide. Once assembled, the fun begins.

Step 1: Determine What Will Be Evaluated

Choosing what to evaluate should be given serious consideration. The resources and time it takes to conduct a rigorous and quality outcomes project can be significant. Prioritizing a list of potential topics to evaluate should be done as a first step in any evaluation program. The process to generate that list of topics and the process to prioritize the list should not be taken lightly. Generate initial ideas with the organization's key stakeholders at the table. One method that can be used is simple brainstorming. In a brainstorming exercise, all ideas are good and written down. Overall, any evaluation conducted should support the organizational mission, vision, and strategic plan. An example brainstorming exercise follows.

Potential Topics for Outcome Evaluations

- Patient adoption of PHR (personal health record)
- Safety of using copy/paste function in EHR
- Effectiveness of allergy alerting
- Reduction of sepsis with new configuration of alerts in EHR with sepsis bundles
- Accuracy of patient-generated data in patient portal
- Patient compliance with vaccinations with alert generated in patient portal
- Financial savings of stopping printing of automated reports

- Reduction of duplicate ordering
- Other ideas?

Measuring and evaluating outcomes from a clinical system implementation or a system enhancement can be as variable as the projects themselves. The evaluation of each project is unique and based on multiple factors including the organizational need, the desired outcome, the data available, and the resources available to perform the evaluation work. A project's outcome may be measured in a number of categories. These include:

- Clinical outcomes
  - Reduction in episodes of ventilator-associated pneumonia with the implementation of electronic, evidence-based order sets and/or appropriate reminders and alerts
  - Increase in compliance with vaccinations or other routine examinations
- Financial outcomes
  - Reduction in or elimination of use of paper/toner
  - Reduction in duplicate processes/systems by centralization of systems
  - Reduction in lab or radiology orders by using duplicate order alerting
- Research outcomes
  - Improved accuracy of data to support research
  - Improved access to data by researchers
- Adoption
  - Increased use of system (or new component) by physicians
  - Increased use of system (or new component) by nurses and other care providers
  - Increased use of patient portal by patients
- User satisfaction
  - End-user satisfaction level with new system or new feature
  - Satisfactory usability of system
- Quality/patient safety
  - Reduction in medication errors
  - Improved accuracy of data for clinical decision-making

- Administrative outcomes
    - Improved administrative report accuracy
    - Improved access to administrative data
- Productivity
    - Reduction in time to document in new system
    - Workflow process streamlined

From these examples, it becomes clear that a "one size fits all" evaluation process to measure the outcome of an implementation or enhancement project does not exist. It must be customized to fit the specific desired and expected outcomes. Regardless, the first step must be the prioritization and organizational agreement on what aspects of healthcare IT should be studied.

Multiple factors should be taken into consideration when deciding which project to undertake. After a list has been generated from a brainstorming session, the next step is to prioritize the list.

There are two ways to add quantification to the prioritization process. (Although neither of these prioritization methods are perfect, they provide a starting point to begin the planning process for your project.) The first is the *nominal group technique*. With this technique, a list of potential topics is distributed to all stakeholders, who rank order each item on a scale of 1 to 5, with 1 being the highest and 5 the lowest. All items must be scored for this to work.

Then all scores for each topic can be summed, and the total values assessed. The topic with the lowest score will be the item felt to be the most important to the organization. In the example in Table 8.1, you can see that the group collectivity felt that the outcome evaluation on the reduction of sepsis is the most important with the lowest (meaning, highest-priority) score of 11. Using this method, a team can easily visualize which topics would be of highest priority.

Table 8.1 Example Nominal Group Technique for Prioritization

Potential Topic	*Person 1*	*Person 2*	*Person 3*	*Person 4*	*Total*
Patient adoption of PHR	5	8	8	6	27
Safety of using copy/paste function in EHR	2	6	7	1	16
Effectiveness of allergy alerting	3	5	4	3	15
Reduction of sepsis with new configuration of alerts in EHR with sepsis bundles	1	7	1	2	**11**
Accuracy of patient-generated data in patient portal	4	2	3	7	16
Patient compliance with vaccinations with alert generated in patient portal	6	1	2	5	14
Financial savings of stopping printing of automated reports	8	4	6	8	26
Reduction of duplicate ordering	7	3	5	4	19

Another tool that can help quantify prioritization of an organization's outcomes work is presented in Table 8.2. This tool can be used to help quantify prioritization by addressing factors including the study's potential to impact quality, safety, and value to the organization. Using a tool such as this allows each stakeholder to weigh in on the topic's importance and results in a score that can be used to determine which outcome evaluation to do first. It includes areas to consider, such as the number of end users impacted, the patient safety impact, the value of the outcomes study to the organization, and how much this study will potentially contribute to the growing body of evidence of EHR use.

Stakeholders can be asked to complete this form with a brief answer to each item as well as their score on a scale of 1 to 10. With all the stakeholders at the table, each rating item can be reviewed and scored. After each potential outcome's evaluation project has been scored, they are compared to see which one scored the highest.

Table 8.2 Reduction of Sepsis with New Configuration of Alerts in EHR with Sepsis Bundles

Rating Item	*Answer*	*Score Guideline*	*Score*
Number of end users impacted by the feature to be studied		1–10 (1 for a small number of users, 10 for all system users)	
Patient safety impact		1–10 (1 for negligible, 10 for significant impact)	
Patient quality of care impact		1–10 (1 for negligible, 10 for significant impact)	
Value of study results to the organization (support of mission and strategic plan)		1–10 (1 for negligible, 10 for significant value)	
Opportunity to publish		1–10 (1 for no chance, 10 for a significant opportunity)	
Meets a regulatory need		1–10 (1 for no regulatory need, 10 for current regulatory need)	

Rating Item	*Answer*	*Score Guideline*	*Score*
Data is easily available for evaluation		1–10 (1 for very difficult, 10 for very easily accessible)	
How much will this contribute to the growing body of evidence-based knowledge for EHR use?		1–10 (1 for negligible, 10 for significant contribution)	
		Total Priority Score =	

Step 2: Determine the Question

After the evaluation topic has been determined, the next step—and sometimes the most challenging step—is to determine the question you are trying to answer. The reason that determining the question is so important is that this initial step in the process lays the foundation for the entire evaluation. A clear, focused question helps the team determine what data will need to be collected and how it ultimately should be reported.

Here are a few examples of questions that can be asked for an outcomes project:

- How many patients have accessed laboratory results via their patient portal over the last 6 months?
- How many patients have entered blood glucose readings into their patient portal over the last 6 months?
- Do patients who enter their blood glucose readings into their patient portal have better control over their diabetes than patients who do not use a patient portal?
- Has implementation of the sepsis alert in the EHR resulted in improvements in timeliness of antibiotic administration for patients determined to be at risk?

- What is the estimated amount of financial savings if automated report printouts were reduced by 50%?
- Has the implementation of the nurse-driven urinary catheter protocol reduced the number of catheter days for patients?
- Have the new admission assessment screens resulted in timesaving and improved support of workflow for nurses?
- Do patients who have scored higher than 20 on the electronic Risk for Readmission tool have a follow-up appointment scheduled with their physician within 72 hours of discharge?
- Has duplicate ordering of chemistry labs been reduced since the duplicate order checking functionality was implemented?

When your evaluation is seeking to make a comparison, the question can use a standardized format for formulating searchable, answerable questions called PICOT (Fineout-Overholt & Johnston, 2005). Table 8.3 defines the acronym with an example question. This standard format was originally developed to answer clinical questions, but in some cases can be used for healthcare IT outcome evaluations.

Table 8.3 Standard PICOT Method Example

Do diabetic patients who have entered their blood glucose readings into their patient portal over the last 6 months have better control over their diabetes than patients who do not use a patient portal?

P: Specific patient population of interest	Diabetic patients
I: Intervention of interest or issue of interest	Access to a patient portal to enter glucose readings by the patient
C: Comparison of interest (that is, intervention or issue)	Patients who enter glucose reading via the patient portal versus those who do not
O: Outcome of interest	Controlled A1C levels
T: Time frame	6 months

As you can see, the data that will need to be collected will differ based on the question being asked. The key is to agree on the question first.

Step 3: Conduct a Literature Search

After a question is determined, a literature review should be conducted. Perhaps others have studied this question in the past, and evidence may already be published that answers your question. Searches should be conducted in peer-reviewed journals by searching available databases such as Cumulative Index to Nursing and Allied Health Literature (CINAHL), PubMed, and Cochrane Reviews. Questions to ask as you review the literature should include:

- Has this topic been studied before?
- What data was collected?
- What were the findings?
- Can we replicate the methods of the study?

A helpful guide that can be used to evaluate the quality of a published study has been created by Talmon et al. (2009): namely, the Statement on Reporting of Evaluation Studies in Health Informatics (STARE-HI). This guide provides criteria upon which to evaluate the study from the title all the way to the appendices. For example, it states that the title should contain three elements: the type of system being evaluated, the study question, and the study design. A good example of a title would be, "An Assessment of the Effectiveness of an EHR's Allergy Alerting: A Retrospective Review."

The study design section of the guide is particularly helpful in determining the rigor of a study. It provides details on what should be addressed, including clear descriptions of the participants, the study flow, outcomes measures, methods for attaining the data, and data analysis. In the results section, STARE-HI lists and describes a number of important areas to evaluate, including the presence of demographic data, unexpected events during the study, study findings and outcome data, and unexpected observations.

TIP

Reviewing literature on your topic of interest using a guide such as STARE-HI will ensure that quality evaluations are considered as you develop your plan to conduct an evaluation of your own.

Step 4: Determine the Needed Data

It will now begin to be clear why agreement on the outcome evaluation question was so important in the beginning stages of planning. In this step, the specific data elements to be collected need to be determined. For example, if your question is *How many patients have accessed laboratory results via their patient portal over the last 6 months?* you will want to consider the following:

What data is needed to answer the question?

- Number of unique patients who have accessed results via their patient portal
- If percentage is desired, then would need count of all patients who have a patient portal account set up as the denominator and the numerator would be those who have reviewed labs.
- If percentage of entire population is desired, then would need denominator of all patients with an encounter in the last 6 months and numerator of those who have reviewed labs.
- Could also provide data on number of times each patient has accessed their labwork via the patient portal
- May also want demographics (age, gender) on the patients who have access to their labwork

Is it available? Can the data be easily queried and pulled into a report or spreadsheet for data manipulation? Yes, these data elements can be provided.

Who will collect it? Will need the expertise from someone with database query skills.

What data collection tool will be used? Will need to use a spreadsheet (Excel).

It is also important to evaluate whether the data you will need to answer your question even exists. At this point, you may realize that the EHR does not contain the data needed, or that it is not technically feasible to get a report out of the system's database for what you need.

Remember that working through this early in the evaluation is important. To obtain the data necessary, a new field in the EHR may need to be added, or a manual process may be required. If the data is related to end-user satisfaction, you may need to create a survey or a method to observe users as they interact with the system. To put it simply, the question, *Where will we get the data we need?* should be addressed early in the evaluation process.

Step 5: Determine the Study Type

Although the gold standard and most rigorous studies are felt to be randomized controlled trials (RCTs), the reality is that these are difficult to conduct in the area of healthcare IT. Imagine attempting to study one group in your hospital using a particular function in the EHR, with a control group that does not use that function. Or think of the challenges with studying a phenomenon within a computerized provider order entry (CPOE) system and compare it with a similar population in your hospital that does not use CPOE.

Because of these challenges, studies on healthcare IT outcomes are typically not RCTs, although there are some that have been published. The majority of studies that evaluate outcomes of healthcare IT are descriptive studies or comparative studies over time: that is, pre-post studies. All of them have limitations, and most note that generalizability is not practical due to the heterogeneity of systems and lack of standard terminologies and study methods.

The point here is that your outcome evaluation does not need to take on the form of a highly sophisticated research project. When determining your study design, first take into account the question you are asking, then the data you are collecting to answer the question. Having a clear understanding of these foundational concepts will lead you to the right study design. Keeping it simple, clear, and straightforward is key to not only ensuring that the evaluation can be conducted, but also that the information gleaned from the assessment can easily be disseminated to an audience who can take action on the results. If you want to make comparisons between two similar groups but are not sure which comparative statistics would be best, we recommend that a statistician is part of your evaluation team.

In Table 8.4, find types of studies and examples.

Table 8.4 Study Types and Examples

Type of Study	*Examples*
Pre-Post evaluation of an intervention	A study of the effectiveness of an alert that displays to nurses when an indwelling urinary catheter has been in place for more than 2 days. Determine pre- and post-number of "catheter days" to look for a downward trend.
Retrospective study	A chart review to determine compliance with timeliness of documentation of STAT antibiotics.
Observational study	A count of the number of clicks needed for a nurse to access and enter a falls risk assessment.
Time/motion study	Time, using a stopwatch, taken for a nurse to enter all data fields for a patient's admission assessment.
Case study	A review of a root cause analysis that involved a near-miss error when a nurse entered an incorrect weight into the EHR and a medication dose was prepared based on that weight.
Randomized control trial	*A Randomized Controlled Trial of the Effect of Real-Time Telemedicine Support on Glycemic Control in Young Adults with Type 1 Diabetes* (Farmer et al., 2005)
Descriptive evaluation of current state	An organization's patient portal has just been launched with a big marketing effort. After 3 months, a descriptive evaluation of adoption is conducted to determine how many patients have created their accounts and used features, such as accessing labs and emailing their providers.

Step 6: Determine the Data Collection Method and Sample Size

At this point of the evaluation, you may already have an idea of how you will obtain the data. In this step, the exact method that will be used to attain the data is clarified.

Whichever method is selected, ensure that there is key stakeholder consensus on both the type of data and the collection method. Data can be obtained to answer your outcome question in a number of ways:

- Data is already available in the EHR database (or other database), and you will need the assistance of someone skilled in running a query or developing a report.
- You will need a manual chart review.
- You will need to observe end users as they interact with the system.
- You will need to conduct a survey.
- You will need a focus group to gather data.

Additionally, you need to determine a sample size or date range to evaluate. Fundamentally, the larger the sample size, the better the study and the better chance at generalizability of the results. Keep in mind that it may not be realistic or necessary to assess 10 years' worth of data when 6 months or even 3 months or maybe even a week will provide an adequate picture of the current situation. Generally, you will need enough observations or incidents to feel comfortable about the conclusions you are attempting to draw from the data collected. The AHRQ Health Information Technology Evaluation Toolkit, mentioned earlier in this chapter, offers a hypothetical example of determining sample size that may be helpful (Cusack et al., 2009).

To help make the decision on sample size, utilize these methods:

- Check sample size and date ranges in previous studies on the same topic (from literature search in Step 3).
- Secure the help of a statistician.
- Use common sense and level of confidence that the volume of observations is adequate to represent the situation under study.
- Secure consensus from key stakeholders.

Step 7: Collect, Analyze, and Display Data

After data has been collected over the agreed-upon time frame, it will need to be presented and displayed in a format that can be comprehended by multiple audiences. Data that represent the results of an outcome evaluation must contain all the information necessary for interpretation. Data can be displayed in graphs, charts, and/or tables; each of these should include the following:

- Title with date range and sample size as appropriate
- Legends that clearly explain the content and colors
- Labels on the x and y axis so the numerical value can be understood
- Other descriptors necessary for interpretation

Qualitative studies may result in written summaries, narrative text, or bullet points that represent the responses to a survey or interview. Table 8.5 gives some examples of display options for different data types.

Table 8.5 Data Display Options

Data Type	*Display Options*
Demographic data (age, gender, marital status, education, race, and so on)	Table, bar chart, pie chart
Descriptive statistics (mean, median, mode, standard deviation)	Table, bar chart, pie chart
Comparative statistics (*p* values, confidence intervals)	Table
Data representing processes over time	Run charts
Qualitative descriptions/summary	Tables, narrative text, bullet point lists

Run Charts

Run charts—graphs of data over time—can be a very valuable tool for assessing the effectiveness of change and are very easy to use. Determining whether lasting improvement has really happened requires observing patterns. Run charts look something like a line graph that plots the number of times something occurs each day or each week. Looking at a run chart, you can easily see when interventions have truly made a lasting improvement by observing the pattern of data over the course of time. The figure below illustrates the concept of a run chart.

You can see an example of a run chart tool from the Institute for Healthcare Improvement (IHI) at http://www.ihi.org/resources/Pages/Tools/RunChart.aspx.

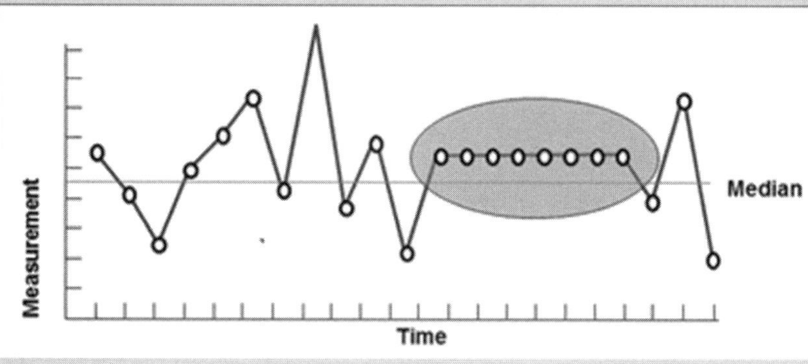

International Six Sigma Institute™ (http://www.sixsigma-institute.org)

Step 8: Document Your Outcome Evaluation

Writing up your evaluation and potentially submitting for publication is the last step in the process. Without comprehensive documentation of your study, the chance that any practice improvements occur becomes unlikely.

Do not keep your work a secret. Talmon et al. (2009) recommended the following headings in a healthcare IT evaluation report: Title, Abstract, Keywords, Introduction, Study Context, Methods, Results, Discussion, and Conclusion. Using the STARE-HI guidelines (described earlier in this chapter) for each section of a report will add strength and rigor, improving chances of publication. The following recommendations for what to include in a healthcare IT evaluation report provide some details regarding each section, but it is highly recommended that the STARE-HI guidelines are reviewed in their entirety.

- Title
- Abstract
- Keywords
- Introduction
    - Scientific background
    - Rationale for the study
    - Objectives for the study
- Study Context
    - Organizational setting
    - System details and system in use
- Methods
    - Study design
    - Theoretical background
    - Participants
    - Study flow
    - Outcome measures or evaluation criteria
    - Methods for data acquisition and measurement
    - Methods for data analysis
- Results
    - Demographic and pertinent study data
    - Unexpected events during the study
    - Study findings and outcome data
    - Unexpected observations
- Discussion
    - Answers to study question
    - Strengths and weaknesses of the study
    - Results in relation to other studies
    - Meaning and generalizability of the study
    - Unanswered and new questions
- Conclusions
- Author's contributions
- Competing interests
- Acknowledgements
- References
- Appendices

Future Directions

Although we are in the midst of changing payment models, a shift in focus from inpatient to ambulatory services, government requirements that continue to impact healthcare IT, and a cry for Big Data, it is clear that technology is going to be a big part of the equation. We have the knowhow, we have the technology, and we have the science. Now we just need the resources with the right skills and also the organizational support to provide focus on this important facet of our clinical systems.

What is Big Data?

Big Data in healthcare refers to electronic health data sets so large and complex that they are difficult (or impossible) to manage with traditional software and hardware. The volume and diversity of the data that organizations have residing in numerous systems including EHR, laboratory, pharmacy, finance, and other clinical systems is overwhelming. And do not forget about data now contained within social networks, such as Twitter, Facebook, and other blogs with social media posts. Accessing all these data sources in a way that allows the analysis of patients and populations in ways never before imagined is exciting; in fact, it is BIG!

Without strong processes in the evaluation of our systems, it will be almost impossible to determine whether healthcare IT is really helping or hindering progress. We need to see growth in the emergence of informatics evaluation teams and the development of organizational programs that support the evaluation process. Outcome evaluation programs need to become the norm—not the exception.

After reading this chapter, we hope that informatics specialists will determine what is important to study, bring the key stakeholders together, and give it a try. Conducting outcome evaluations in healthcare IT does not need a grant or a team of highly skilled researchers: It just needs your passion and the tools. We hope this chapter has provided just that.

Conclusion

As the U.S. federal government's Meaningful Use program begins shifting toward a more outcomes-oriented focus in Stage 3, we will not have a choice but to focus on outcomes. Learning how to conduct these types of studies becomes imperative as evidence is created, disseminated, and applied to practice. We need to get to a point in the evolution of the EHR where we are not continually using the trial-and-error method of configuration and implementation. With those of us in the informatics field pushing toward evidence-based methods to conduct outcome evaluations and disseminate the findings, we will begin to see better products and improved outcomes that live up to expectations.

References

Cusak, C., Byrne, C., Hook, J., McGowan, J., Poon, E., & Zafar, A. (2009). *Health information technology evaluation toolkit.* Agency for Healthcare Research and Quality, 2009 Update. (AHRQ Publication No. 09-0083-EF). Retrieved from http://healthit.ahrq.gov/sites/default/files/docs/page/Evaluation%20Toolkit%20Revised%20Version.pdf

Farmer, A., Gibson, O., Dudley, C., Bryden, K., Hayton, P., Tarassenko, L., & Neil, A. (2005). A randomized controlled trial of the effect of real-time telemedicine support on glycemic control in young adults with Type 1 diabetes. *Diabetes Care, 28*(11), 2697–2702.

Fineout-Overholt, E., & Johnston, L. (2005). Teaching EBP: Asking searchable, answerable clinical questions. *Worldviews on Evidence-Based Nursing, 2*(3), 157–160.

Healthcare Information and Management Systems Society (HIMSS) (2014). *The HIMSS health IT value suite.* Retrieved from http://www.himss.org/ValueSuite.

Institute of Medicine (IOM). (2012). Health IT and patient safety: Building safer systems for better care. Washington, DC: The National Academies Press.

International Six Sigma Institute™ (n.d.). *Six Sigma DMAIC process-measure phase-measurement system.* Retrieved from http://www.sixsigma-institute.org/Six_Sigma_DMAIC_Process_Measure_Phase_Measurement_System.php

Nykanen, P., Brender, J., Talmon, J., de Keizer, N., Rigby, M., Beuscart-Zephir, M., & Ammenwerth, E. (2011). Guideline for good evaluation practice in health informatics (GEP-HI). *International Journal of Medical Informatics, 80*(12), 815–827.

The Office of the National Coordinator for Health Information Technology (ONC). (2013). *Update on the adoption of health information technology and related efforts to facilitate the electronic use and exchange of health information: A report to Congress.* Retrieved from http://www.healthit.gov/sites/default/files/rtc_adoption_of_healthit_and_relatedefforts.pdf

Poon, E., Cusak, C., & McGowan, J. (2009). Evaluating healthcare information technology outside of academia: Observations from the National Resource Center for Healthcare Information Technology at the Agency for Healthcare Research and Quality. *Journal of the American Medical Informatics Association, 16*(5), 631–636.

Talmon, J., Ammenwerth, E., Brender, J., de Keizer, N., Nykanen, P., & Rigby, M. (2009). STARE-HI – Statement on reporting of evaluation studies in health informatics. *International Journal of Medical Informatics, 78*(1), 1–9.

"Working ten hour days allows you to fall behind twice as fast as you could working five hour days."

–*Isaac Asimov*

Essential Tools for Project Management

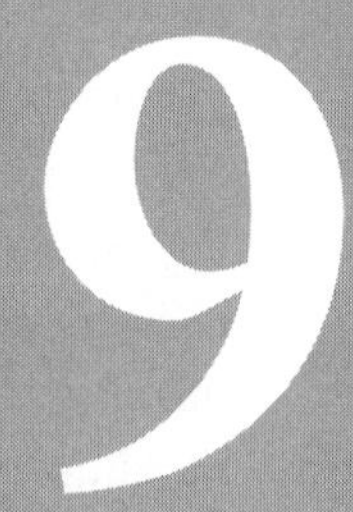

Lisa Anne Bove, DNP, RN-BC

OBJECTIVES

- Define project management.
- Highlight three project management tools.
- Describe how project management tools influence time, budget, and value.

Healthcare is changing at a very fast pace. With the Institute of Medicine (IOM) report, *To Err is Human*, and the American Recovery and Reinvestment Act (ARRA) of 2009, electronic medical records (EMRs) and electronic health records (EHRs) implementation and optimization projects abound. Both initiatives have focused attention on the expected value of EMRs. The IOM report (2000), which primarily focused on patient safety, identified specific applications including computerized provider order entry (CPOE) and Bar Code Medication Administration (BCMA) that would improve outcomes and reduce errors. ARRA included many initiatives, including what is now known best as "Meaningful Use." This program, now managed by the Centers for Medicare and Medicaid Services (CMS), provides financial incentives for the "meaningful use" of certified EHR technology to improve patient care. The financial incentives of Meaningful Use are provided in three stages, with increasing requirements for participation (CMS, 2014). Because this program does not pay for the implementation of EHR technology, many organizations expect project management to help make the implementations as quick (and cost-effective) as possible.

Informatics clinicians are often called upon to implement EHRs with or without the training needed to be a project manager and bring in a project on time and on budget while managing expectations. Clinicians often make good project managers given that they already have many of the skills that make a good project manager: the ability to plan, communicate, and "generate a spirit of cooperation while coordinating diverse activities" (Houston & Bove, 2007). Without some basic project management training, however, clinicians do not necessarily know how to apply their nursing skills to projects. The goal of this chapter is to help the informatics clinician successfully implement projects that will help improve patient outcomes.

The Focus of Project Management: Projects

To comprehend project management, one should understand what a project is. A *project* is a temporary endeavor with a "defined beginning and end" (Houston & Bove, 2007; p. 2). Software implementations are good examples of projects. They often start with the decision to implement a certain application and end when the application *goes live* (is in use).

Projects have a specific *scope of work,* which defines what will be completed within the project's duration. Often, scope is tied to requirements defined before choosing to do the project. Scope drives the work to be done and needs to be closely managed in order to complete the project successfully.

All projects require resources. *Resources* generally are the teams working on the project but can also be tools (that is, software or a building) and funding. The units or specialties involved in an implementation would be considered among the project's resources. Typically, the people working on the project do not report directly to the person managing the project—the *project manager.*

Project managers are responsible to see that the scope of work is done on time and on budget and meets the defined expectations and quality. Project managers guide the resources to complete the assigned tasks. However, the resources report to other managers. Project managers manage only the tasks related to the project—not the overall activities of the employee. Often, the project manager is the "enabler" rather than the "doer" for the work required to complete the project.

NOTE

Projects should not be confused with standard operations, which are ongoing efforts without clear end points; or the tasks to "keep the lights on."

Often, projects fail. A project is considered to be a "failure" when it is late, over budget and/or "...it has not delivered what was required, in line with expectations" (Mind Tools, n.d., "Definition" section, para. 1). According to *Harvard Business Review*, "[O]ver half of all projects fail" (Matta & Ashkenas, 2012, p. 123). After an interactive workshop at the American Medical Informatics Association (AMIA) annual conference in 2009, Drs. Kaplan and Harris-Salamone concluded that projects fail "due to sociological, cultural, and financial issues, and hence are more managerial than technical" (Kaplan & Harris-Salamone, 2009, p. 292). KPMG (a U.S. audit, tax, and advisory services firm) found that more than two-thirds of organizations that it surveyed had experienced at least one project failure in the previous year, and more than one-half did not consistently achieve the intended project results (Barlow, Woolley, Rutherford, & Conradie, 2013). And even though these results were from a survey of organizations in New Zealand, they are similar to those found in other organizations. For example, PricewaterhouseCoopers looked at more than 10,000 projects from 200 companies in various industries and found that only 2.5% of the companies successfully completed 100% of their projects (Hardy-Vallee, 2012). *Harvard Business Review* looked at more than 1,400 IT projects and found that the average cost overrun was 27%, and one in six projects had schedule overruns of almost 70% (Flyvbjerg & Budzier, 2011).

Generally, projects fail for three reasons:

- Failure to plan requirements (scope)
- Failure to complete the work (on time)
- Failure to deliver something that is worthwhile (expectations)

Project Management

One way to reduce the risk of project failure is by using project management. No matter the size, all projects can benefit from the use of project management. The Project Management Institute's (PMI) published *A Guide to the Project Management Body of*

Knowledge (PMBOK Guide), which defines project management as "the application of knowledge, skills, tools, and techniques to project activities to meet the project requirements" (PMI, 2013, p. 4). Houston (2011, p. 10) simplified this definition to, "[P]roject management ensures the projects are completed right."

Project management can help to minimize delays and risks, while managing tasks and interaction between groups—and therefore increasing the likelihood of project success. Gartner (a U.S. information technology research and advisory firm; www.gartner.com) identified a number of recommendations to optimize the success of projects, including:

- Carefully monitor costs include resources.
- Understand and manage the business expectations and functionality sought by the project.
- Hold project status and review meetings and confirm the project's alignment with business strategy. (Mieritz, 2012)

These are similar to other recommendations. According to Kropf and Scalzi (2007), University Hospitals in Cleveland, Ohio instituted changes in IT governance and project management that resulted in an increase of on-time and on-budget projects of more than 40% in 3 years. The KPMG survey previously cited also identified that within high-performing businesses the projects:

- Used a detailed business case that was in alignment with the organizations strategy
- Had an effective sponsor who provided clear direction for the project
- Had project managers who used a consistent project management methodology throughout the entire project
- Actively managed project risks
- Reported issues early
- Tracked expected benefits

Phases of a Project

Project managers following a standard methodology break projects into phases or stages or process groups. Although there are a number ways to break the project into stages, they should follow a general guideline similar to that of the nursing process. The American Nurses Association (ANA) defines the five steps of the nursing process as assessment, diagnosis, planning (outcomes), implementation, and evaluation (2014). The phases of project management are initiation, planning, execution, control, and closure (PMI, 2013). In project management, the initiation phase includes assessment and essentially diagnosis; execution and control are the implementation phase; and the closure phase matches the evaluation phase of the nursing process.

ANA Nursing Process	PMI Project Management Phases
Assessment	Initiation
Diagnosis	Planning
Implementation	Execution, Control
Evaluation	Closure

Initiation

During the initiation phase, the project is defined and approved; the project manager, resources, and stakeholders are identified; and the project charter is created.

Planning

During the planning phase, the detailed project plan is created. This project plan includes more than the work breakdown structure (WBS), which is often known as the "work plan" or "timeline." Instead, it includes all the definitions and plans to manage the project successfully, including scope, communication, issues, risk management, and change management plans. Find further detail on WBS later in the chapter. A number of questions need to be part of the planning process (see Table 9.1).

Table 9.1 General Planning Questions

Planning Step	*Questions as Part of Planning*
Plan the success (breath 1)	• How will the project help the organization's strategic goals or priorities? • What will happen if the organization does not do this project? • What does a successful project look like to the stakeholders?
Plan the project (breath 2)	• What activities need to be done? • What is the estimated duration of each activity and stage? • What are the needed resources?
Get buy-in from stakeholders (breath 3)	• Are the stakeholders committing team members? • Are the stakeholders committing to the duration? • Is the project approved?

Planning is a big part of a project manager's work. Per a quote attributed to Benjamin Franklin, "If you fail to plan, you are planning to fail!" Taking the time to plan how the project will be carried out and how to manage risks, issues, and change requests is crucial to project success. During the planning phase, the project manager creates most of the tools that will carry the project to successful completion.

Execution and Control

During the execution phase, the work of the project is done. The control phase, also known as the "monitor and control" phase, includes the activities that the project manager needs to complete in order to track and report on the project, including status reports, tracking issues, analyzing change requests, and risk monitoring.

Closure

The last phase—the closure phase—in a project management plan is often overlooked, as is evaluation in the nursing process. During the closure phase, the project documents such as budget are completed, "lessons learned" are documented, and metrics are collected for the project. This phase starts after the go-live event and includes sign-off from the stakeholders that the requirements have been met. The closure phase is vitally important to a project because without this step, the project may never be considered completed. Stakeholders need to understand that the project is complete, although there may be future work that stemmed from the initial project. Additionally, the closure phase helps to define successes as well as challenges of the project that can be improved upon during the next project.

Applying Project Management Skills

Using the tools available in project management will increase the likelihood that a project will be successfully completed on time and on budget. Clinician do not need to be project managers to use these tools; and often, clinicians use or have used one or more of these tools even when not functioning as a project manager. Project managers need to identify information for each project, and answering the following questions can help the project manager put together the detailed project plan and support documents:

- Why does this project need to be done? (project charter with objectives)
- What needs to get done? (scope)
- When does it need to completed? (timeline)
- Who will complete the activities? (resources)
- How will the project be accomplished? (detailed work plan, communication, issues, risk management and change management plans)
- Where is the project in relation to the timeline and outcomes? (status reports)

These are questions that any leader needs to answer for operations activities, but following a standard project management methodology will help improve the likelihood of project success.

Stakeholder Management

One of the first activities that should be completed in a project is to identify stakeholders for the project. Matta and Ashkenas (2012) defined stakeholders as those who will be affected by the project's activities or outcomes and/or contribute resources including staff, tools, and money. Stakeholders should work with the project manager to help define the metrics or success measures. They should also sign off on major activities such as scope documents, training, testing plans, and other activities that impact users. After all the stakeholders are identified, they should be assessed for their attitude about the project and for any support or barriers they may put up against the project.

At times, it is easy to identify most if not all the groups or persons that may be impacted by a project. Other times, identifying all the stakeholders can be difficult. Surveying all the key hospital groups can help identify stakeholders and the impact from the project. By asking the stakeholders identified, the project manager can identify other stakeholders. Truly understanding who the stakeholders are and how they feel about the project will help the project manager better manage the project.

Putting together the information discovered—a *stakeholder analysis*—will assist the project manager to successfully manage the project. Ask your stakeholders what will happen if the project is completed or not completed. Ask your stakeholders what they expect as a result of the project.

Put together a grid that identifies who is responsible for an activity versus the person or group that has the ability to approve decisions. One such grid is an *RACI diagram* (Kantor, 2012); see more detail in Table 9.2:

- **R:** Responsible
- **A:** Accountable
- **C:** Consulted
- **I:** Informed

Table 9.2 RACI Defined

Criteria	*Description*
Responsible (R)	• Person who is working on the activity • Usually there is one person responsible, but this could also be a team.
Accountable (A)	• Person (or committee) ultimately accountable for the correct and thorough completion of the deliverable or task • Must sign off (approve) on work that Responsible provides: yes/no authority • There is only one Accountable specified for each task or deliverable.

Criteria	*Description*
Consulted (C)	• Person whose opinions are sought in advance of the decision or action and with whom there is two-way communication
Informed (I)	• Persons who are kept up-to-date on progress, often only on completion of the task or deliverable, and with whom there is just one-way communication

The RACI diagram is used to help determine how project decisions are made (see Table 9.3) by stakeholders. Typically, among project stakeholders, you find:

Chief Medical Officer

Chief Nursing Officer

Chief Medical Informatics Officer

Chief Nursing Informatics Officer

Program Manager

Project Managers

Vendors

Table 9.3 Sample RACI Diagram

RACI	*CMO/CNO*	*CMIO/CNIO*	*Program Manager*	*Project Managers*	*Vendor*
Clinical Standardization Plan	A	C	R	R	N/A
User Engagement	C	A	I	R	N/A
Project Life Cycle Plan	I	C	AR	R	C

continues

Table 9.3 Sample RACI Diagram *(continued)*

RACI	*CMO/CNO*	*CMIO/CNIO*	*Program Manager*	*Project Managers*	*Vendor*
Learning Plan	A	R	C	C	C
Testing Plan	I	C	AR	C	C
Super User Identification Plan	C	AR	C	r	N/A
Metrics/ Measure of Success	A	R	R	R	C

After stakeholders have been identified, project governance should be defined from among them. Include persons at a level of authority and decision-making who can really make the decision: that is, have the authority and knowledge rather than those who are available. Include people at the same level so all voices are heard. Bring only the issues that the governance body needs to give input on and bring it in a way they understand and can make a decision about. Establish thresholds requiring governance approval up-front. These thresholds, for example, could include a 5% or more increase in costs, any change in scope, additional resources, greater than 10% change in major milestone dates, and/or issues likely to impact requirements. Bring the issue as a question with options and ask for a recommendation or decision.

For example, you could mandate that an issue must go to a steering committee if there is substantially less functionality or quality (project manager judgment) if cost is greater than 20% of approved total budget; if schedule is showing a 5% delay of approved completion date or 2 weeks, whichever is less; and/ or if there is 10% fewer approved business case benefits (for example, net present value [NPV], return on investment [ROI], and so on) expected. All these items should be reported at each steering committee meeting and included in the project manager's status report.

Project Management Tools

Every project manager has a set of tools to use during the project. These tools make up the project management methodology. Larger, more complicated projects require more and more complex tools, but every project should have the minimum tool set.

Project Charter

The purpose of the project charter is to document the project and get sign-off and agreement from the stakeholders. Lowenhaupt & Friedman (2003, p. 137) further described the purpose of the project charter as follows:

- "Document agreement between client organization, team sponsor, project team, team leader, and project manager.
- Provide a clear statement of purpose of the implementation project and what the team is committed to deliver.
- Define the project roles and responsibilities.
- Provide the baseline for scope and expectation management."

The *charter* documents the overall project methodology. All the project sponsors should sign the charter as their agreement of the project plan, scope, roles, and organization. Charters do not need to be lengthy documents; rather, they should be concise statements of the plan. The content of the charter should include all the following:

- **Project purpose and goals:** a paragraph or two describing what the project is for and what it is expected to accomplish. This should be a general description of the project such as "implement BCMA in all inpatient nursing units" or "collect new quality measures in the emergency department." In addition to the project purpose, a description of what the project is intended to accomplish should be included. In the example of BCMA, a project goal could be to scan 95% of medications or reduce medication errors.
- **Project scope:** what is and is not part of the project. This should also include all the departments or units that are included or excluded from the project's scope.

- **Project assumptions:** the expectations that guide the project effort. Assumptions can include resource duration, prerequisites, software functionality, building codes, and other basis for the project plan.
- **Project approach:** a description of how the project will be implemented. This section usually has a description of the high-level milestones, such as planning, analysis, build, testing, training, and go-live activities.
- **Project reporting structure:** describes the hierarchy of responsibility and often include a project organization structure (see Figure 9.1).
- **Project roles and responsibilities:** a description of who is part of the project, including teams, stakeholders, leaders, and third-party vendors (see Table 9.4).

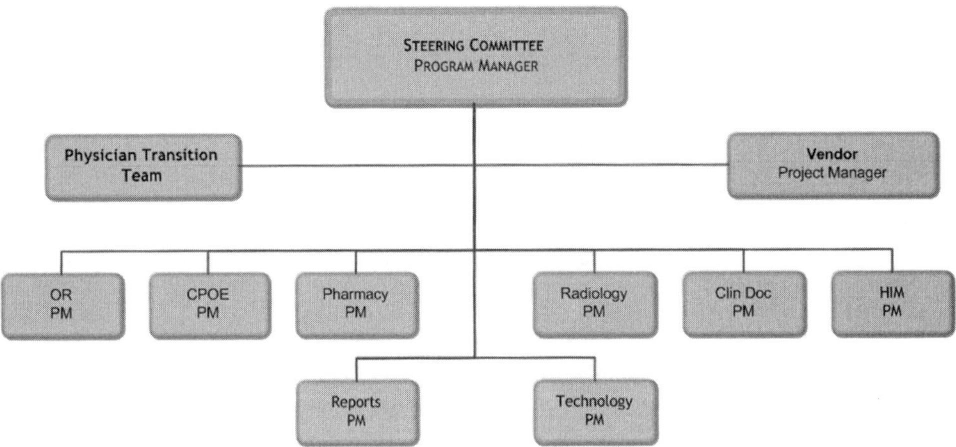

FIGURE 9.1 Sample organization chart.

Table 9.4 Sample Roles and Responsibilities

Role	*Responsibility*
Executive Sponsor	Champions program for the organization Willing to approve the business case Chairs the project steering committee Secures project funding
Business Owners (CNO, Directors of Patient Access, Accounting, Lab, Radiology, Pharmacy, and so on)	Commits user resources Translates and communicates business needs
Clinical Advisory Group	Provides oversight and decisions for clinical applications activities, issues, and risks
Information Systems (IS) Director	Provides project oversight and guidance Manages project team resources Provides and manages project resources Manages project budgets
Project Manager	Creates and drives project timelines Identifies and manage project issues and risks Directs work efforts of project team toward milestones
Testing Coordinator	Drafts the overall program testing plan Defines testing scripts Manages development of the testing scripts Manages the integrated testing activities
Analysts	Builds the system Responsible for completing all assigned project-related tasks and activities Identifies and reports issues Updates project manager on work progress

continues

Table 9.4 Sample Roles and Responsibilities *(continued)*

Role	*Responsibility*
Informatics	Validates clinical information Identifies clinical process to help define future state Responsible for completing all assigned project-related tasks and activities Identifies and reports issues and risks Updates project manager on work progress
Trainers	Provides training to end users Provides go-live support
Vendor Project Managers	Provides project management tools, methodology, and standards Coordinates resources including vendor implementation consultants (ICs)

The charter stands as a document throughout the project, and any changes are captured in other documents, such as the change requests.

Scope Management Plan

To keep projects on time and on budget and meet requirements, project managers need to closely manage scope. One tool that needs to be part of any project is the *scope management plan*, which helps to "ensure the project includes the processes required to ensure that the project includes all the work required, and only the work required" (PMI, 2013, p. 2).

Scope management has been identified as one of the problems with the recent roll out of the Health Insurance Marketplace (Thomas, 2014). One of the biggest issues with scope is *scope creep*, which is uncontrolled changes in scope (Babu, 2005). Scope creep affects every project and needs to be carefully managed. Sometimes scope creep happens because of unclear, undefined, or changing requirements; sometimes it just occurs because someone is trying to do something above and beyond for a stakeholder.

Although changes in requirements certainly can occur, the scope management plan defines how new or changing requirements should be managed. The *scope management plan* defines the detailed scope and how change requests should be managed, including who has the authority to approve changes.

One of the best ways to bring forward a potential change in scope is through a *decision document*, which identifies the change requested along with the benefits and risks of doing or not doing the change (see Table 9.5). The document should be completed by the requestor and created by using the risks and benefits form the stakeholder's point of view. Two or three options including not doing the change should be presented. The project manager can also include a recommendation from among the options based on the overall project risks and metrics. The person requesting the change should generate the decision document. The Steering Committee or accountable leader is then tasked with deciding if the benefits of the change request are worth the impact to the project. If the change is approved, the project manager then needs to modify the project plan by adding time and/or resources, or reducing scope in other areas to absorb the change.

Table 9.5 Sample Decision Document

	Approved Scope	*Alternative #1*	*Alternative #2*
Options	Move Nutrition Department to paper like the Legacy hospitals.	Expand use of EHR to include Nutrition documentation (entity build).	Expand use of EHR to include Nutrition documentation at all facilities (enterprise build).
Description	Nutrition Department is currently fully automated on electronic documentation. The Legacy hospitals are currently on paper for all Nutrition documentation.	Nutrition Department is currently fully automated on electronic documentation. Approximately five forms will need to be assessed and potentially built.	Nutrition Department is currently fully automated on electronic documentation. The Legacy hospitals are currently on paper for all Nutrition documentation. Approximately five forms will need to be assessed and potentially built for all entities.

continues

Table 9.5 Sample Decision Document *(continued)*

	Approved Scope	***Alternative #1***	***Alternative #2***
Benefit (B)	Meets standard (Legacy hospitals). No additional build resources or time will be needed.	Nutritionists, nurses, and physicians will have automated information to support CPOE, workflow, and patient safety. Should help increase physician acceptance of system conversion. Facility will not be required to "go backward."	All hospitals will be automated and have the same solution. Nutritionists, nurses, and physicians will have automated information to support CPOE, workflow, and patient safety. Should help increase physician acceptance of system conversion. Facility will not be required to "go backward."
Risks (R)	Potential reduction in adoption Nutritionists will need to return to paper for documentation. Physicians and nurses will need to look in multiple places for information. Nutritionists and nurses may need to double document so that information is available for orders and so on.	New build requires design, build, and testing; may extend timeline. Despite the addition of the forms, nurses and physicians will have a new system to get used to. Does not meet standard and will potentially require re-do when the Legacy hospitals are added. May impact other projects	All hospitals would need to be involved in the design and go-live dates. New build requires design, build, and testing; may extend timeline. Despite the addition of the forms, nurses and physicians will have a new system to get used to. Will impact other projects
Resources (C)	No additional build resources or time will be needed.	Will require additional build analyst and operations staff time at facility May require additional hardware	Will require additional build analyst and operations staff time across the organization May require additional hardware

	Approved Scope	*Alternative #1*	*Alternative #2*
Summary	Benefit: Low Risk: Low Cost: Low Organization priority: Low	Benefit: High Risk: Low Cost: Medium Organization priority: Low	Benefit: High Risk: Medium Cost: High Organization priority: Low

Work Breakdown Structure and Timeline

Many people see the project plan as the most difficult part of project management. Although some of the tools available are complicated, a simple timeline with activities, due dates, and person responsible is sufficient to run many projects.

As mentioned earlier, formal project management classes teach a concept called a *work breakdown structure* (WBS). The WBS defines the work that needs to be done broken down in doable chunks. For an implementation project, the major tasks could be plan, build, test, train, activation, and so on. For each one of these, the project manager would list activities that need to be completed in order to complete the task. Breaking down the major tasks into doable activities helps to drive the duration. For example, if you need to train 200 nurses on BCMA, and each class is 4 hours long; and if three classes per day are offered, and each class has 10 seats, the staff could potentially be trained in about 7 days after the materials are created and the schedule is published.

TIP

Sometimes starting with the known tasks is easier than starting with the more difficult tasks, such as how long will it take to build all the tables needed.

For the WBS, each one of the major tasks (such as training) should then be broken into smaller tasks, such as curriculum design, schedule development, classroom set-up, and actual training. Each project manager has her own way of organizing this task. Most project managers will include the project team and stakeholders to help identify all the activities needed. When the project manager (along with the team and stakeholders, if possible) starts the WBS, they just list tasks first without an attempt to organize them. Then, after most of the tasks have been identified, the project manager will organize them into groups or phases or by resource (see Table 9.6). Activities can be separated by resource needed to complete the task and/or by prerequisites to the task. In larger projects, no task should be longer than two to four weeks in duration so it can be tracked and managed. After the tasks have been organized, the last step is to sort them in date order and create the timeline.

Table 9.6 Sample Work Breakdown Structure

Unorganized Tasks	*Organized Tasks*
Service Pack 7 To TST	**Service Pack 7**
Service Pack 7 Testing	Service Pack 7 To TST
Service Pack 7 Live	Service Pack 7 Testing
Service Pack 8 To TST	Service Pack 7 Live
Service Pack 8 Testing	**Service Pack 8**
Service Pack 8 Live	Service Pack 8 To TST
Pharmacy V24 To Rx TRN	Service Pack 8 Testing
Pharmacy V24 Testing w current interface	Service Pack 8 Live
Pharmacy V24 Testing w new interface	**Pharmacy V24**
Pharmacy V24 Training	Pharmacy V24 To Rx TRN
Pharmacy V24 Live	Pharmacy V24 Testing w current interface
CPOE Order Set Build & Validation	Pharmacy V24 Testing w new interface
CPOE Medication Testing	Pharmacy V24 Training
CPOE Integrated Testing (current interface)	Pharmacy V24 Live
CPOE Pharmacy Training	**CPOE**
CPOE Physician User Acceptance Testing	CPOE Order Set Build & Validation
CPOE Pilot Live	CPOE Medication Testing
CPOE Rollout (after SP8)	CPOE Integrated Testing (current interface)

Unorganized Tasks	*Organized Tasks*
	CPOE Pharmacy Training
	CPOE Physician User Acceptance Testing
	CPOE Pilot Live
	CPOE Rollout (after SP8)

Communication

Good stakeholder and team communication can increase the chances of project success. This communication starts with the charter and the communication plan in which the project manager outlines what will be communicated, who will get regular communication, and how often formal communication will occur. The main purpose of communication is to get the right information to the right people at the right time and in a useful format. There should be no surprises; a lack of communication actually sends a message that some will interpret as hiding information. More communication is better, not less, but communication needs to be valued by the recipient. The project manager needs to communicate in a way the stakeholder understands and/or can use, such as updates on metrics, issues requiring input, and milestone updates.

Dashboards

Stakeholders should have access to information about the project. The project manager (or IT) can create a shared space for those who want more information, and project documents can be posted to this site. For formal communication with stakeholders, however, using a dashboard style report is often very well received by stakeholders. Dashboards can include the following:

- Project progress toward milestone completion (% complete)
- Overall status (using red-yellow-green highlights)
- Key issues
- Key risks with any available mitigation plans
- Upcoming milestones

Dashboards should be designed with the person or group receiving the information. Different dahboards may be necessary for different groups (see Figures 9.2, 9.3, and 9.4).

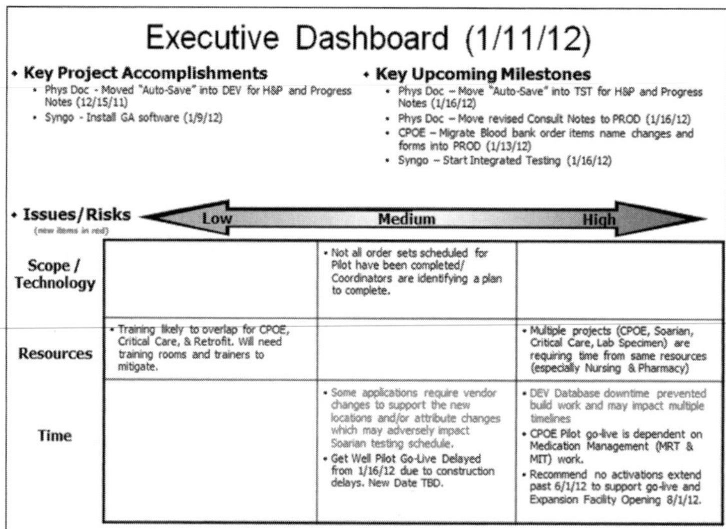

FIGURE 9.2 Sample executive dashboard.

Scope Item	!	Description (If the status is red, decisions or actions needed from project leadership will be indicated)
Deliverables	G	
Costs	G	
Schedule	Y	
Resources	R	

FIGURE 9.3 Sample overall project dashboard.

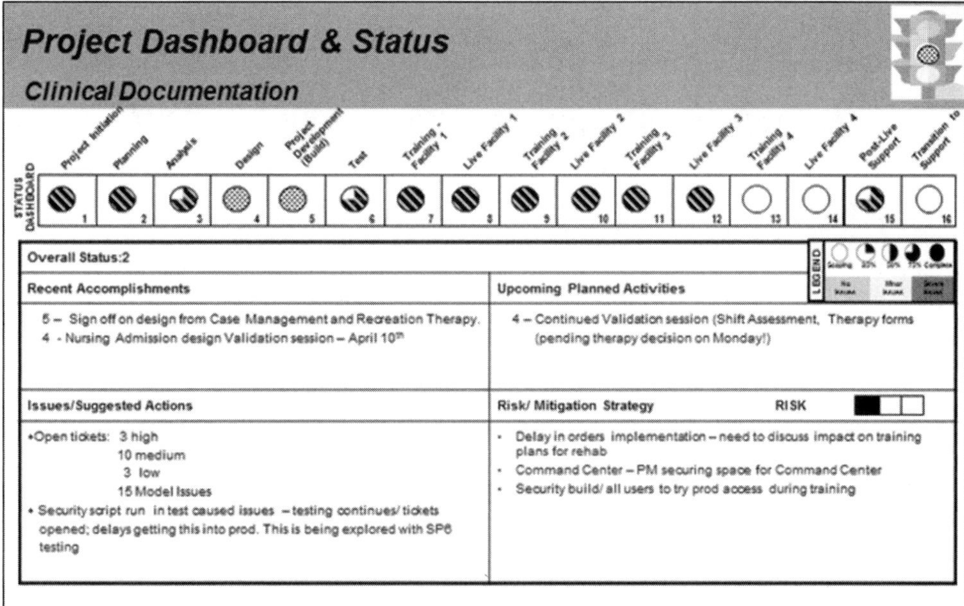

FIGURE 9.4 Sample detailed project dashboard.

Status Reports

Project managers need to complete status reports and submit them at regular intervals. For projects less than 6 months in duration or during periods of rapid project activity, status reports should be submitted weekly. For projects of a longer duration, monthly status reports may be sufficient. Establishing these reporting frequencies is part of the communication plan and/or charter. Status reports do not need to be lengthy but do need to provide useful information. At a minimum, status reports (see Figure 9.5) should include information about the following:

- What was accomplished since the last reporting period?
- What are the planned activities by the next reporting period?
- Are there any priority issues and risks?

MILESTONE STATUS– MILESTONES PAST DUE OR DUE IN THE NEXT 30 DAYS

Status Color Legend: Green = On Target.

Yellow = Milestones at risk but will be resolved by team.

Red = Seriously off track – milestones at risk without external assistance and/or multi-team mitigation strategy.

Major Milestones	Target Start Date	Target End Date	Status Indicator	Status	Color Status
Assessments/ POC		31-Oct-2013	In Process	59%	□
Gap Analysis Assessments	06/01/13	1-Sep-2013	Complete	100%	●
Gap Analysis POC	09/01/13		Complete	100%	●
Design	09/01/13	15-Oct-2013	Complete	100%	●
Build: TST	09/01/13	15-Oct-2013	In Process	100%	●
Build: TRN	10/01/13	15-Dec-2013	In Process	95%	●
Build: PRD	10/01/13	1-Mar-2014	In Process	13.1%	●
Pat Record/Clin Sum	09/01/13	20-Dec-2013	In Process	77.0%	●
CSP/WFE Reports/Print View/Discharge Workflow	09/01/13	20-Dec-2013	In Process	15%	□
Test	10/01/13	20-Dec-2013	In Process	96%	●
Sign Off	10/01/13	20-Dec-2013	In Process	8%	□
Security: TST	10/01/13	15-Oct-2013	In Process	16%	□
Security: PRD	10/01/13	1-Feb-2014	Not Started	17%	●

KEY MILESTONES COMPLETED - THIS REPORTING PERIOD

1. Lab Tests passed from LAB to Clinicals

WORK COMPLETED - THIS REPORTING PERIOD

1. Trouble shooting and working on critical care issues as they arise specific to Respiratory. Held call with Respiratory management and staff to address issues.
2. Assigned testing of assessments that have gone through user validation
3. Testing of documents in TRAIN
4. Assigned CS to analyst
5. Call/meetings participated in during the week
   a. Program Meeting
   b. Reports Project Meeting
   c. Clin Doc Project Meeting
6. Managed project plans updated Sharepoint

WORK TO BE COMPLETED – NEXT REPORTING PERIOD

1. Move information into TRAIN
2. Finish outstanding build of assessments
3. Sign off on reports
4. Receive outstanding items from informatics to complete build of assessments/reports/workflow—Meeting scheduled

ISSUES REQUIRING ESCALATION

#	Issue	Impact	Recommended Action/Mitigation	Date Needed	Escalate To:
1	Outstanding orderables for Lab	Delaying the build of the orders	To receive the orders on 12/13 however there are questions on the information that are needed answered	12/13/13	Jane
7	Surgical Documentation	Facility will use the documentation that is currently in the system.	George has engaged informatics to assist with process mapping.	12/15/13	George

RISKS REQUIRING ESCALATION

#	Risk	Impact	Recommended Mitigation	Escalate To:
2	Communication between teams	What is needed for like for like	Stay firm with the needs for the communication from the team. Continue scheduled meetings	CNO's
3	Scope creep	Will cause the project to be too big to be able to meet the go live of 4/1. Particularly	Firm boundaries for the scope creep and a due diligence to	Jack

FIGURE 9.5 Sample project status report.

Future Directions

More and more, project success can be attributed to the use of project management methodology. Studies by KPMG, McKinsey, the Standish Group, Gartner, and PricewaterhouseCoopers have all identified the costs of projects that do not finish on time, on budget, and on value (Barlow et al., 2013; Bloch, Blumberg, & Laartz, 2012; IT Cortex, n.d.; Mieritz, 2012; Hardy-Vallee, 2012). Many of these same studies as well as others have identified that project management and the use of a standard consistent methodology greatly increases the likelihood of project success.

Although hospitals have lagged behind other industries in adopting project management methodologies and creating a project management office, more and more organizations are embracing project management, at least for IT projects. Although project managers often report to the IT or facilities department, clinicians need project management skills to help manage projects. Nursing schools are adding project management classes or lessons to courses at the bachelor's, master's, and doctorate levels. Certification classes in informatics often included basic project management education. Full-day and multiple-day continuing education courses are also offered across the country. As project management becomes more the norm in facilities, informatics clinicians may fill the role of project managers more often.

References

American Nurses Association (ANA). (2014). The nursing process. Retrieved from http://www.nursingworld.org/EspeciallyForYou/What-is-Nursing/Tools-You-Need/Thenursingprocess.html

Babu, S. (2005). Scope creep is not only inevitable; it's natural. Retrieved from http://www.projectperfect.com.au/downloads/Info/info_scope_creep_mgmt.pdf

Barlow, G., Woolley, P., Rutherford, L., & Conradie, C. (2013). Project management survey report 2013. Retrieved from http://www.kpmg.com/NZ/en/IssuesAndInsights/ArticlesPublications/Documents/KPMG-Project-Management-Survey-2013.pdf

Bloch, M., Blumberg, S., & Laartz, J. (2012). Delivering large scale IT projects on time, on budget and on value. Retrieved from http://www.mckinsey.com/insights/business_technology/delivering_large-scale_it_projects_on_time_on_budget_and_on_value

Centers for Medicare and Medicaid Services (CMS). (2014, April). Electronic health record (EHR) frequently asked questions (FAQs). Retrieved from http://www.cms.gov/Regulations-and-Guidance/Legislation/EHRIncentivePrograms/Downloads/FAQs_Apr_2014.pdf

Flyvbjerg, B., & Budzier, A. (2011, September). Why your IT project may be riskier than you think. *Harvard Business Review.* Retrieved from http://hbr.org/2011/09/why-your-it-project-may-be-riskier-than-you-think/ar/1

Hardy-Vallee, B. (2012, February 7). The cost of bad project management. *Gallup Business Journal.* Retrieved from http://businessjournal.gallup.com/content/152429/cost-bad-project-management.aspx

Houston, S. (2011). *The project manager's guide to health information technology implementation.* Chicago, IL: HIMSS.

Houston, S., & Bove, L. A. (2007). *Project management for healthcare informatics.* New York, NY: Springer.

Institute of Medicine (IOM). (2000). *To err is human: Building a safer health system.* Washington, DC: The National Academies Press. Retrieved from http://www.iom.edu/Reports/1999/To-Err-is-Human-Building-A-Safer-Health-System.aspx

IT Cortex. (n.d.). Failure rate: Statistics over why projects fail. Retrieved from www.it-cortex.com/Stat_Failure_Rate.htm

Kantor, B. (2012, May 22). How to design a successful RACI project plan. *CIO.* Retrieved from http://www.cio.com/article/706836/How_to_Design_a_Successful_RACI_Project_Plan?page=1&taxonomyId=3013

Kaplan, B., & Harris-Salamone, K. (2009). Health IT success and failure: Recommendations from literature and an AMIA workshop. *JAMIA, 16*(3), 291–299.

Kropf, R., & Scalzi, G. (2007). *Making information technology work: Maximizing the benefits for health care organizations.* Chicago, IL: Health Forum/AHA Press.

Lowenhaupt, M., & Friedman, D. (2003). How to organize. Retrieved from http://mthink.com/article/how-organize/

Matta, N., & Ashkenas, R. (2012). Why good projects fail anyway. In Harvard Business Review, *Guide to project management* (pp. 123–126). Boston, MA: Harvard Business Review Press.

Mieritz, L. (2012). *Gartner survey shows why projects fail.* Retrieved from http://thisiswhatgoodlookslike.com/2012/06/10/gartner-survey-shows-why-projects-fail/

Mind Tools. (n.d.). Why do projects fail? Retrieved from http://www.mindtools.com/pages/article/newPPM_58.htm

Project Management Institute (PMI). (2013). *A guide to the project management body of knowledge (PMBOK guide)* 5th ed. Newtown Square, PA: Project Management Institute.

Thomas, E. (2014). Project management lessons from HealthCare.Gov. Retrieved from http://www.cioinsight.com/it-management/project-management/project-management-lessons-from-healthcare.gov.html#sthash.GTmpFjaP.dpuf

"The fantastic advances in the field of electronic communication constitute a greater danger to the privacy of the individual."

—*Earl Warren, 14th Chief Justice of the United States*

10

Security and Privacy Concepts in Healthcare IT

Susan Martin, RN, BSN, JD

Ensuring the accuracy and confidentiality of sensitive medical information is so vital to what we do every day as clinical informaticists. Patients, providers, and even insurance companies are counting on us to "get it right." This responsibility can feel like a daunting task, learning what is required and where to begin. Do you remember the saying, "It takes a village to raise a child?" It is also true when it comes to protecting our clients' privacy and health information: It takes a village. Do you know everyone in your village? Do you understand their role and yours? This chapter introduces core concepts of information technology (IT) security and information privacy and the roles of many professionals engaged in data protection.

Information privacy is concerned with establishing rules that govern collecting and handling personal information, which can include medical information. Across individual physician practices or large integrated healthcare systems, it is impossible to guarantee that information contained in an electronic health record is 100% private. Rules that govern medical information include security controls built into the system and also privacy practices defining who may access medical information. Security engineers practice a concept of *defense in depth*, building multiple security controls to protect sensitive data systems like moats

OBJECTIVES

- Informaticists will be knowledgeable of the laws and regulations that govern the protection of ePHI.
- Informaticists will be knowledgeable of the administrative, technical, and physical security controls that safeguard ePHI.
- Informaticists will be able to describe the roles and responsibilities of other IT professionals that protect the data in clinical applications.
- Informaticists will be knowledgeable of best practices for safeguarding health information and have resources to evaluate practices in their organization.

with drawbridges or watch towers with cannons surrounding a castle to protect against invaders. The security controls include administrative, physical, and technical safeguards that address human factors as well as configuration settings that may contribute to loss of data. Each safeguard adds a layer to make the entire system secure and ensure privacy.

This chapter will provide some background on the regulatory frameworks for safeguarding health information in clinical information systems. Primarily, three U.S. federal privacy laws apply to medical information held by public and private organizations in the United States. Federal agencies providing clinical care to military veterans, active duty military personnel, and dependents and participants in clinical research studies must follow the Privacy Act (PA) of 1974 and the Federal Information Security Management Act (FISMA) of 2002. Healthcare organizations that bill patients and/or their insurance plan for services provided must also comply with the Fair Credit Reporting Act (FRCA) of 1970 and also the Health Insurance Portability and Accountability Act (HIPAA) of 1996 when collecting, storing, and transmitting identifiable health information and applicable state privacy laws. You can read about these acts in more detail later in this chapter.

Application security and network security are critical to safeguarding medical information in healthcare organizations. This chapter will help clinical informaticists to understand how network and application security controls protect data in both wired and mobile devices. Organizations with multiple users dispersed across several locations and clinical applications present additional challenges to protect data across several networked environments. Clinical informaticists are responsible for providing a list of recommended best practices for protecting health information and practical tips to consider when implementing new information systems.

Protecting Medical Information?

The field of clinical informatics is concerned with medical and personal information use in healthcare by clinicians. Practicing as a clinical informatics professional (informaticist) requires an understanding of the data collected and their uses, data users, integration of business systems, and application of information technology in healthcare settings. The information is sensitive, so ensuring the security and privacy of patient information is paramount for everyone who touches the data. In addition to the clinical informatics professional, a host of other IT professionals work together in designing, implementing, and deploying safe and usable health information systems and technology. This section will provide an overview of other IT roles and IT management activities for protection of data in clinical applications.

Network Administrator

Healthcare in the twenty-first century requires the integration of medical and personal information from several applications, each with a specific purpose. Applications may include an electronic health record (EHR), a billing system, or laboratory and radiology systems. For the most part, these applications are located on the hospital or provider office network and share information related to patient transactions through authorized interfaces or secure connections.

The *network administrator* is responsible for designing, installing, configuring, maintaining. and repairing network infrastructure and application components. The primary role includes designing perimeter and internal security through the configuration of firewalls, virtual private networks (VPN) concentrators, and security appliances for access to vital business applications. The network may be a single wired local area network (LAN) or may include a wireless network to support the use of handheld medical devices and tablets, allowing the clinician to bring the patient's record to the bedside. The connection between the wireless barcode scanner, handheld medical devices (such as a glucose monitor), or tablet to the electronic medical record system should be configured to use HTTPS, Wi-Fi Protected Access encryption (WPA), or a virtual private network (VPN) to protect data from interception by unauthorized persons during transmission within the organization.

Healthcare organizations that enable providers to connect electronically with patients and families by the provision of personal health records, the adoption of patient portals, or the use of mHealth applications take advantage of the Internet.

TIP

Read more about mHealth—mobile health—in Chapter 17 of this book.

Patients increasingly demand timely access to their medical information from their home, office, or public locations using Wi-Fi over the Internet. Unfortunately, accessing an EHR from unsecure devices—think personal computers (PCs) and smartphones—can introduce security risks to an organization's network. The network administrator may significantly reduce associated risk by configuring a DMZ and employing an intrusion detections system (IDS) to monitor traffic. The application web servers are located in the DMZ, where external traffic from the Internet is scanned for intrusions known to shut down the network or introduce malware with the intent of stealing sensitive information. The DMZ adds another defensive layer that restricts direct access to the clinical databases located behind internal firewalls. After authentication, the user's information may be viewed via the web servers located in the DMZ.

System Administrator

A *system administrator* is responsible for the configuration, upkeep, and reliable operation of computer systems; especially multi-user computers, such as servers in a healthcare setting. The system administrator may boast that his role is "building security" into a system by configuring and maintaining minimum security standards, installing patches to close gaps in security, reviewing system logs of user login and user activity, and reporting malicious or suspicious activity to the information security official (ISO).

The system administrator will often have responsibility to create and maintain user accounts. In a large enterprise with an Active Directory (AD) environment, the system administrator uses group policy objects (GPOs) to provide centralized management and configuration of operating systems (OS), applications, and user settings. The GPO defines registry-based policies: security options to close ports and disable unnecessary protocols and services that add a security risk to the environment. All organizations must prepare for those planned and unexpected downtimes when the system is not available to users.

Another important job of the system administrator includes generating and retaining application backups used to restore the clinical system as part of the organization's contingency plan or disaster recovery plan after the network and critical infrastructure are restored. In small organizations, the system administrator may have a dual role as the network administrator and monitor network to ensure security and availability to users.

Application Administrator

An *application administrator* is responsible for the administration of one or more clinical applications. Such responsibilities typically include application configuration, account management, installation of software upgrades, and user support. In addition to account management, the application administrator may also be responsible to design access controls so that authorized accounts provide users access to only the information and functions needed to perform their job. Role-based access controls, which limit the access that users have to data based on their job responsibilities, are an important first step for data protection and breach prevention.

The system administrator role has the most privileges and access in the system, but that role should be limited to a small number of identified persons, such as the application administrators, after access controls are developed as a collaborative effort among the clinical informatics team, organizational leadership, and health information management department. After individual roles are established from which to grant access and functional privileges based on the user's job—prescriber, nurse, patient care technician, scheduler, billing verification—the application administrator's focus becomes managing memberships within the roles and verifying that each role's permissions are properly configured.

Information Security Official

HIPAA regulations require healthcare operations to designate an information security official (ISO) responsible to oversee the covered entity's compliance with information security requirements. The ISO implements policies and procedures to prevent, detect, contain, and correct security violations. An ISO must conduct a thorough assessment of the potential risks and vulnerabilities to the confidentiality, integrity, and availability (CIA) of electronic protected health information (PHI) and introduce security measures sufficient to reduce risks and vulnerabilities. Although the ISO is responsible for information security, he relies on the network, system, and application administrators to maintain physical and technical controls that protect health information.

Privacy Official

Similarly, HIPAA regulations also require the designation of a privacy official responsible for the development and implementation of privacy policies and procedures. The privacy official's duties include creating, posting, and distributing the notice of information/privacy practices; and in facilities with direct treatment providers, securing and recording each patient's acknowledgement of receiving the notice of privacy practices; implementing the patient's right to access, review, and request amendment to their health records; request additional protection for, or confidential communications of, particularly sensitive health information; and handle any complaints from patients (or staff) about possible HIPAA violations.

Security and Privacy Regulatory Frameworks

This section provides a high-level overview of the afore-mentioned FCRA, PA, FISMA and HIPAA and also their contributions to safeguarding health information in clinical information systems. Each of these regulatory frameworks includes core elements from the Code of Fair Information Practices Principles (FIPP), which is a widely accepted framework of principles that affect individual privacy. The cornerstone of fair information practices, notice, and choice is also embodied in the PA, FCRA, and HIPAA. See Table 10.1.

Table 10.1 Code of Fair Information Practices Principles

Fair Information Practices Principle	*Description*
Transparency	Organizations should be transparent and notify individuals regarding collection, use, dissemination, and maintenance of personally identifiable information (PII).
Individual Participation	Organizations should involve the individual in the process of using PII, and to the extent practicable, seek individual consent for the collection, use, dissemination, and maintenance of PII. Organizations should also provide mechanisms for appropriate access, correction, and redress regarding use of PII.

Fair Information Practices Principle	*Description*
Purpose Specification	Organizations should specifically articulate the authority that permits the collection of PII and specifically articulate the purpose or purposes for which the PII is intended to be used.
Data Minimization	Organizations should collect only that PII directly relevant and necessary to accomplish the specified purpose(s), and retain PII only for as long as is necessary to fulfill the specified purpose(s).
Use Limitation	Organizations should use PII solely for the purpose(s) specified in the notice. Sharing PII should be for a purpose compatible with the purpose for which the PII was collected.
Data Quality and Integrity	Organizations should, to the extent practicable, ensure that PII is accurate, relevant, timely, and complete.
Security	Organizations should protect PII (in all media) through appropriate security safeguards against risks, such as loss, unauthorized access or use, destruction, modification, or unintended or inappropriate disclosure.
Accountability and Auditing	Organizations should be accountable for complying with these principles, providing training to all employees and contractors who use PII, and auditing the actual use of PII to demonstrate compliance with these principles and all applicable privacy protection requirements.

Fair Credit Reporting Act

The Fair Credit Reporting Act (FCRA), Public Law No. 91-508, was enacted in 1970 to promote accuracy, fairness, and the privacy of personal information assembled by credit reporting agencies (CRAs). The Fair and Accurate Credit Transactions Act of 2003 restricts CRAs from reporting medical information in reports that will be used for employment, credit transactions, or insurance transactions unless the consumer consents to such disclosures. Creditors are prohibited from using consumer medical information in deciding whether to grant or extend credit to a consumer. Medical information is extended additional protection when it has been provided electronically for certain information exchanges, including those related to insurance transactions and disclosures authorized by the U.S. Department of Health and Human Services (HHS). For instance, medical information obtained from a consumer reporting agency (CRA) appears in a coded form that does not identify the medical provider.

Privacy Act

The Privacy Act (PA) of 1974, 5 U.S.C. § 552a, establishes a code of fair information practices that governs the collection, maintenance, use, and dissemination of information about individuals that is maintained in systems of records by federal agencies. The law was created in response to concerns about how the federal government's computerized databases might impact an individual citizen's privacy rights. It requires government agencies to provide individuals with access to review any records kept about them and request an amendment of records that are not accurate, not timely, or may be incomplete. The Privacy Act also places limits on sharing an individual's data among government agencies and further limits disclosures of identifiable information outside of the agency. The law requires agencies to follow FIPPs when gathering and handling personal data. The information systems of the National Institutes of Health (NIH), the Centers for Medicare and Medicaid Services (CMS), the Food and Drug Administration (FDA), the Department of Defense (DoD), and the Veterans Administration (VA) are subject to the Privacy Act.

Federal Information Security Management Act

The Federal Information Security Management Act (FISMA), enacted by Congress in 2002, requires each federal agency to develop, document, and implement an agency-wide program to provide information security for the information and information systems that support the operations and assets of the agency. The FISMA framework is further defined by the standards and guidelines developed by the National Institute of Standards in Technology (NIST). Due to the increasing threats to the security of electronic data available on the Internet, FISMA includes measures taken to protect a computer or computer system against unauthorized access or attack. Although FISMA currently applies to federal agencies using medical information, NIST standards and publications can be valuable resources for healthcare organizations with specific questions about IT security.

Health Insurance Portability and Accountability Act

A third regulatory framework for health information came from Congress in HIPAA of 1996. HIPAA is the probably the most familiar mandate that hospitals are required to train their staff on the law and its specific application within their organization. Healthcare organizations are required to provide notice of their information practices to the patients they serve.

Under HIPAA, the HHS Office of Civil Rights (OCR) set national standards for the security of electronic protected health information in the HIPAA Security Rule. The HIPAA Security Rule extends many fair information practices to healthcare settings and codifies requirements for administrative, physical, and technical safeguards of electronic protected health information. The HHS website provides materials where clinical informatics professionals may gain insight on the implementation of the security standards prescribed in the HIPAA Security Rule:

http://www.hhs.gov/ocr/privacy/hipaa/administrative/securityrule/securityruleguidance.html

The HIPAA Privacy Rule establishes national standards to protect individuals' medical records and other personal health information and applies to health plans, healthcare clearinghouses, and those healthcare providers that conduct certain healthcare transactions electronically. The rule requires appropriate safeguards to protect the privacy of personal health information, and sets limits and conditions on the uses and disclosures that may be made of such information without patient authorization. The rule also gives patients' rights over their health information, including rights to examine and obtain a copy of their health records and to request corrections.

Informatics in Action

In 2009, Congress modified HIPAA, requiring healthcare providers, healthcare plans, and healthcare clearinghouses to report breaches and unauthorized access of protected health information (PHI) to the HHS OCR. The analysis of data posted at www.hhs.gov/ocr/privacy/hipaa/administrative/breachnotificationrule/breachtool.html from 2009–2013 reveals that theft is the most common cause of a reported breach (83%), followed by hacking/IT incidents (6%) and loss of unencrypted devices storing patient information. By reviewing how medical information is exposed, security and privacy professionals learn where to focus attention on technical solutions and educational efforts that can reduce future exposure.

NIST published *An Introductory Resource Guide for Implementing the Health Insurance Portability and Accountability Act (HIPAA) Security Rule (SP 800-66 Revision 1)* in October 2008 to assist covered entities in understanding and properly using the set of federal information security requirements adopted by the Secretary of Health and Human Services (HHS) under the Health Insurance Portability and Accountability Act of 1996. You can review it at

http://csrc.nist.gov/publications/nistpubs/800-66-Rev1/SP-800-66-Revision1.pdf

Basic Safeguards of IT Security

A major focus of information security is preventing authorized and unauthorized individuals from accessing, creating, or modifying information inappropriately. Security controls applied to the application and surrounding IT infrastructure can greatly reduce the impact or probability of security threats and vulnerabilities affecting any organization's information systems. The security controls required will depend on certain factors, such as the sensitivity of the information; the organization's mission; and impact on the mission if the information becomes unavailable, is modified, or is stolen. There are basic safeguards of IT security that can be found across organizations of all sizes.

As noted in the previous section, the HIPAA Security Rule and Federal Information Security Management Act (FISMA) of 2002 provide minimum security requirements to healthcare organizations by establishing standards for administrative safeguards, physical safeguards, and technical safeguards designed to protect electronic health information.

It is important for healthcare organizations to implement reasonable and appropriated physical safeguards for their information systems as well as related equipment and facilities.

Administrative Safeguards

Administrative actions, policies, and procedures can manage the selection, development, implementation, and maintenance of security measures to protect electronic protected health information (ePHI). Additionally, these safeguards manage the conduct of the covered entity's workforce in relation to the protection of that information. Examples of administrative safeguards include:

- **Risk analysis:** Create an accurate inventory of systems containing ePHI, followed by a thorough assessment of the potential risks and vulnerabilities to the data as it flows throughout the organization. Threats to information systems can be human, natural, environmental, internal, and external. A risk analysis can identify specific security risks, the probability of occurrence, and the magnitude of risk to the organization.
- **Risk management:** Identify and implement security measures to reduce risk to a reasonable and appropriate level based on the organizational circumstances. Involve executive leadership in the risk-mitigation decisions to define what risk level is reasonable and appropriate for its environment and business processes.
- **Sanctioning:** Apply appropriate sanctions against workforce members who fail to comply with the organization's security policies and procedures. To deter noncompliance, ensure that workforce members understand the consequences of failing to comply with security policies and procedures.
- **Information system activity review:** Examine audit logs, access reports, and security incident tracking reports to determine whether any ePHI is being used or disclosed in an inappropriate manner.
- **Accessibility:** Ensure that workforce members have appropriate access to the ePHI required to perform their assigned job functions based on job descriptions and/or supervision procedures. This includes procedures to terminate access when workforce members leave or change job functions. Limit access to ePHI to authorized workforce members.

- **Security and privacy awareness training:** Educate on security policies related to login monitoring, password management, guarding against malicious software, reporting security incidents, and user activities that affect the security of ePHI.

Physical Safeguards

Physical measures, policies, and procedures can protect a covered entity's electronic information systems and related buildings and equipment from natural and environmental hazards and unauthorized intrusions. Examples of physical safeguards include:

- **Access controls:** Door locks, electronic card readers, security officers, security cameras, and video monitoring limit unauthorized access to the electronic information systems and facilities in which they are housed.
- **Downtime operations policies and procedures:** Having contingency plans, disaster recovery plans, and alternate locations directs the workforce responsible for data restoration in the event of an emergency and provides steps for continued operations using manual procedures. An alternate location is where information systems and data will be available in the event a natural disaster to the primary data location makes it unusable for a prolonged time.
- **Backup power supply, backup heating/cooling sources.** Allows for the continued operation of clinical applications in the data center.
- **Place workstations with health information in locations not accessible to the public.** Reduces access to unauthorized individuals.
- **Policies and procedures for the disposal of hardware and electronic media containing ePHI.** Renders the data unusable and/or inaccessible after it leaves the facility, thus preventing unauthorized exposure.
- **Data backup and offsite storage plan.** Creates a retrievable, exact copy of electronic health information to restore operations in the primary data location when the downtime ends.

Technical Safeguards

The technology executed by information systems and the policies and procedures for its use can also protect and control access to health information.

- **Assignment of unique name and/or number for identification and tracking of user activity.** Allows organization to detect unauthorized user when monitoring system logs.
- **Automatic logoff procedure that terminates an electronic session after a predetermined time of inactivity.** Prevents unauthorized user from accessing ePHI on a workstation when it is left unattended.
- **Encryption and decryption of ePHI that utilizes PKI encryption.** Encrypted data reduces the probability that anyone other than the receiving party who has the key to the code can convert data to plain, readable text.
- **Configuration of audit controls for recording and examining information system activity.** Useful when determining if a security or privacy violation has occurred.
- **Authentication procedures that verify a person seeking to access ePHI is in fact who he/she claims before being allowed access to the data.** Examples include complex passwords; personal identification number (PIN); smart card badge or personal identity verification (PIV) card; token; or something unique to the individual, such as biometrics (fingerprints, voice patterns, facial patterns, iris patterns). These prevent unauthorized users from accessing ePHI on local workstations or from remote locations.
- **Integrity controls and encryption of ePHI when transmitted through email, over the Internet, or via some form of private or point-to-point network when appropriate per organizational policy.** Ensures the data sent is the same as the data received and that it has not been improperly modified during transmission.

> Hospitals are increasingly requiring multi-factor authentication when accessing the EHR from home or an off-site medical office.

IT Security and Privacy Professionals Jargon

Security and privacy professionals involved in healthcare are passionate about protecting their organization's medical information. Unfortunately, the acronyms and technical terms used may be a foreign language to many clinical informaticists. Hopefully, Table 10.2 will help informaticists to bridge the language gap and understand the "geeky" jargon used by the IT professionals in their organization.

Table 10.2 Glossary of IT Security Acronyms and Technical Terms

Acronym	*Description*
Active Directory (AD)	*Active Directory (AD)* is a directory service that Microsoft developed for Windows domain networks and is included in most Windows Server operating systems as a set of processes and services. An AD domain controller authenticates and authorizes all users and computers in a Windows domain type network—assigning and enforcing security policies for all computers and installing or updating software. Active Directory is a centralized and standardized hierarchical organization that provides a single point of access for system administration (management of user accounts, clients, servers, and applications, for example) to reduce redundancy and errors. In most hospitals, the user's AD credentials (user ID and password) can be used to log in to the network as well as AD-enabled applications like the EHR.
Biometrics	Technology can be used to define an individual's unique identity, often for security purposes. Examples include fingerprinting and voice, facial, iris, and handwriting patterns.

Acronym	*Description*
Contingency plan/disaster recovery (CP/DR)	*CP* refers to interim measures to recover information system services after a disruption. Interim measures may include relocation of information systems and operations to an alternate site, recovery of information system functions using alternate equipment, or performance of information system functions using manual methods. The HIPAA Security Rule requires covered entities to have a documented CP and test the plan at organizationally defined intervals. A *DR* plan is a documented process or set of procedures to recover and protect a business IT infrastructure in the event of a natural, environmental, or man-made disaster. After Hurricane Katrina hit the Gulf states in 2005, hospitals and medical practices everywhere have increased their focus on developing a plan to restore information technology to access medical records and continue providing necessary healthcare services.
Demilitarized Zone (DMZ)	The general idea is that you put your public-facing servers in the "DMZ network" so that you can separate them from your private, trusted network. Patient portal web servers are located in the DMZ to provide a layer between web traffic and the EHR.
Group Policy Object (GPO)	*GPO* is A feature of the Microsoft Windows NT family of operating systems that control the working environment of user accounts and computer accounts. Group Policy provides the centralized management and configuration of operating systems, applications, and users' settings in an AD environment.
HTTPS	*HyperText Transfer Protocol Secure* is a protocol for secure communication over a computer network, with especially wide deployment on the Internet. The main motivation for HTTPS is to prevent wiretapping and man-in-the-middle attacks.

continues

Table 10.2 Glossary of IT Security Acronyms and Technical Terms *(continued)*

Acronym	*Description*
Intrusion Detection System (IDS)	An *IDS* is a device or software application that monitors network or system activities for malicious actions or policy violations and produces reports to a management station. IDS primarily come in two forms: There are network-based (NIDS) and host-based (HIDS) intrusion detection systems. Although some organizations configure their IDS to block an intrusion attempt, others configure it as a monitoring system. The management reports are analyzed with goals of identifying possible incidents, logging information, and developing corrective actions to add protection from future attacks.
Malware	*Malware* is a general term used to refer to a variety of forms of hostile or intrusive software used by hackers to disrupt computer operations, gather sensitive information, or gain access to private computer systems. Malware includes computer viruses, worms, trojan horses, ransomware, spyware, adware, scareware, and other malicious programs. Malware is frequently introduced in healthcare environments through human activities, such as visiting websites with links designed to introduce malicious code, opening suspicious emails, clicking links in a phishing scam, and loading files using a USB thumbdrive from an infected computer. The IDS looks for malware signatures when scanning external traffic coming into the organization's network.
Man-in-the-middle (MITM) attack	A *man-in-the-middle attack* is a type of cyber-attack where a malicious actor inserts him/herself into a conversation between two parties, impersonates both parties and gains access to information that the two parties were trying to send to each other. A man-in-the-middle attack allows a malicious actor to intercept, send, and receive data meant for someone else, or not meant to be sent at all, without either outside party knowing until it is too late. Most Wi-Fi Protected Access environments have cryptographic protocols that include some form of endpoint authentication specifically to prevent MITM attacks.

Acronym	*Description*
Multifactor Authentication	*Multifactor authentication* is using two or more forms of identification to authenticate a user. Single factor authentication (commonly used) employs a unique username and password combinations known to the user. For more security, multifactor authentication adds at least one more form, such as a physical token or biometrics that only the user possesses.
Personal Identity Verification (PIV) card	A *PIV card* is a smart card badge issued as part of a background investigation that verifies a person's identity and contain electronic certificates permitting access to healthcare facilities and login to the facility's network.
Public key infrastructure (PKI) encryption	*Encryption* is the process in which information is turned into letters and numbers to be rendered unreadable by unauthorized persons. Providers are required by HIPAA to use encryption as a means of protection for their patients' ePHI. *PKI* is a comprehensive system required to provide public-key encryption and digital signature services in the electronic transmissions of sensitive data. The goals are to manage keys and certificates through a PKI, maintaining a trustworthy networking environment, while providing an automatic and transparent system to the user. A PKI enables the use of encryption and digital signature services across a wide variety of applications that include an EHR and email.
Virtual private network (VPN)	A *VPN* extends a private network across a public network, such as the Internet. It enables a computer to send and receive data across shared or public networks as if it is directly connected to the private network, while benefiting from the functionality, security, and management policies of the private network. A VPN is created by establishing a virtual point-to-point connection through the use of dedicated connections, virtual tunneling protocols, or traffic encryptions. The most important thing you need to know about a VPN: It secures your computer's Internet connection to guarantee that all of the data you're sending and receiving is encrypted and secured from prying eyes.
Wi-Fi Protected Access (WPA) and Wi-Fi Protected Access II (WPA2) encryption	*WPA* and *WPA2* are two security protocols and security certification programs developed by the Wi-Fi Alliance to secure wireless computer networks used to secure transmissions from mobile devices in clinical areas to the clinical systems within the internal network.

continues

Table 10.2 Glossary of IT Security Acronyms and Technical Terms *(continued)*

Acronym	*Description*
Windows registry	The *Windows registry* is a hierarchical database that stores configuration settings and options on Microsoft Windows operating systems. It contains settings for low-level operating system components and for applications running on the platform that have opted to use the registry. The kernel, device drivers, services, security account manager (SAM), user interface, and third-party applications can all make use of the registry and simplify workstation administration. Backup and restoration is also simplified, because the registry can be accessed over a network connection for remote management/support, including from scripts, using the standard set of APIs, as long as the remote registry service is running and firewall rules permit this.

Recommended Best Practices and Checklist

There is so much to remember when implementing or maintaining clinical information systems. Whether you work in a small medical practice or a large healthcare system with multiple hospitals and care delivery centers, the recommended best practices for safeguarding health information are similar. Organizations vested in the protection of health information have created materials to assist IT professionals and clinical informaticists in understanding common requirements. Several good resources are listed below for your review.

The Department of Health and Human Services (DHHS) provides a terrific resource on the HHS HealthIT.gov website: *CyberSecurity 10 Best Practices for the Small Healthcare Environment* (ONC, 2014). The security checklist assesses if your organization is following prescribed practices to support proper information security. See Table 10.3.

Table 10.3 Security Checklist Questions from HealthIT.gov

Recommended Practice	*Questions from the Checklist*
Practice 1: Password	• Does organization have password policies and trained staff on the requirements? • Does staff have unique username and passwords that are strong, not shared, written down, or displayed on the screen? • Are passwords changed routinely and not re-used? • Are default passwords changed during product installation?
Practice 2: Anti-Virus	• Does organization have policies requiring the use of anti-virus software and trained staff on recognizing the symptoms of viruses or malware on their computer, what to do to avoid virus/malware infections, and how to report it? • Is anti-virus software installed and operating effectively on each computer and receiving automatic updates from the manufacturer? • Do handheld or mobile devices that support anti-virus software have it installed and operating?
Practice 3: Firewall	• Does organization have polices in place prescribing the use, configuration, and operation of firewalls and firewall logs? • Does staff understand the operation of the firewall and agree not to hinder its operation? • Are all computers protected by a properly configured firewall?
Practice 4: Access Control	• Does organization have polices prescribing access controls for users? • Are staff trained on access control policies and agree to abide by them? • Is every user account tied to a currently authorized individual? • Are users only authorized to access information needed to perform their duties? • Have files been set to restrict access only to authorized individuals? • Are computers running healthcare-related applications available for other purposes?

continues

Table 10.3 Security Checklist Questions from HealthIT.gov (continued)

Recommended Practice	*Questions from the Checklist*
Practice 5: Physical Access	• Does organization have polices prescribing physical safety and security of devices that make up the EHR system? • Are staff trained on physical access policies and agree to abide by them? • Does organization have an inventory of devices containing PHI and can be accounted for? • Are computers protected from environmental hazards and located in secure areas limited to authorized individuals? • Are computers running EHR systems shielded from unauthorized viewing? • Is equipment located in high-traffic areas physically secured?
Practice 6: Network Access	• Does organization have polices prescribing network configuration and access? • Are staff trained on network use policy and agree to abide by it? • Is access to the network restricted to authorized users and devices? • Are guest devices prohibited from accessing networks containing PHI? • Do wireless networks use appropriate encryption? • Are computers free of peer-to-peer applications and public instant messaging services are turned off?

Recommended Practice	*Questions from the Checklist*
Practice 7: Backup & Recovery	• Does organization have policies prescribing backup and recovery procedures? • Does staff understand the recovery plan and their assigned duties during recovery? • Are system restore procedures and a copy of the recovery plan stored off-site? • Are all critical files documented and listed in the backup configuration? • Are backups run as scheduled and tested periodically for ability to restore data accurately? • Are back up media physically secured, encrypted if stored offsite, and made unreadable before disposal? • Are multiple backups retained as a failsafe?
Practice 8: Maintenance	• Does organization have polices prescribing EHR system maintenance procedures? • Do staff with system maintenance responsibilities understand and agree to the policies and procedures? • Are computers that are part of the EHR system free of unnecessary software and data files, updated or patched regularly as recommended by the manufacturer, and have remote file sharing and printing disabled? • Are vendor remote maintenance connections documented and fully secured?
Practice 9: Mobile Device	• Does organization have polices prescribing use of mobile devices? • Does all staff understand and agree to abide by mobile device policy and procedures? • Are mobile devices configured to prevent unauthorized use? • Are mobile devices containing or accessing PHI encrypted? • Are all connections between authorized mobile devices and EHRs encrypted?

Additionally, the American Health Information Management Association (AHIMA) provides an excellent resource on their website: *Information Security – An Overview. Appendix A: Information Security Checklist for Healthcare Professionals. (Updated January 2014)*

http://library.ahima.org/xpedio/groups/public/documents/ahima/bok1_050559.hcsp?dDocName=bok1_050559

The Office of the National Coordinator for Health Information Technology (ONC) also released Safety Assurance Factors for EHR Resilience (SAFER) guides that aim to reduce risk to the safety and safe use of EHRs at

http://www.healthit.gov/safer/

Finally, the HHS Health Resources and Services Administration has developed a Health IT Implementation toolbox listing nine steps to implementing EHRs. Step 8 describes the law and the information you need to know about ensuring privacy and security. The list is available on their website at

http://www.hrsa.gov/healthit/toolbox/healthitimplementation/implementationtopics/ensureprivacysecurity/ensureprivacysecurity.html

Other Online Resources

The Fair Credit Reporting Act of 1970

http://www.consumer.ftc.gov/sites/default/files/articles/pdf/pdf-0111-fair-credit-reporting-act.pdf

The Privacy Act of 1974

www.justice.gov/opcl/privacy-act-1974

The Health Insurance Portability and Accountability Act of 1996.

www.hhs.gov/ocr/privacy/hipaa/administrative/statute/

The HIPAA Privacy Rule

www.hhs.gov/ocr/privacy/hipaa/administrative/combined/hipaa-simplification-201303.pdf

The HIPAA Security Rule

www.hhs.gov/ocr/privacy/hipaa/administrative/securityrule/securityrulepdf.pdf

The HHS Office of Civil Rights Health Information Privacy website

www.hhs.gov/ocr/privacy/hipaa/administrative/breachnotificationrule/breachtool.html

References

Office of the National Coordinator for Health Information Technology (ONC). (2014) CyberSecurity: 10 Best Practices for the Small Health Care Environment. Retrieved from http://www.healthit.gov/providers-professionals/cybersecurity

"We can only see a short distance ahead, but we can see plenty there that needs to be done."

–Alan Turing

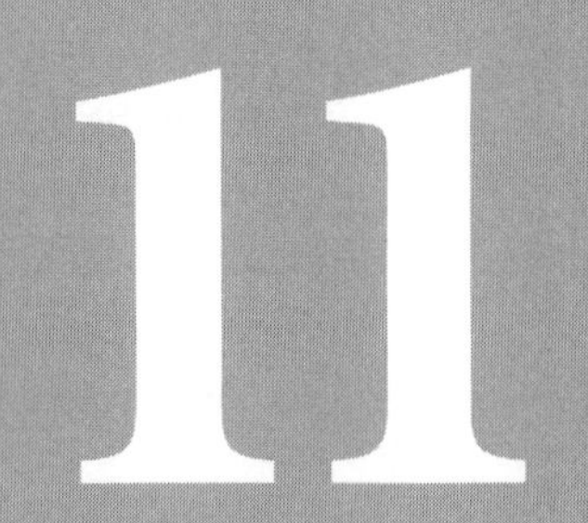

Healthcare Clinical Decision Support

Lincoln S. Farnum, MS, RRT, CPHIMS

OBJECTIVES

- Describe the various types of clinical decision support.
- List various objections to and arguments for the use of clinical decision support (CDS).
- Describe the importance of building a CDS development team.
- List the key tasks for CDS deployment.

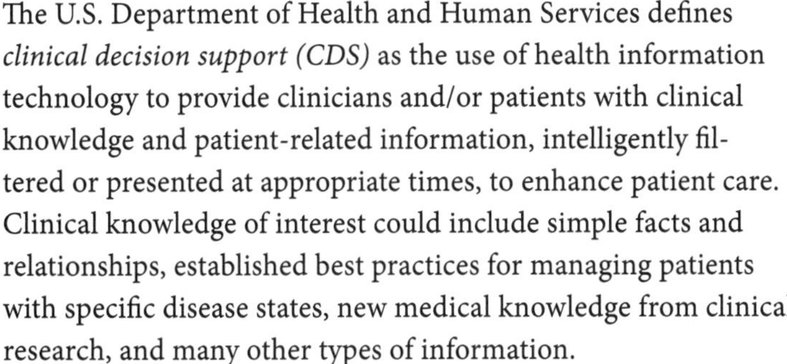

The U.S. Department of Health and Human Services defines *clinical decision support (CDS)* as the use of health information technology to provide clinicians and/or patients with clinical knowledge and patient-related information, intelligently filtered or presented at appropriate times, to enhance patient care. Clinical knowledge of interest could include simple facts and relationships, established best practices for managing patients with specific disease states, new medical knowledge from clinical research, and many other types of information.

http://www.hrsa.gov/healthit/toolboxHealthITAdoptiontoolbox/EvaluatingOptimizingandSustaining/decisionsupport.html

Although this definition is admittedly rather nonspecific, it makes sense to consider CDS as an array of methods and techniques to provide pertinent, actionable information to the user—in this case a clinician, patient, or other interested stakeholder—at a time when that information might make a difference in the speed, quality and/or delivery of clinical care.

The *point of care*—that period of time when a clinician is rendering care, writing medical orders, and investigating or documenting symptoms—has typically been considered the moment of maximum return on investment in CDS. There are many other points in the delivery of clinical care that provide opportunities for support as well. CDS can take the form of synchronous alerts or reminders presented to the clinician while ordering (for example, "This patient has a documented allergy to penicillin.") or be presented in the form of emails or even snail-mail (for example, "Please don't forget your appointment tomorrow."). CDS systems can monitor physiologic parameters in the ICU and issue providers early warning of deteriorating clinical conditions. *Order sets* (prewritten groups of orders) can facilitate consistent care processes, and checklists help synchronize care and avoid errors of omission.

The CDS system developed at the Regenstrief Institute in Indianapolis, Indiana, which is computer-based and incorporates the following:

- Decision support provided automatically as part of provider workflow
- CDS delivered at the time and location of decision-making
- Actionable recommendations provided

The CDS system is well accepted by providers and has been documented to improve patient safety and the quality of healthcare delivered (Friedlin, Dexter, & Overhage, 2007; Overhage, Tierney, Zhou, & McDonald, 1997).

Although CDS can be of great help in an environment as complex as healthcare, it carries some risk. Providing meaningful alerts and clinical information poses many challenges in timing, accuracy, currency, and providing information free of bias or commercial intent. When planning any CDS deployment, it is helpful to thoroughly consider the implications of the support not just from clinical and ethical but from legal perspectives as well.

CDS is also cause for more general concerns, such as dehumanizing medical decisions based on automated advice or the "de-skilling" effect of repeatedly reminding a provider of some set of facts: A simple, real-world example is how everyday math skills have become eroded by the use of handheld calculators. Providers might consider CDS to be a threat to their clinical judgment and experience or inflexible to complex situations, or they might have concerns for the legal ramifications of accepting or not accepting the offered advice. Providers and patients alike might have inadequate time to read and fully consider and understand the information offered by the support. Some providers fear that CDS might lengthen patient encounters or the length of a clinician's workday. CDS is also resource-intensive, not just to develop and deploy but to evaluate and maintain as well. Like any system, go-live is only one point in the software development life cycle, and its development and maintenance costs must be weighed against other opportunities.

Modern medicine has become so complex that it is humanly impossible for unaided healthcare professionals to possess all the information needed to deliver medical care with the efficacy and safety made possible by the current scientific knowledge, and this situation will only worsen with the enormous quantities of data we can now generate through genetic sequencing in the post-genomic era. As medical knowledge evolves and clinical care becomes more advanced, we hope to see—especially in wealthy countries—increases in the efficiency and quality of our healthcare services, although in many cases, these promised improvements remain unrealized. The growth in our understanding and management of diseases has far exceeded our abilities to apply that knowledge in practice (Open Clinical White Paper, 2000).

Accordingly, even the most professional and committed clinicians cannot avoid gaps in their knowledge—or always apply that knowledge in the right way, at the right time. This has consequences in terms of avoidable mortality, morbidity, and the use of resources such as ordering inappropriate tests and procedures and missing returned results or being unable to "connect the dots" because of the complexity or fragmentation of various clinical data, (Open Clinical White Paper, 2000).

The need for supportive tools in the delivery of clinical care, lack of consistency of and the inherent limitations in resources, the danger of errors and harm, and the concomitant growth in data volume and complexity provides excellent opportunities for informatics professionals to improve healthcare processes and delivery through clinical decision support. In this chapter, we will consider methods for successful CDS implementations and provide guidance in the application of CDS to the practitioner and informatics specialist.

Background

Early efforts at CDS were largely directed toward assisting in the process of diagnosis during a patient encounter. These early systems failed to gain sufficient support from clinicians to see their routine introduction and use in the market.

DXplain was one of these systems. Developed by Barnett and colleagues at the Massachusetts General Hospital/Harvard Medical School Laboratory of Computer Science beginning in 1987, DXplain (http://lcs.mgh.harvard.edu/projects/dxplain.html) is used in the process of diagnosis by taking a set of clinical findings as input and then producing a ranked list of possible diagnoses. It provides justification for the list of differential diagnoses; makes suggestions for further investigations; can provide a description of more than 2,000 different diseases, signs, and symptoms; and provides recent references for each. In spite of its age, DXplain is still in routine use at a number of hospitals and medical schools, mostly for clinical education purposes. Some of its limitations are that it is a standalone system and requires user input of signs and symptoms rather than extracting them from a clinical database. Additionally, it never really fit into the clinical workflow (Bartold & Hannigan, 2002).

Efforts to better integrate CDS into clinical databases and workflow saw systems developed such as the Health Evaluation through Logical Processing (HELP) system operational at LDS Hospital in Salt Lake City. HELP is a complete, knowledge-based hospital information system inclusive of patient registration functions, pharmacy management capabilities, order entry and charge capture, nursing documentation, and ICU monitoring. It also supports a robust decision support system. Concepts developed with the HELP system have shown that clinical care can be provided with such a system, computerized decision support is feasible, computerized decision-support can aid in providing more cost-effective and improved patient care, and clinical user attitudes toward computerized decision support can be positive and supportive (Gardner, Pryor, & Warner, 1999).

The Regenstrief Institute created its own homegrown clinical information system with integrated CDS (Regenstrief Medical Record System [RMRS]). From its beginning, RMRS included mechanisms for writing rules for generating reminders to physicians based on clinical data, including laboratory results, visit diagnoses, coded medications, and vital signs collected from encounter forms. Over time, other non-reminder CDS capabilities were built in to support cost savings, clinical research, drug-drug interactions, drug-problem contraindications, drug-allergy checking, insurance-based formulary control, and medical necessity checking.

Important lessons from a quarter of a century of using RMRS include that computerized reminders can change clinical behavior, reduce errors, increase compliance to clinical guidelines, and having a strong and persistent effect on clinical care (Berner, 2007). A number of other early homegrown CDS systems saw significant use. Each system developed its own unique features and met with varying degrees of success, but all contributed to the understanding that the application of CDS can be of significant value in the delivery of clinical care (Berner, 2009; Overhage et al., 1997).

Uses and Types of CDS

The concept of CDS can be confusing because it consists of many different types of support. The term *CDS* is really an umbrella term that represents any functionality configured in the clinical system that helps care providers make better decisions. This section will review the different types of CDS and provide some examples of each.

As discussed previously in this chapter, common uses of CDS include assistance with differential diagnoses and the application of rules and clinical guidelines, such as vaccination schedules. Order sets are also a common feature of CDS. They can save time by applying individual prescribers' preferences, reflect and adhere to clinical guidelines, and ensure appropriate and consistent levels of care. Medication ordering uses CDS in a variety of ways to avoid drug-drug, drug-allergy, and drug-food reactions. It is used in dose calculations, especially for medications with critical dosing requirements, such as chemotherapy. It directly saves resources by alerting prescribers to duplication of orders and of orders that might be contraindicated for certain diagnoses or clinical trials. (Farnum, Cimino, DiPatrizio, & Goldspiel, 2011).

Additionally, CDS can monitor databases, looking for laboratory or physiologic parameters out of specified ranges, and alert care providers. Clinical documentation templates can help ensure that appropriate documentation is completed for regulatory and reimbursement purposes and to check data entered for accuracy and completeness. It becomes apparent that CDS can take on many forms with almost limitless boundaries.

Less commonly but with increasing frequency, CDS has been designed to optimize critical care processes. The LDS Hospital HELP system was modified to follow ventilator protocols in the care of patients with Acute Respiratory Distress Syndrome (ARDS), which is a commonly fatal condition often seen in cases of acute bacterial sepsis. Through HELPs use, LDS realized a significant decrease in staff response times to changes in patient condition and impressively increased survival rates (41% versus 9.5% for patients meeting protocol criteria) (East, Henderson, Morris, & Gardner, 1989). HELP was also used to monitor and prevent overuse of antibiotics and monitor for adverse drug events (Classen, Pestotnik, Evans, & Burke, 1992).

In Table 11.1, the various types of CDS are listed along with examples for each type.

Table 11.1 CD Types and Examples

CDS Type	*Examples*
Medication alerts	Drug allergy
	Drug-drug interaction
	Drug-food interaction
	Drugs that require knowledge of lab values prior to administration
	Recommend less-costly substitutes for very costly medications
	Antibiotic monitoring and recommendations
Documentation support	Notification of potentially incorrect data being entered
	Notification that key documentation is incomplete
	ICD, SNOWMED codes entered based on documentation keywords
	Discharge order entered with discharge documentation
Appointment alerts and reminders	Appointment reminders
	Vaccination reminders
	Mammogram reminders
	Colonoscopy reminders
Order sets (evidence-based)	Sepsis bundle order sets
	Thromboembolism protocol orders
	Research protocol order sets
	Chemotherapy order sets

CDS Type	*Examples*
Reports and real-time dashboards	A real-time nurse manager dashboard that displays number of days a urinary catheter has been in place
	Clinical documentation completion dashboard
	Patient list report documenting length of stay
	Patients without advance directives
	Percentage of patients provided smoking cessation counseling
Access to knowledge tools within EHR	Links to PubMed by documentation keywords
	Links to ClinicalTrials.gov by protocol code
	Links to UpToDate by medication name
Diagnostics recommendations	Recommendations based on documentation or ICD codes for follow up or additional diagnostics
	Recommendations for routine diagnostics based on demographics (colonoscopy for >50 years old)
Treatment recommendations	Compression hose for patients not on anticoagulants
	Anticoagulants for patients at risk for stroke
	Cholesterol management based on Framingham calculations

More examples of CDS to consider include the following:

> *Report:* querying a clinical database rather than auditing a manual chart to get information to make decisions. This can be at point of care (*synchronous*) or retrospectively (*asynchronous.*)

> *Documentation alert:* use of clinical alerts to manage data quality by comparing height and weight values entered for patients to previously entered values (and/or comparing to nomograms) and preventing the user from entering significantly divergent values (perhaps inadvertently substituting pounds for kilograms or inches for centimeters, or transposing patient height and weight values.)

Alert: requesting information regarding the reason for not following CDS recommendations. For example, if a clinician does not provide an influenza vaccine recommended by the CDS, the clinician is asked to justify the decision with a reason. This might be intended to promote adherence to regulatory provisions such as Meaningful Use, to document user performance, or to support clinical research.

Appointment alerts: providing preventive care recommendations during an encounter, rather than as monthly reports that list all the patients in need of services. Moving decision support to the point of care provides both opportunities for performance improvement and the ability to perform procedures while the patient is actually present.

Drug/lab alerts/order sets: recommendations executed by other actions, such as a computerized provider order entry (CPOE) system recommending peak and trough drug levels in response to an order for aminoglycoside, and the clinician simply clicking an Okay button to order the recommended tests. Recommending groups of orders provides an electronic checklist by which important follow-on orders are more easily captured and less easily missed.

Treatment recommendation: providing a recommendation, not just an assessment. For example, the system recommends that the clinician prescribes antidepressants for a patient rather than simply identifying the patient as being depressed.

Clinical documentation support: Opportunities for decision support are rich in clinical documentation, both in diagnosis and treatment. Medical orders and ICD 9 (and 10) codes specific to key words can be automatically entered into the system based on entry of the documentation supporting them. This saves time and improves diagnostic accuracy and reimbursement.

Treatment recommendation: this can include a recommendation for diabetic foot exam by providing data from randomized controlled trials that show benefits of conducting the exam. Keyword links to PubMed and other clinical data sources can provide guidance and clinical justification for tests and procedures and the use of their resources.

Reminders: generate and send postcards to patients to inform them of overdue preventive care services; easily performed from claims data, reminding patients of overdue preventive services that can minimize the cost of expensive treatment later. CDS can also send reminders for patient appointments and provide tailored educational materials.

Reports: Clinicians are sent emails every 2 weeks that summarize their compliance with CDS recommendations for the care of patients with diabetes or other chronic conditions. This supports long-term care and population health initiatives, increases consistency within a product line, and provides performance metrics against which to measure care or perform clinical research.

Usability Issues and CDS Frameworks

Usability in CDS, as in other aspects of EHR use, can be very difficult to define and evaluate. *Human factors engineering*, which is the study of designing equipment and devices that fit the human body and its cognitive abilities, intersects with convenience and "just feeling right" in determining what makes CDS usable. With that in mind, approaching CDS through generally agreed-upon principles is a good first step to designing systems with high usability, and the following frameworks are intended to provide that guidance.

NOTE

The Five Rights of CDS should not be confused with the Five Rights of Medication Administration.

The Five Rights of CDS

According to the Agency for Healthcare Research and Quality (AHRQ) (Berner, 2009), the Five Rights model for Clinical Decision Support (CDS) can facilitate significant improvements in healthcare outcomes when used effectively, and if we communicate the following:

> *The right information:* The information presented to the end-user—or in some cases, the patient—should be evidence-based, derived from a set of recognized guidelines, or based on a national performance measure. In the case of a 55-year-old patient, an alert is generated informing the physician that the patient needs to be screened for colon cancer. The alert is based on the performance measure NQF-0034, which is a national measure developed by the National Committee for Quality Assurance (NCQA). Furthermore, this performance measure is based on a set of guidelines developed by the American Cancer Society that stipulates who, from the general population, should be screened for colon cancer on a regular basis (U.S. Preventive Services Task Force, 2008).
>
> *To the right person:* It is important to make sure that the right information gets to the right person, who can then take action. The right person can be a nurse, physician, physical therapist, or in some cases, significant other. Using the preceding example, the right person is the physician who receives the alert and advises the patient to schedule a colonoscopy. It is important to note that CDS interventions can sometimes change care team roles. In this example, if the patient is resistant to advice from the physician, the information may be best conveyed by a significant other or sibling who can use persuasion to help ensure patient compliance. The primary concept here is to present information only to those individuals who can take action. An example of a poorly presented alert is one that a nurse receives to adjust medication dosing for a patient. This type of information is problematic because the nurse is not the provider who performs the medication dosing adjustment, and the information is likely to be lost or miscommunicated.

In the right CDS intervention format: CDS may be implemented in various formats: alerts, order sets, protocols, and patient-monitoring systems. It is therefore important for implementers to clearly identify the issues and problems that they are trying to solve and choose the best format to achieve the desired outcome. Furthermore, when developing a CDS program, implementers should create an inventory of CDS tools that are currently available, tools that need to be developed, and tools that can be purchased through a vendor. In the opening example of screening for colon cancer, say that a practice wishes to identify patients at risk for major illnesses and encourage them to adopt preventive measures. The simplest solution is to use an alert that non-intrusively informs the physician of a patient's predisposition to an illness: in this case, colon cancer.

Through the right channel: CDS interventions can be delivered electronically through an EHR, a personal health record (PHR), computerized physician order entry, or an app running on a smartphone or device. Paper transfer might be necessary, perhaps in flow sheets, forms, and labels. In the earlier example, if the physician is the right person, the EHR may be the best platform for delivering the alert. Conversely, if a significant other is the right person, then the right platform may be a text messaging app or a simple postcard with discounted co-pay for the procedure or some other inducement.

At the right time in the workflow: CDS interventions that are presented at the right time feel natural, and they offer guidance when that guidance can best be used. For example, when a patient is on an aspirin regimen, and a provider is ordering an anticoagulant, the right time for an alert to appear is at order selection, before the order is filled out and entered—not after. In the colon cancer screening example, a passive alert might signal that the patient is eligible for colonoscopy. If it is not acted upon before the provider closes the chart, an active alert might remind her to encourage scheduling the procedure.

Obviously, the Five Rights are an ideal for which we strive. In practice, it is tremendously difficult to anticipate at any particular moment exactly what the user will most benefit from knowing and how to communicate that in the best way possible. A successful methodology is to identify specific opportunities based on acknowledged user need and provide interventions targeted to address those critical moments.

Alert presentation is critical to positive user responses, and the CDS developer should remain conscious of the range of user situations that must be anticipated and addressed in any situation. For example, a simple alert to identify a typographic error in data entry might find the user extremely distracted, frustrated, under significant time constraints, or unable to reproduce the situation in which the patient measurement was performed. Each of these situations can produce a different user response to the alert, and this is critical to anticipate while attempting to evaluate the alert for effectiveness.

Additionally, clinicians are often bombarded with alerts (this is sometimes called "alert fatigue") and may often not read more than the first few words of the alert. In the sequence of events that begins with attempting to enter a patient note, when the alert presents to the user, he may respond by noticing the error and returning to correct it or by proceeding and filing the datum in question regardless, or he may just delete the alert. If Return is selected to reenter the datum, he may reenter the value more carefully or instead choose to reenter a value calculated to satisfy the alert just to make it go away. Retrospectively, each of these actions can be intuited by examining the electronic record, and this is routinely done to evaluate the effectiveness of alerts. Measurements of responses of *quit*, *changed*, or *overridden* can be calculated and assessed. Based on these examinations, in the effort to maximize accuracy and minimize alert fatigue, the alert firing parameters, timing, and message structure can all be fine-tuned to optimize the alert's sensitivity and specificity (Haerian, McKeeby, DiPatrizio, & Cimino, 2009).

The Ten Commandments of CDS

Bates et al. (2003) studied the impact of decision support across a broad array of domains and found a number of common elements important to success. They named these factors the Ten Commandments of CDS. Informatics specialists should keep them in mind as CDS opportunities are identified and designed in order to best ensure user acceptance and maximize the intended effect of CDS.

1. **Speed is everything.** Clinicians require that CDS respond in real time to the dynamic circumstances of clinical care and will not wait. Having to wait for decision support will effectively invalidate it in the eyes of its users.
2. **Anticipate needs and deliver in real time.** CDS users require support be delivered when the question presents. Decision support cannot be adequately provided retrospectively.
3. **Fit into the user's workflow.** Making the user stop and look somewhere else during a critical workflow will both discredit the decision support and invite the introduction of unintended circumstances into clinical care workflow processes.
4. **Little things can make a big difference.** Small changes in the flow of screens, the presentation of information, and the usability of CDS can have great impact on its success. Do not overlook small factors such as appearance, wording, or placement in system deployment.
5. **Recognize that physicians will strongly resist stopping.** Clinicians act on their thoughts. Interrupting their thoughts is neither useful nor practical. CDS must be delivered in-line and presented in a manner not requiring the user to stop what she is doing.
6. **Changing direction is easier than stopping.** A change in direction will be accepted more positively than stopping. Guiding user responses into the appropriate channel is a superior tactic to stopping and requiring a restart.
7. **Simple interventions work best.** Although one may provide references to decision support, messages requiring significant reading or explanation will not be positively accepted. Find a critical point and address it; leave the educational materials for later.
8. **Ask for additional information only when you really need it.** In an effort to avoid stopping the user and interrupting workflow, ask for additional information only when specifically required to perform a function—and only if it is unavailable elsewhere.
9. **Monitor impact, get feedback, and respond.** Users know more about our systems than we designers do. Be sure to monitor the effects created by the systems, ask users how it works for them, and respond by making system improvements based on gathered data.

10. **Manage and maintain your knowledge-based systems.** All CDS needs to be current and up to date. Giving users decision support with outdated information or inappropriate suggestions for care is likely to result in the general disregard and ignoring of all subsequent CDS suggestions/decisions.

Convene a CDS Committee

CDS is a clinical methodology of great significance and complexity. However, satisfying the stakeholders, end users, clinicians—and increasingly patients—involves a number of process-oriented initiatives as well as technical ones. Limited resources in the clinical environment require consensus about which clinical areas CDS can most positively affect to obtain the best return on investment. In addition to resource allocation issues, practitioners and other stakeholders may disagree as to the need or appropriateness of various CDS implementations. CDS is resource-intensive and can carry significant political and legal implications as well as clinical ones. There are quite often differences of opinion between medical staff members about how CDS should or should not be applied and managed. This can limit and stifle CDS development in the very areas where it might make its biggest impact.

To address potential challenges, it is considered best practice to convene a CDS development committee composed of not only IT leadership informatics specialists but also influential and forward-thinking members of the medical staff and clinical areas, such as pharmacy and nursing. Needs assessments, proposals, and CDS prototypes should be presented to the committee, and development efforts should proceed based on their consensus. This provides both direction and support for the development effort and can assist in preventing special interests from derailing valuable projects either for their own interests or to avoid implementation in specific areas.

The CDS committee should also include the CDS development team, which will ideally consist of a clinical expert—typically, a care provider intimately familiar with the clinical domain to be addressed—and a knowledge base administrator. The clinical expert can liaise with clinical users to help identify opportunities and needs and then develop process flows from which the CDS applications can be developed. The *knowledge engineer* is the coder or programming manager for CDS implementations, depending on project scope. The role typically requires a strong programming background and may or may not include a clinical component. Finally, the knowledge base administrator will actively maintain applicable knowledge bases and catalog and manage CDS applications to avoid conflicts and redundancies between CDS deployments and other applications (Balko, 2008). The CDS development team can consist of one to many individuals in these roles, but all should be an integral part of the CDS committee to help guide it toward its desired goals.

Specification Form for CDS Intervention Design

You can use this worksheet example in Table 11.1 (Osheroff et al., 2012) to ensure that you have considered the core components during CDS design and to also help make sure that all clinical and technical team members are aware of the key elements. This worksheet can become a living document fostering discussion about issues and evolve in response to those discussions.

Table 11.1 CDS Design Worksheet Example

CDS Intervention Name	***Heparin in Post-Op Orders***
Description	When post-op order sets are displayed, an item to order heparin (for thrombosis prophylaxis) will always be included.
Clinical Leader	Dr. Howard Klott, vascular medicine
Technical Leader	Jennifer Rose, IT
EHR Application Affected	CPOE
Intervention Type	Order set modification
Workflow Step	Order set initiation (post-op)
Specifically Triggered By	Order set user (ordering provider)
Logic (in plain English) to determine whether intervention is presented	Order set type: Post-op Except: patient already on any form of heparin, warfarin, or dabigatran Except: patient with history of GI bleed, intracranial hemorrhage, subarachnoid hemorrhage, or hemophilia

continues

Table 11.1 CDS Design Worksheet Example *(continued)*

CDS Intervention Name	***Heparin in Post-Op Orders***
Data Items Needed (where found in system)	Order set type Problem list Medications list
Notification Type, If Any	None (synchronous display)
Presentation Type	Order set item
Who is primary user of intervention?	Ordering clinician
Summary Statement	Thromboembolism prophylaxis
Supporting of Knowledge to Be Presented	Postoperative thrombosis prophylaxis for all patients not on anticoagulation and without significant bleeding risk has been shown to reduce overall net vascular complications by 32%
Evidence Source	Anderson and Wilkins' review of post-op clotting complications ASC recommendations on post-op anticoagulation
Offered Action Items	Order unfractionated heparin 5,000 units subcutaneously twice per day Order enoxaparin 1mg/kg subcutaneously twice per day Order warfarin, start at 5mg/day Order PTT Order INR
Feedback Channels and Plan	Contact information for responsible department already exists on order set

Reprinted with permission.

Tasks Checklist for CDS Implementation

Although implementing CDS from scratch in your healthcare environment may seem a daunting prospect with a challenging and complex set of requirements, like any other project, it is composed of a list of separate and discrete tasks. The following checklist (used with permission) from Osheroff et al.'s *Improving Outcomes with Clinical Decision Support: An Implementer's Guide* (2012) can serve as a primer to effecting the necessary organizational and system changes.

Develop a shared broad understanding of CDS as an operational imperative

- Establish a strong/shared foundation around basic concepts (for example, CDS definition and scope) and approaches for yourself and your team to underpin your efforts to develop a successful CDS program and interventions.
- Begin outlining, or refining, a set of initial strategic victories to be pursued.
- Begin building a shared vision among key participants (for example, physicians, nurses, implementers, practice managers, office staff, and patients, to the extent that CDS affects their care) about CDS's role in enhancing the practice's clinical and operational performance.
- Likewise, begin building a shared, broad perspective on a CDS toolkit: for example, many potential content and intervention types, recipients, delivery channels, and workflow opportunities (that is, the CDS Five Rights approach for improving outcomes with CDS configurations that optimize the aforementioned factors).

Document a plan for CDS-related assessments, decision-making processes, oversight, and execution

- Why, what, how, who, and when of CDS approach and activities are documented.
- CDS program is appropriately integrated with quality and HIT planning and execution.
- Oversight for various strategic and tactical decisions (such as initiation and review of interventions of various types) is in place.

- All key participants are engaged (or represented) in CDS program decision-making process and oversight, and each recognizes personal advantages from the CDS activities.
- CDS is approached as a shared effort with intervention recipients as part of collaborative improvement culture.
- Primary champions are identified, representing "a collection of respected figures in various positions, such that everyone else will listen to at least one of them"—and richly engaged in the process.
- Mechanism for ongoing communication is identified and begun.
- Staff, consultants, and/or vendor personnel are available to fill essential roles needed for CDS program success: design, development, implementation, and evaluation.
- Documented plan used for prioritizing CDS-mediated improvement objectives, based on internal/external drivers (for example, Meaningful Use, Patient-Centered Medical Home Certification, clinical quality measures).

Address other key CDS program building blocks: Systems, workflow, and measurement

- Consider tools and expertise in workflow analysis.
- Develop capabilities and tools for measuring intervention effects on clinical quality and user satisfaction.
- Technology and organizational infrastructure catalogued and its implications are understood (what you can do easily, what requires a greater or different type of effort).

Utilize a proactive and systematic process for acquiring, validating, and updating CDS content

- Knowledge management policies are in place, along with tools and processes to enforce policies.
- Explicit approach (in-house or outsourced vendor personnel or consultants) for managing the CDS content portfolio's life cycle (scope, currency, consistency) in place.

Understand the foundational considerations for effective CDS interventions

- Apply your CDS program's systematic approach to prioritizing improvement targets to select specific focal points for your CDS intervention efforts.
- Understand the components of the CDS Five Rights and how each is applicable to the development of effective CDS interventions.
- Understand the several major types of CDS interventions that can be delivered via information systems and other channels. Understanding these different types, and their advantages and disadvantages, is critical in selecting and designing optimal interventions to accomplish specific goals.
- Understand the general life cycle of a CDS intervention; keep pertinent clinical and office staff engaged throughout this cycle.
- Selecting the optimal intervention for the need: Intervention type is the best choice for the objective.
- Intervention(s) are focused on an improvement priority, driven by the CDS decision-making process.
- Intervention type (alerts, reminder, order set, documentation templates, and so on) is the best choice for the objective; among appropriate intervention types, final choice reflects balance between ease of implementation, acceptability, and impact (these may be tuned based on your organization's experience and comfort level).

Specifying (or configuring) interventions: Intervention is optimally designed to fit workflow and clinical objective and vetted by stakeholders

- Intervention design:
    - Critical elements of the intervention are included (easy to understand the reason; necessary supporting data and knowledge to make a decision; easy access to action items; mechanisms to document medical and patient reasons for exceptions, such as a patient's refusal of treatment).
    - Intervention content coordinated with related clinical quality/performance measure(s) as appropriate.
    - Intervention is optimized to support workflow and desired outcomes; CDS Five Rights are addressed, and unhelpful disruption is minimized.

    - Intervention behaves as expected, providing useful and appropriate information needed to support desired decisions, actions, and outcomes; consider implications of possible future care process or data changes.
    - Intervention contains ability to measure user response and process change.
- Vetting interventions with stakeholders, and testing before go-live:
    - All parties key to intervention success are engaged at appropriate stage; an early shared vision is developed among end users and other participants about needs, goals, and strategies related to interventions; interventions are done *with* end users, not *to* them.
    - Intervention content thoroughly tested for usability and safety before deployment in live environment; explicit responsibility for owner to approve final version of intervention before deployment; backup and failsafe measures in place as appropriate.

Deployment plan is in place

- All stakeholders and all users are prepared for intervention launch: for example, via communication, training, and user support.
- Capability is in place to address altered workflows and care delivery needs (for example, providing more procedures, testing, or medications that may result from successful CDS intervention).
- Capacity is in place to obtain user feedback and to deal rapidly with immediate concerns.

Measure results and continuously refine the program

- Plan is in place for identifying, tracking, and addressing intended and unintended intervention behaviors and effects.
- Plan is in place for reporting intervention effects to pertinent stakeholders and supporting continuous monitoring and improvement.
- Victories and exceptional efforts are tracked, frequently communicated, and leveraged to sustain performance and set up enthusiasm for future CDS interventions.

- Owners or responsible parties are identified for CDS interventions and their content; processes are in place to maintain and update intervention, periodically and as needs arise.

Conclusion

The resource commitment required to implement CDS is considerable. The CDS committee's time, the efforts of the CDS development team, the deployment effort, evaluation effort, maintenance, and the need to keep supporting documentation current all carry significant costs. Even when deploying clinical decision support is the right thing to do from a clinical perspective, CDS also has to make sense for the organization. Cost savings, improvements in quality, a decreased length of stay, and a decrease in medication errors are all possible with effective CDS (Chaiken, 2003). Documenting these will help justify the resource costs of deploying CDS and provide a rationale for any change management requirements engendered by the CDS applications.

CPOE is a key success factor for CDS implementations. The "point of care" is almost literally those moments during which medical orders are entered and initiated or documentation is entered, and it is during those pivotal moments that decision support can make a critical difference to the user and the patient. The CMS Meaningful Use requirements recognize and acknowledge this in requiring a combination of CPOE and CDS to qualify for enhanced reimbursement and to avoid penalties. Although medication ordering is an important use of and has often received a lion's share of energy and interest in CDS, order sets, care pathways, and clinical reminders (such as vaccination messages) are all relatively less complex and completely appropriate uses of CDS.

An EHR is another success factor. When clinical information is contained in a database and available to CDS applications, alerts, reminders and suggestions can be provided in real time. As previously discussed, the right data at the right time by the right communication method delivered quickly is vitally important to successful decision support. The integration of multiple clinical areas is another advantage of an EHR. Having medications, laboratory results, clinical documentation, and order entry all available on the same platform allows much greater flexibility and accuracy and increases the potential benefits of CDS.

When researching CDS needs within a clinical environment, looking to the body of documented CDS successes is an appropriate first step. The mix of systems, databases, and clinical requirements between providers and provider organizations is such that not all CDS applications in the literature will be applicable to every clinical environment or combination of systems. Based on a needs assessment, begin by performing a system and process inventory and determine which avenues of approach are most feasible based on documentation of previous successes. Although one facility's success is not necessarily indicative of another's, it just makes good sense not to reinvent CDS from scratch when it is not necessary. Study and rely on others' successes as a starting point and look for easy wins, that is, visible successes able to be achieved with minimal resources and likely to produce positive political influence. Keep in mind that a few small successes in an institution can help pave the way and build organizational and clinical support for more ambitious initiatives.

Institutions employing CDS must reach internal consensus regarding which decision support features, rules, and alerts to use, and must also determine the most appropriate place to insert them into clinical processes. The clinician users of such systems must actively provide feedback that system maintainers rapidly and regularly address in order to attain an optimal approach to using CDS (Bates et al., 2003).

Finally, as with most other information technology initiatives, stakeholder involvement is primary to success in CDS implementations. Doing things with stakeholders will always be more successful than doing things to them. Providing CDS to caregivers is a process fraught with the potential to create distractions and interruptions in workflow, political ill-will, and the even more serious effects on patients from inappropriate suggestions, outdated information, or poor timing. Although these dangers must be acknowledged and fully appreciated, the potential for improvements in the quality, safety, and consistency of clinical care from CDS is so significant that practically, ethically, and now perhaps legally as well (Weed, 1999), we must identify appropriate applications of CDS and prepare ourselves to proceed with applying them to the development, maintenance, and improvement of the systems and processes on which we depend for clinical care.

References

Balko, J. (2008). *CDS made ridiculously simple.* Phoenix, AZ: Eclipsys Corporation.

Bartold, S., & Hannigan, G. G. (2002). DXplain. Invited review. *Journal of the Medical Library Association, 90*(2), 267–268.

Bates, D., Kuperman, G. J., Wang, S., Gandhi, T., Kittler, A., Volk, L., ... Middleton, B. (2003). Ten commandments for effective clinical decision support: Making the practice of evidence-based medicine a reality. *Journal of the American Medical Informatics Association, 10*(6), 523–530.

Berner, E. (2007). *Clinical decision support systems, theory and practice,* 2nd ed. NewYork, NY: Science+Business Media, LLC.

Berner, E, (2009). *Clinical decision support systems: State of the art.* Rockville, MD: AHRQ. Report No. 09-0069-EF.

Chaiken, B. P., (2003).Clinical ROI: Not just costs versus benefits. *Journal of Healthcare Information, 17*(4), 36–41. Retrieved from http://www.docsnetwork.com/articles/BPC03134.pdf

Classen, D. C., Pestotnik, S. L., Evans, R. S., & Burke, J. P. (1992). Description of a computerized adverse drug event monitor using a hospital information system. *Hospital Pharmacy, 27,* 774–783.

East, T. D., Henderson, S., Morris, A. H., & Gardner, R. M. (1989). Implementation issues and challenges for computerized clinical protocols for management of mechanical ventilation in ARDS patients. SCAMC, Inc. *AMIA annual symposium proceedings,* 538–587. PMCID: PMC2245793

Farnum, L., Cimino, J., DiPatrizio, G., & Goldspiel, B. (2011). Improving adherence to research protocol drug exclusions using a clinical alerting system. *AMIA annual symposium proceedings.* 257–266.

Friedlin J., Dexter P., & Overhage, M. (2007). Details of a successful clinical decision support system. *AMIA annual symposium proceedings,* 254–258.

Gardner, R. M., Pryor, T. A., & Warner, H. R. (1999). The HELP hospital information system: Update 1998. *International Journal of Medical Informatics, 54*(3), 169–182. PMCID: PMC2655822

Haerian, K., McKeeby, J., DiPatrizio, G., & Cimino, J. (2009). Use of clinical alerting to improve the collection of clinical research data. *AMIA annual symposium proceedings,* 218–222. PMCID: PMC2815392

Open Clinical White Paper. (2000, October 25). The medical knowledge crisis and its solution through knowledge management. Retrieved from http://www.openclinical.org/docs/whitepaper.pdf

Osheroff, J., Teich, J., Levick, D., Saldana, L., Velasco, F., Sittig, D., ... Jenders, R. (2012). *Improving outcomes with clinical decision support: An implementer's guide,* 2nd ed. Chicago, IL: HIMSS.

Overhage, J. M., Tierney, W. M., Zhou, X. H., & McDonald, C. J. (1997). A randomized trial of "corollary orders" to prevent errors of omission. *Journal of the American Medical Informatics Association. 4*(5), 364–375.

U.S. Preventive Services Task Force. (2008). *Screening for colorectal cancer: U.S. Preventive Services Task Force recommendation statement.* AHRQ Publication 08-05124-EF-3, October 2008. Agency for Healthcare Research and Quality, Rockville, MD.

Weed, L. L. (1999). Opening the black box of clinical judgment – An overview. *British Medical Journal, 319*(7220), p. 1279.

"It ain't what you don't know that gets you in trouble. It's what you know for sure that just ain't so."

–Mark Twain

Use of Standard Terminologies in Healthcare IT

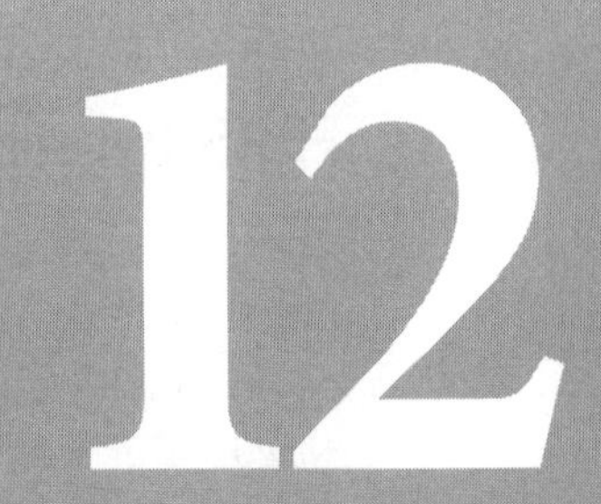

Luann Whittenburg, PhD, RN-BC, FNP-BC, CPHQ, CPHIMS
Amy K. Jacobs, MSN, RN-BC

OBJECTIVES

- Identify the 12 nursing terminologies recognized by the American Nurses Association.
- Describe the benefits of using structured data to represent the complexity of nursing care and knowledge in computer systems.
- Describe a method to demonstrate the nursing contribution to the health of individuals.
- Describe the informatics and technology impact on nursing practice and care outcomes.
- Name a nursing terminology standard for the efficient information retrieval of nursing care.

Nurses communicate professional assessments about patients to other nurses and providers through nursing documentation. Nurses document observations about nursing decisions, interventions, actions, advocacy, and outcomes in the communication tool for health information exchange (Institute of Medicine [IOM], 2001): electronic health record (EHR) systems.

Since 2000, U.S. federal policy has been promoting changes in healthcare delivery performance among synthesizers of healthcare in order to obtain transparency in healthcare quality. The Office of Management and Budget (OMB) asserts that models of care in the United States are not aligned with the objective to provide the right care to the right patient at the right time.

According to Kane and Siegrist (2006), nursing consumes 30% of the hospital operating budget, yet the impact of nursing on patient care outcomes is invisible. Nurses are discovering that an electronic health information record system (HIRS) is unlikely to be a direct replica of traditional medical records (Moen, Gregory, & Brennan, 2007; Smolij & Dun, 2006). A standard coded, structured nursing documentation standard is needed to exchange nursing communication to bring transparency to the contributions of nursing to patient care continuity and the quality of health outcomes. This chapter describes the purpose, value, and benefit of implementing nursing terminology in nursing documentation systems.

HIRS Implementation

The *HIRS* is a communication tool that involves completely different physician/nurse processes to describe and document care delivery and coordination. The IOM Committee on the Quality of Health Care in America 2001 report ("Crossing the Quality Chasm: A New Health System for the 21st Century") concluded that only a HIRS with time-relevant access to appropriate healthcare knowledge will give clinicians the information required to make well-informed decisions (2001). Many nursing informatics professionals envision a HIRS that is patient-centric, in which healthcare information follows the patient, such as information access to a patient's complete history, including medical records, medication history, laboratory results, and radiology, among other patient-centric information. The HIRS implementation is expected to eliminate clinical errors due to handwriting, automate checks on patient medication doses and lab results (too high or too low), and provide alerts for harmful interactions among therapies, drugs, and allergies.

Structured Data

Structured data is required for standard terminologies and is a collection of codes, words, measurements, observations or descriptions, values (numbers), or measurements that can be processed by computers. Data can be words and descriptions such as *nursing diagnoses*, *outcomes*, *interventions*, and *actions*. See Figure 12.1.

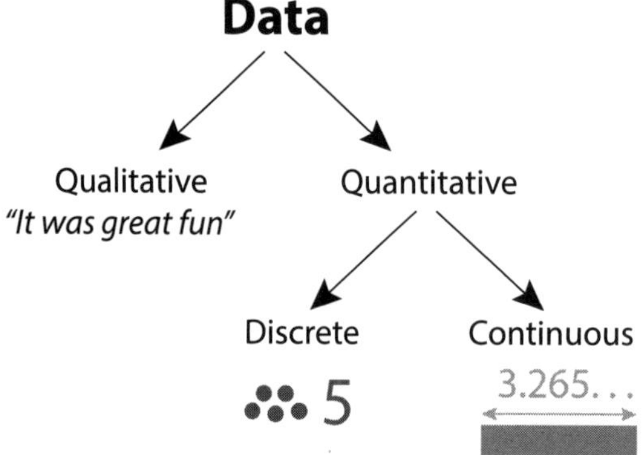

FIGURE 12.1 Examples of structured data types (© 2012 MathsIsFun.com [Data, n.d.]).

Structured data is the first step in the implementation of standard nursing terminologies required to promote evidence-based practice. The use of a nursing terminology standard in a HIRS provides a common representation of pertinent documentation by nursing and allied health professionals to allow the retrieval of documentation, which could then be exchanged between and among healthcare systems for care continuity and outcomes analysis. Structured data in healthcare information systems strengthens clinical decision support by standardizing data. Without structured data, there is a duplication of information, and *data interoperability* (the internal and external exchange of data) declines. Without standardized data, hospital operating costs may increase due to a loss of critical information for disease-management interventions or the avoidance of nosocomial illness. The use of structured nursing terminology allows the reuse of information from disparate locations, enables communication about the patient's care and care plan with others, and creates nursing data for evidence-based research and practice.

Nursing Data Systems

In most HIRS, the standard nursing terminology implemented—sometimes called the *system nomenclature*: that is, the nursing body of knowledge or data dictionary—is proprietary with pre-existing structure or ontology frameworks. The *ontology* is a pre-existing framework that explains the relationship between concepts. These proprietary frameworks may significantly influence nursing documentation by constraining nursing documentation fields (Snyder, Weston, Fields, Rizos, & Tedeschi, 2006; Turpin, 2005). Due to the highly structured design of today's healthcare systems, nursing practice may be determined by ontology framework configuration and workflow constraints. If nurses cannot select the ontology framework, nursing care becomes the data structure rather than a flexible tool to enable nurses to improve nursing interventions and practice.

Use of Standard Terminologies

The selection of an ontology framework for nursing sufficient to support nursing and allied health professional documentation is a crucial decision. The American Nurses Association (ANA) has recognized 12 nursing terminology standards. Thede and Schwiran (2011, para. 1) reflected that "[C]apturing nursing's independent contributions requires the use of standardized terminologies that reflect the uniqueness of nursing care." Yet, what is a "standard," and what criteria did the ANA use to approve the 12 terminology standards? These standards provide the ontology and may effect the collection of nursing information. The International Organization for Standardization (ISO) defines a *standard* as a document that provides requirements, specifications, guidelines, or characteristics that can be used consistently to ensure that materials, products, processes, and services are fit for their purpose (ISO, n.d.: para. 2): "[S]tandards ensure that products such as health information record systems and services are safe, reliable and of good quality. For business, they are strategic tools that reduce costs by minimizing waste and errors, and increasing productivity."

The following list contains the initial seven desiderata for the design of a controlled healthcare terminology (sometimes known as a "vocabulary") (Cimino, Hripcsak, Johnson, & Clayton, 1989):

- **Domain completeness:** the ability to accommodate appropriately all necessary concepts. Schemes should not limit depth or breadth of hierarchies. Compositional approaches allow complex concepts to be represented.
- **Unambiguous:** Terms should clearly represent only a single concept. Synonyms should be pure.
- **Non-redundancy:** There must be only one way of representing a concept in the vocabulary, or equivalences between alternative representations should be detectable.
- **Synonymy:** More than one term (synonym) may describe the same concept.
- **Multiple classifications:** Entities from the vocabulary should be placed in more than one hierarchy location if appropriate. For example, *Carcinoma of the colon* is both a *Malignant disease* and a *Large intestinal disease.*
- **Consistency of views:** Cimino, Hripcsak, Johnson, and Clayton (1989) identified the problem of multiple classification being inconsistent or incomplete and that qualifiers or modifiers might vary between different parts of the hierarchy.
- **Explicit relationships:** The nature of relationships between concepts in the vocabulary structure should be explicit and usually subclass.

Subclass Relationships

A subclass (also known as a 'subtype', 'derived', or 'child') relationship inherits information from another class (also known as 'is a', 'super', or 'parent' classes). "Almost all active SNOMED CT concepts are the source of at least one |is-a| relationship. The only exception is the root concept |SNOMED CT Concept| which is the most general concept. The |is a| relationship states that the source concept is a subtype of the destination concept" (International Health Terminology Standards Development Organisation [IHTSDO], 2014, p. 16)

The use of a subclass allows information capture at several levels of detail to suit individual uses. For example: "the concept |pneumococcal pneumonia| is a subtype of |bacterial pneumonia| which has a defining relationship that specifies that the |causative agent| is |streptococcus pneumoniae| and this allows the organism causing this disease to be analyzed" (IHTSDO, 2014, p. 7).

Cimino (1998) produced 12 desiderata for controlled medical vocabularies in the 21st century:

- **Content:** To most users, "What can be said?" is more important than "How can it be said?" Omissions are readily noticed, and timely, formal, and explicit methods for plugging gaps are required.
- **Concept orientation:** The unit of symbolic processing is the concept, and each concept in the vocabulary should have a single, coherent meaning.
- **Concept permanence:** A concept's meaning cannot change, and it cannot be deleted from the vocabulary.
- **Meaningless concept identifier:** Concepts typically have unique identifiers (*codes*), and these should be nonhierarchical to allow for later relocation and for multiple classification.
- **Polyhierarchy:** Multiple classification. Entities from the vocabulary should be placed in more than one hierarchy location if appropriate. For example, *Carcinoma of the colon* is both a *Malignant disease* and a *Large intestinal disease.*
- **Formal definitions:** Semantic definitions of concepts: for example, *Streptococcal tonsillitis* = *Infection* of *tonsil* caused by *streptococcus.*
- **No residual categories:** Traditional classifications have rubrics that include *NOS, NEC, Unspecified, or Other*, whose meaning may change over time as new concepts are added to the vocabulary. These are not appropriate for recording data in an electronic health record.

- **Multiple granularities:** Different users require different levels of expressivity. A general (family) practitioner might use the term *myocardial infarction*, while a surgeon may record *acute anteroseptal myocardial infarction*.
- **Multiple consistent views:** Although there may be multiple views of the hierarchy required to support different functional requirements and levels of detail, these must be consistent.
- **Representing context:** There is a crucial relationship between concepts within the vocabulary and the context in which they are used. Cimino defines three types of knowledge:
    - *Definitional:* How concepts define one another
    - *Assertional:* How concepts combine
    - *Contextual:* How concepts are used
- **Graceful evolution:** Vocabularies must be designed to allow for evolution and change in order to incorporate new advances in healthcare and to correct errors.
- **Recognize redundancy:** Where the same information can be expressed in different ways, a mechanism for recognizing equivalence is required.

Zielstorff (1998), a nursing informatics pioneer, published "Characteristics of a Good Nursing Nomenclature from an Informatics Perspective." The characteristics included "… domain completeness, granularity, parsimony, synonymy, non-ambiguity, non-redundancy, clinical utility, multiple axes, and combinatorial" (Zielstorff, 1998, p. 2). Using coded nursing terminology standards, nurses are able to determine which nursing interventions achieve the expected outcome. As the profession systematically collects electronic information about nursing care, nursing and allied health professionals acquire evidence-based practice knowledge of nursing interventions that occur for patient populations. This information may be useful in determining the cost of nursing services, planning for nursing resource allocation, and constructing nursing and interprofessional plans of care.

Granular/ity

1. An expression of the relative size of a unit. The smallest discrete information that can be directly retrieved. In security, it is the degree of protection. Protection at the file level is consider coarse granularity, whereas protection at the field level is finer granularity.
2. Refers to a high degree of detail. In particular, a vocabulary that is highly granular provides names and definitions for the individual data elements within the context of a broader concept.

From *HIMSS Dictionary of Healthcare Information Technology Terms, Acronyms and Organizations* (Whittenburg, 2013, p. 62)

The ANA (2008) defines nursing informatics as a "specialty that integrates nursing science, computer science, and information science. This integration is accomplished through the use of information structures, information processes, and information technology" (ANA, 2008, p. 65). The Committee for Nursing Practice Information Infrastructure (CNPII) is the governing body within the ANA responsible for recognizing and accepting standardized nursing terminology and data sets.

Currently, the ANA has recognized seven nursing terminologies, two nursing data element sets, and three multidisciplinary terminologies for the documentation of nursing practice in the ANA scope of practice (ANA, 2012). "The data element sets and terminologies are foundational to standardization of nursing documentation and verbal communication that will lead to a reduction in errors and an increase in the quality and continuity of care. It is through standardization of nurse documentation and communication of a patient's care that the many nurses caring for a patient develop a shared understanding of that care. Moreover, the process generates the nursing data needed to develop increasingly more sophisticated decision support tools in the electronic record and to identify and disseminate best nursing practices" (ANA, 2006, para. 1).

American Nurses Association Committee for Nursing Practice Information Infrastructure

The ANA has long been involved in nursing practice with its mission to advance and protect the profession of nursing. The ANA recognizes the use of seven nursing terminologies, two nursing data element sets, and three multidisciplinary terminologies as standards for the documentation of nursing practice in *Nursing Informatics: Scope and Standards of Practice* (ANA, 2008).

The terminologies and data sets recognized by the ANA are approved by the ANA Committee for Nursing Practice Information Infrastructure (CNPII), which is the governing body responsible for recognizing and accepting standardized terminologies and data sets. All terminology recognition requests to the ANA are voluntary. When terminology recognition is requested, the CNPII conducts an evaluation for conformance to criteria. The CNPII approval criteria require that the terminology development "…supports the nursing process by providing a clinically useful terminology" (Thede & Sewell, 2010, p. 203). These criteria ensure recognized terminologies will be able to document nursing care within each of the six steps of the nursing process: Assessment, Diagnosis, Outcomes Identification, Planning, Implementation, and Evaluation.

Other CPNII required criteria (Thede & Sewell, 2010) are:

- Unambiguous concepts
- Documented use in practice
- Valid and reliable concepts
- Identified group responsible for maintaining and revising

In response to ongoing nursing documentation requirements to address regulatory, compliance, quality measures, and rule sets, the recognized CNPII nursing terminologies and data sets approved increased from 1992 to 2000. Each of the ANA–recognized terminologies was initially developed to meet specific professional nursing needs: For example, the Perioperative Nursing Data Set (PNDS) was developed to meet the nursing needs for the documentation of pre-, post-, and intra-operative nursing care.

Although each terminology supports the nursing process, the criteria do not require each terminology to include the full six steps of the nursing process. The first four nursing terminologies were recognized in 1992, which included the Clinical Care Classification System (CCC) (formerly known as HHCC), NANDA-I, Omaha System, and NIC; the remaining three nursing terminologies (ICNP®, NOC, and PNDS); two data sets (NMDS and NMMDS); and three multidisciplinary terminologies (ABC, LOINC®, and SNOMED CT) followed.

The ANA recognized standard terminologies and data sets for use in nursing practice documentation are discussed below. The nursing terminologies, classifications, and data element sets are listed below in alphabetical order by standard category type: nursing terminologies, nursing data sets, and multidisciplinary terminologies.

Clinical Care Classification System™

The Clinical Care Classification (CCC) System™ allows nurses to communicate the nursing diagnoses of patients, the nursing interventions performed, and resulting care outcomes. The CCC System is a "research-based, coded terminology standard that identifies the discrete data elements of nursing practice—the essence of care. The CCC System includes a holistic framework and coding structure of diagnoses, interventions, and outcomes for assessing, documenting, and classifying care in all healthcare settings" (Hunter & Bickford, 2011, p. 183).

The CCC research project was conducted under a federal grant from the Health Care Financing Agency (HCFA), now the Centers for Medicare and Medicaid Services (CMS), to develop a methodology for classifying patient and measuring outcomes. The research project represented every state in the United States, including Puerto Rico and the District of Columbia (Saba, 1992). The CCC System uses the six steps of the nursing process to describe nursing practice in a coding structure designed for retrieving data from computer information systems (Hardiker, Bakken, Casey, & Hoy, 2002). For more information, see

www.sabacare.com

www.clinicalcareclassification.com

International Classification for Nursing Practice (ICNP®)

The International Classification for Nursing Practice (ICNP®), developed and maintained by the International Council of Nurses (ICN), "provides a unifying framework into which local language and existing nursing vocabularies and classifications can be cross-mapped to enable comparison of nursing data across organizations, across sectors within health care systems, and among countries" (Coenen, 2003, para. 6). The ICNP® "is a combinatorial terminology for nursing practice that facilitates cross-mapping of local terms as well as existing vocabularies and classifications. The ICNP® includes nursing phenomena (nursing diagnoses), nursing actions, and nursing outcomes" (Hunter & Bickford, 2011, pp. 183–184). The ICNP® terminology is available in several languages (ICNP, 2014).

Information on translations is updated regularly and available at

http://www.icn.ch/pillarsprograms/icnpr-translations/

www.icn.ch

NANDA International

NANDA-I is a "nursing diagnoses classification developed to describe the important judgment of nursing in providing nursing care for individual, families, groups, and communities. These judgments, or diagnoses, are the basis for selection of nursing outcomes and interventions. The terminology is updated every two years" (Hunter & Bickford, 2011, p. 184–185). For more information, see

www.nanda.org

Nursing Interventions Classification (NIC)

The Nursing Interventions Classification (NIC) is a "comprehensive research-based, standardized classification of interventions that nurses perform and use for clinical documentation, communication of care across settings, integration of data across systems and setting, effectiveness research, productivity measures, competency evaluations, reimbursement, and curricular design" (Hunter & Bickford, 2011, p. 185). In NIC, an intervention is defined as "...any treatment, based upon clinical judgment and knowledge that a nurse performs to enhance patient/client outcomes. The NIC terminology includes interventions that nurses do on behalf of patients, both independent and collaborative interventions, both direct and indirect care" (Hunter & Bickford, 2011, p. 185). For more information on NIC, see

www.nursing.uiowa.edu

Nursing Outcomes Classification (NOC)

The Nursing Outcomes Classification is a "comprehensive, standardized classification of patient/client outcomes developed to evaluate the effects of nursing interventions. For NOC, an *outcome* is a measureable individual, family, or community state, behavior, or perception that is measured along a continuum and is responsive to nursing interventions" (Hunter & Bickford, 2011, p. 185). For more on NOC, see

www.nursing.uiowa.edu

Omaha System

The Omaha System is a "comprehensive practice and documentation tool used by multidisciplinary healthcare practitioners in any setting, from the time of client admission to discharge. The Omaha System includes an assessment component (Problem Classification Scheme), an intervention component (Intervention Scheme), and outcomes component (Problem Rating Scale for Outcomes)" (Hunter & Bickford, 2011, p. 185). For more on the Omaha system, see

www.omahasystem.org

Perioperative Nursing Data Set (PNDS)

The Perioperative Nursing Data Set describes "perioperative nursing practice with a subset of terms that specifically describe perioperative nursing diagnoses, nursing interventions, and patient outcomes in surgical settings from preadmission until discharge" (Hunter & Bickford, 2011, p. 185). For more on PNDS, see

www.aorn.org

Nursing Minimum Data Set (NMDS)

The Nursing Minimum Data Set (NMDS) is a "...minimum set of essential data elements that are necessary to describe clinical nursing practice. The USA NMDS consists of a set of 16 data elements intended to be used in all settings where nurses provide care.

Initially conceptualized in 1977, the USA NMDS has served as a foundation for the development of nursing minimum data sets throughout the world" (USA NMDS, n.d., para. 1).

These essential data elements are categorized into three general groups: (1) nursing care, which includes nursing diagnoses, nursing interventions, nursing outcomes, and a measure of nursing intensity; (2) patient or client demographics, which includes personal identification, date of birth, sex, race and ethnicity, and residence; and (3) service elements, which includes administrative type data—for example, a unique number for the principal nursing care provider; a unique health record number of the patient or client, admission, or encounter date; and discharge or termination date (USA NMDS, n.d.).

A few of the benefits of NMDS include that ability to compare nursing care and resources data across local, regional, national, and international levels; enhance nursing care documentation, and comparative research on nursing care (Schwiran & Thede, 2012; Werley, Devine, Zorn, Ryan, & Westra, 1991).

To read more about NMDS, see

www.nursing.umn.edu

Nursing Management Minimum Data Set (NMMDS)

The Nursing Management Minimum Data Set (NMMDS) "contains 18 data variables, categorized into 3 categories: environment, nurse resources, and financial resources, "used to inform the decision-making process of nurse executives related to leading and managing nursing-services delivery and care coordination" (USA NMDS, n.d.; Hunter & Bickford, 2011, p. 183).

The NMMDS is a research-based data set developed by Huber and Delaney. The NMMDS provides data that reflects discipline specific requirements. This data enables nursing leaders and healthcare administrators to compare, analyze, and benchmark nursing requirements and productivity within and across organizations. Research demonstrates that the NMMDS data elements influence both patients (adverse events, and morbidity and mortality) and staff (retention, satisfaction, and well-being) (Huber, Delaney, Crossley, Mehmert, & Ellerbe, 1992).

To read more about NMMDS, see

www.nursing.umn.edu

Alternative Billing Codes (ABC)

The Alternative Billing Codes "contains terminologies describing alternative medicine, nursing, and other integrative healthcare interventions. These codes include the type of provider and the recognized level of licensed practitioner by state" (Hunter & Bickford, 2011, p. 185). For more on ABC, see

http://abccodes.com

Logical Observation Identifiers Names and Codes (LOINC®)

The Logical Observation Identifiers Names and Codes (LOINC®) is a set of universal names and codes for identifying laboratory and clinical observations. The laboratory portion of the LOINC® database contains the following categories: chemistry, hematology, serology, microbiology (including parasitology and virology), and toxicology; as well as categories for drugs and the cell counts, antibiotic susceptibilities, and others. The clinical portion, which contains classes that are pertinent to nursing, includes entries for vital signs, hemodynamics, intake/output, electrocardiogram, obstetric ultrasound, neonatal APGAR measures, vaccination records, cardiac echocardiogram, urologic imaging, gastroendoscopic procedures, respiratory measures and ventilator management, selected survey instruments (for example, the Glasgow Coma Score, PHQ-9 depression scale, CMS-required patient assessment instruments), and other clinical observations (LOINC, 1994-2014; Martin & Scheet, 1992; Saba & Zuckerman, 1992).

The nursing content in LOINC® focuses on the assessment phase of the nursing process and also includes goals and outcomes. Some examples of these nursing assessment measurements include, but not are limited to, falls risk, pain status, skin integrity, patient performance of activities of daily living, family coping, and patient and family knowledge regarding the disease process. These nursing assessment codes in LOINC® are then mapped to the applicable nursing diagnoses and nursing interventions from two other ANA recognized terminologies: the Omaha System and the Home Health Care Classification system (now CCC System) that are also incorporated into the LOINC® database (Martin & Scheet, 1992; Matney, Bakken, & Huff, 2003; Saba & Zuckerman, 1992).

Find more on LOINC® at

www.loinc.org

Systematized Nomenclature of Medicine Clinical Terms (SNOMED CT)

The Systematized Nomenclature of Medicine Clinical Terms (SNOMED CT) is a "core terminology providing a common language that enables a consistent way of capturing, sharing, and aggregating health data across specialties and sites of care" (Hunter & Bickford, 2011, p. 185). SNOMED CT was a joint development between the NHS in England and the College of American Pathologists (CAP). It was formed in 1999 by the convergence of SNOMED RT and the United Kingdom's Clinical Terms Version 3 (formerly known as the Read Codes).

SNOMED itself was started in 1965 as SNOP (Systematized Nomenclature of Pathology), and later extended into other medical fields. In 2007, the SNOMED CT intellectual property rights were transferred from the CAP to the SNOMED SDO in the formal creation of the IHTSDO" (IHTSDO, n.d., para. 1-3). Standardized nursing language concepts and terminologies recognized by the ANA have been added to SNOMED CT and include NANDA-I Taxonomy II, NIC, NOC, Omaha System, and the CCC. The relationship link between terminologies and SNOMED CT are provided in mapping tables that identify the source terminology (Park, Lu, Konicek, & Delaney, 2007). To read more, see

www.ihtsdo.org

How to Incorporate Standard Terminologies

Now we need to consider how to introduce the standardized nursing terminologies described above in health information record systems. The benefits of a standard terminology (Thede & Schwiran, 2011) include:

- Better communication among nurses and other healthcare providers
- Increased visibility of nursing interventions
- Improved patient care
- Enhanced data collection to evaluate nursing care outcomes
- Greater adherence to standards of care
- Facilitation of assessment of nursing competency

TIP

The realization of these benefits is critical for the professional nurse; until nurses record what nurses do, documentation cannot support nursing research or reflect the contribution of nursing to patient quality of care outcomes (Thede & Schwiran, 2011).

Figure 12.2 is a sample diagram to begin the process of incorporating nursing terminology standards in electronic health record systems. The purpose is demonstrating how to organize an ontology mapping to define the relationships between the terminology concepts. By creating a diagram, the informatics nurse or reader can quickly identify the one to many relationships between major concepts, subcategories, and qualifiers in the nursing terminology. Figures 12.2 and 12.3 use the CCC Nursing Diagnoses and Nursing Interventions to guide the reader in conceptualizing the CCC relationships.

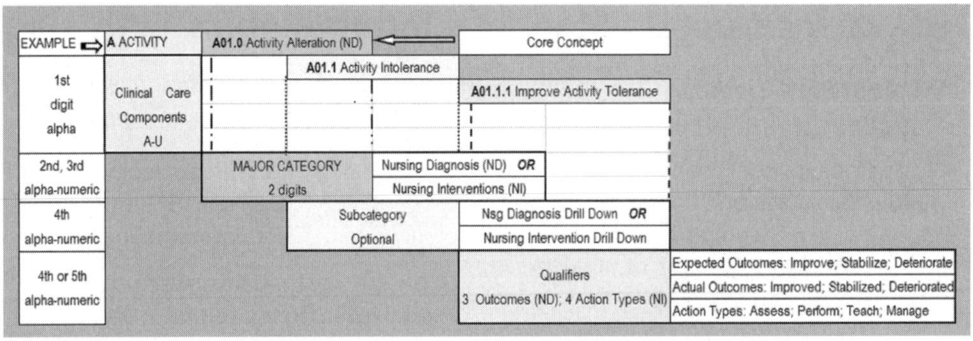

EXAMPLE ⇨ A ACTIVITY
A01.0 Activity Alteration (ND)
Core Concept
A01.1 Activity Intolerance
A01.1.1 Improve Activity Tolerance
1st digit alpha
Clinical Care Components A-U
2nd, 3rd alpha-numeric
MAJOR CATEGORY 2 digits
Nursing Diagnosis (ND) *OR*
Nursing Interventions (NI)
4th alpha-numeric
Subcategory Optional
Nsg Diagnosis Drill Down *OR*
Nursing Intervention Drill Down
4th or 5th alpha-numeric
Qualifiers
3 Outcomes (ND); 4 Action Types (NI)
Expected Outcomes: Improve; Stabilize; Deteriorate
Actual Outcomes: Improved; Stabilized; Deteriorated
Action Types: Assess; Perform; Teach; Manage

FIGURE 12.2 Diagram of CCC Building Blocks (© 2010 Kate A. O'Toole, RN, BSN, MSMOB, CNOR).

In Figure 12.3, look at Nursing Diagnosis: Activity Intolerance (A01.1). This diagnosis may link to several Nursing Interventions. For example: the Diagnosis of Activity Intolerance (A01.1) could map to Activity Care (A01.0), Energy Conservation (A01.2); Mobility Therapy (A03.0), Ambulation Therapy (A03.1), Assistive Device Therapy (A03.2), Transfer Care (A030.3), or other Nursing Interventions. The CCC Core Concepts and Subcategories have a one-to-many relationship with the qualifiers of Nursing Diagnoses and the modifiers of Nursing Interventions. In Figure 12.3, the Nursing Intervention of Mobility Therapy (A03.0) could link to 2 Action Type Modifier: Assess/Monitor (A03.0.1), and/or Manage/Refer (A03.04), depending upon the nursing approach taken to meet the patient's needs.

NOTE

For every CCC of Nursing Intervention/Action hierarchy, an Action Type Modifier is always combined with the core or subcategory concept. This is how the CCC System was developed for implementation. The CCC action types can also be used to determine nursing time, cost, and resources.

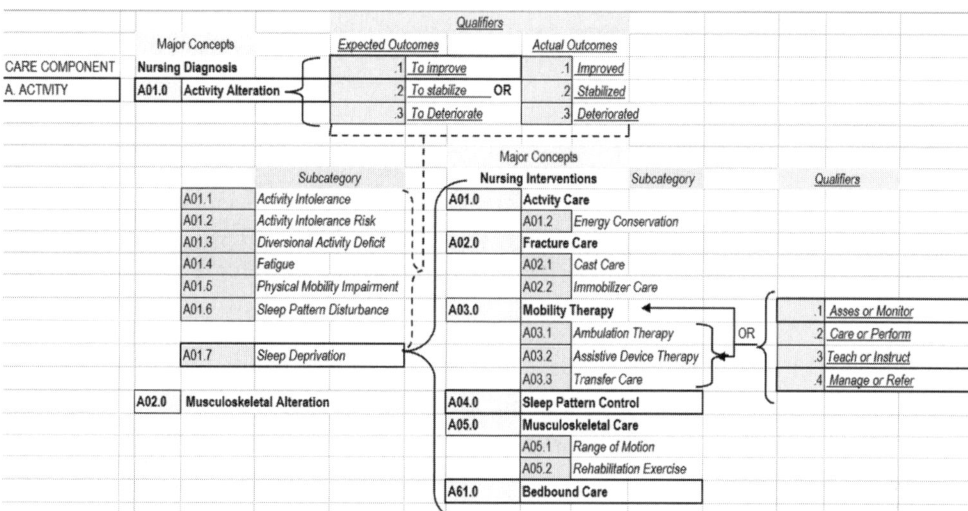

FIGURE 12.3 Expanded diagram of relationship between CCC Nursing Diagnoses and Nursing Interventions (© 2010 Kate A. O'Toole, RN, BSN, MSMOB, CNOR).

Another innovative method for the incorporation of a nursing terminology standard in an EHR system was the development of a contextual hierarchy for the MEDCIN® Engine (see Figure 12.4). MEDCIN® is a system of standardized medical terminologies for point-of-care use in health information systems. MEDCIN® includes more than 300,000 clinical data elements encompassing symptoms, history, physical examination, tests, diagnoses, and therapy. MEDCIN® has the capability to cross-map to leading codification systems, such as SNOMED CT, CPT, ICD-9-CM/ICD-10-CM, DSM, LOINC®, RxNorm, CDT, and the CCC for nursing and allied health.

The method used to integrate the CCC into MEDCIN® was to create separate hierarchies for the nursing diagnoses, nursing interventions, and nursing actions. The three hierarchies were then cross-referenced by using a separate data table (clinical index) that reflected the interrelationships between the hierarchies. This mechanism allowed for viewing the nursing terminology in a contextual hierarchy, which supported the coding integrity of a combinatorial nursing terminology using a poly-hierarchy structure. In MEDCIN®, the creation of the separate hierarchies and the use of a clinical index to form a contextual hierarchy proved to be an appropriate method to integrate the CCC standard for use by nurses and allied health professionals in health information systems.

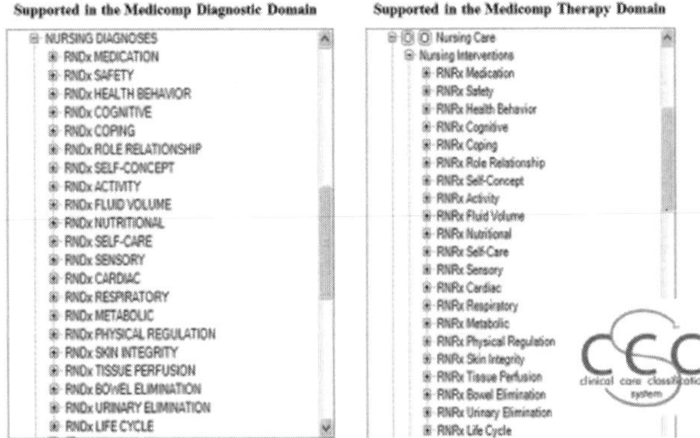

FIGURE 12.4 Clinical Care Classification (CCC) in MEDCIN® (© 2014 Medicomp Systems).

At the point of care, MEDCIN® displays relevant CCC nursing diagnoses, using medical diagnoses or any other patient signs or symptoms in a patient encounter or admission assessment (see Figure 12.5). A subsequent MEDCIN® display (Figure 12.6) is focused on the nursing interventions relevant to a nursing diagnosis with the proper CCC code, allowing for aggregated data analysis.

Component	Map to Potential Nursing Diagnosis
Respiratory	
▪ Pt states is having no shortness of breath	
▪ Respiratory WNL: Breath sounds clear/vesicular throughout all lung fields and bronchial over major airways, no adventitious breath sounds, respirations unlabored, equal chest excursion with inspiration, no coughing, no sputum/secretions	
▪ Pt states feels	
Short of breath	
Fatigued	
Other: ___	
▪ Pt is	
Dusky	
Cyanotic	
Restless	Gas Exchange Impairment
Irritable	
Confused	
Somnolent	
▪ Respiration/breathing characteristics:	
Regular	
Irregular	
Shallow	Breathing Pattern Impairment
Deep	
Absent	
Biot's	
Cheyne-Stokes	
Kussmaul's	
Stridorous	
Expiratory grunt	
Nasal flaring	

FIGURE 12.5 Sample of point-of-care nursing assessment using the CCC (© 2010 S. Taylor).

Nursing Interventions and Action Types:
For Nursing Diagnosis - Respiratory Alteration - Stabilize: (L26.0.2)

Intervention – Pulmonary Care (L36.0.2)

Definition: Actions performed to support the pulmonary hygiene

Nursing Action – Assess respiratory status

Nursing Documentation:

- Document patient findings: dyspnea, abnormal breath sounds, restlessness, confusion

FIGURE 12.6 Example of point-of-care nursing interventions and actions (and documentation detail) in MEDCIN® (© 2014 Medicomp Systems).

The nursing functionality in MEDCIN® is designed specifically to support the data entry functions of a nurse, as well as resourcing and productivity measures. The CCC nursing diagnoses, interventions, action types, and order protocols are interlinked to appropriate clinical diagnoses as part of MEDCIN®. When nursing content is enabled, the nursing content is accessible in the search and browse menus. Nursing content is found in the diagnoses and therapies domains of the MEDCIN Engine®. When browsing to find nursing content, diagnoses can be found in the "Nursing Diagnosis" section of the diagnoses domain in the MEDCIN® hierarchy. Similarly, nursing interventions and actions can be found in the "Nursing Care" section of the therapy domain. Browsing can also be used to derive action documentation detail from the nursing actions for inclusion in the health information workspace.

How to Incorporate the Nursing Process

Although nursing terminology is designed to support the data entry and documentation of nurses, incorporating a nursing terminology into a health information record system requires the incorporation of the nursing process. The systematic incorporation of the nursing process is the crucial component for optimal and integrated use of a nursing terminology standard. The nursing process is the set of criteria that the ANA uses to recognize terminology standards; therefore, the nursing process is the ontology of the professional nurse and must be incorporated into the electronic HIRS to realize the value and benefit of using a nursing terminology for documentation and research.

The ontology of a HIRS affects the collection of nursing information. Nurses typically collect patient data to elicit information to guide nursing actions during care; therefore, the nursing process operationalizes and demonstrates the art and science of nursing. The ANA professional standards and competencies for nurses are based on the six steps of the nursing process:

- Assessment
- Diagnosis
- Outcome Identification
- Planning
- Implementation
- Evaluation

"The six steps of the nursing process describe the component level of nursing care and encompass all significant actions taken by nurses to provide care to patients/clients, and forms the basis for clinical decision making" (Saba, 2007, p. 152). The ANA professional standards allow nurses to practice nursing in a manner that individualizes care to meet a patient's unique needs and situation given that the nurse establishes a caring relationship with patients and families to deliver nursing care. The competent level of nursing care is demonstrated by the nursing process.

The nursing process (ANA, 2010) components are often defined as follows:

- **Patient-centered:** Focused on patient care and adapted to meet patient needs and concerns
- **Goal-oriented:** Interventions are determined by the nursing diagnoses and chosen for the purpose of achieving the nursing outcome.
- **Universally applicable:** As a framework, is appropriate for any patient, of any age, with any clinical diagnosis, at any point on the health continuum and in any setting (for example, school, clinic, hospital, or home) and across all nurse specialties (for example, hospice, maternity, pediatric, etc.)
- **Cognitive process:** Involves nursing judgment and decision-making. The nurse is required to apply nursing knowledge systematically and logically to interpret, analyze, and use data to determine the appropriate plan of care based on

> knowledge of the physical, biological, and behavioral sciences. As part of academic preparation, nurses have biochemistry, biophysics, microbiology, anatomy, physiology, psychology, and sociology courses. This basic knowledge of the sciences enables nurses to recognize patient problems and determine how the patient's health is disrupted by a health problem.

With a nursing terminology standard and the nursing process, now the health information record system needs a nursing plan of care to assess and document the nursing diagnoses/problems of a patient—not only the patient's medical problem. Now a plan of care process begins with the point-of-care application of the ANA nursing process: A nurse must assess the patient, determine the patient's symptoms, assign a nursing diagnosis(es), and then plan nursing interventions. The following sections present an algorithm for the generation of a plan-of-care data tree in MEDCIN® (Medicomp Systems, 2013).

Data Collection

Health information record data used to build the plan of care is currently obtained from MEDCIN® history pool upon clicking the Review Plan of Care button from the Admission, Discharge, and Transfer (ADT) screen with a patient selected. The following data is retrieved from the history pool and passed to the nurse module:

- Data is filtered to include only encounters at or subsequent to the admit date.
- Data is retrieved from the history pool
- A record is included if it has a prefix of "Ordered."
- A record is included if the concept indicates a nursing concept.

Data Tree Build

The following steps are used to build the plan of care data tree:

1. The tree is cleared and initialized with three nodes: Clinical Orders, Active Nursing Diagnoses, and Inactive Nursing Diagnoses.

2. The list of findings is isolated to:
   - Orders (non-nurse findings) with a prefix of "Ordered"
   - Nursing diagnoses (RNDx) that have a CCC code assigned
   - Nursing interventions (RNIx) that have a CCC code assigned
   - Nursing actions (RNAx) that have a complete seven-character CCC code assigned
3. The provider's orders are added as child nodes to the Clinical Order node. These nodes are presented as a two-column table, with the first column containing the encounter date of the finding, and the second column containing the text of the finding.
4. The RNDx items are ordered ascending by the four Care Patterns of the CC: Functional, Physiological, Psychological, and Health Behavior. The last instance of the finding is added as a child node to either the Active Nursing Diagnoses node or the Inactive Nursing Diagnoses node, depending on whether the RNDx is the last instance with "resolved" Outcome (Actual Outcome) or not; an RNDx with one of the CCC outcome prefixes (improved, stabilized, or deteriorated) is considered to be inactive. The caption includes the CCC code, a concept description, CCC Care Pattern, and text that indicates the expected outcome (assigned goal) or actual outcome.
5. For each RNDx added, a list of items is obtained from the therapy domain that includes core RNIx concepts linked in MEDCIN® to the RNDx.
6. For each RNDx added, RNIx concepts are filtered by encounter time and examined so that only the most recent instance of an RNIx is considered. The RNIx is added as a child node to any RNDx where there is a match in the list of core RNIx assigned to the RNDx. This means that if the intervention is present in the index of more than one nursing diagnosis, it will be presented in the plan of care with each. The caption of the entry will include the CCC code and the text (name) of the intervention.
7. For each RNIx added, RNAx concepts are filtered by encounter time and examined so that only the most recent instance of an RNAx is considered. The RNAx is added as a child node to any RNIx where there is a match in the list of RNAx assigned to the RNIx. This means that if the action is present in the index of more than one

nursing intervention, it will be presented in the plan of care with each. The caption of the entry will include the CCC code and text of the nursing action type: Assess, Perform, Teach, or Manage.

Data Management

As of this writing, the following user actions are permitted with any data item in the plan of care presentation:

- The user can drag any data item and drop it on either the note view or the outline view. A dropped item will be entered into the current encounter.
- If the user has Cite Mode turned on, the user can add any item to the current encounter simply by clicking the item, using the left mouse button.
- Clicking an item using the right mouse button will pop up a context menu for selection of various options. For example, right-clicking a nursing diagnosis allows the user to get a list of nursing interventions linked to the nursing diagnosis for entry into the Plan of Care (see Figure 12.7). Also from the context menu are options to link any nursing interventions to the diagnosis, flow sheet the diagnosis, add a diagnosis note, and resolve the diagnosis.

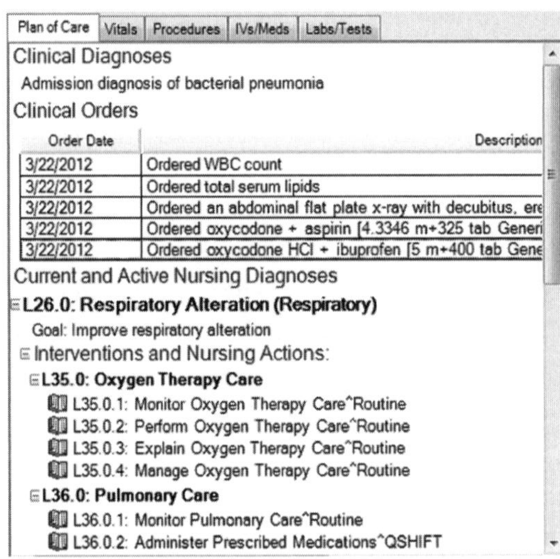

FIGURE 12.7 Sample plan of care in MEDCIN® (© 2014 Medicomp Systems).

Informatics in Action

Fran is 62 years of age and works full time as a cashier at a local grocery store. Fran has just been diagnosed with essential hypertension (HTN). Her identifiable risk factors were her age, family history of HTN in her deceased father, and a reportedly high intake of sodium. You note that her systolic blood pressure (BP) on the last three visits has been between 146 mm Hg and 154 mm Hg. Her diastolic BP was within normal limits (WNL).

Further discussion reveals that Fran continues to eat a diet rather high in sodium and calories, but she is walking 30 minutes 3 days per week. She denies any shortness of breath. Your physical findings reveal the following: a body mass index (BMI) of 25.0 and an apical heart rate of 82 beats per minute and regular. After Fran has been seated for 5 minutes in a chair, feet on the floor and arms supported at heart level, her BP measures 152/82 mm Hg on the right.

Today's blood lab results reveal that her glucose, hematocrit, potassium, creatinine, calcium, and urine studies were all WNL, and a fasting lipid profile was pending. Her practitioner conducts an examination including: auscultation for carotid, abdominal, and femoral bruits; palpation of the thyroid gland; listening to her heart and lungs; palpating her abdomen for the presence of masses and aortic pulsation; examining the lower extremities for edema; and concluding with a neurological assessment. An inspection of her retinas does not reveal changes consistent with HTN.

The practitioner writes a prescription for the diuretic and tells Fran that if this and prescribed lifestyle modifications do not bring her BP to goal, she will likely have to add a second medication. Before she leaves, the practitioner asks you to meet with Fran to make sure she understands the treatment plan and goals of therapy and to update the patient-centered interprofessional care plan.

Nursing Plan of Care

Figure 12.8 is a three-panel layout that reflects the workflow for building a Nursing Plan of Care. The Nursing Diagnoses Prompt Panel reflects the contextual hierarchy related to the clinical diagnosis of Hypertension. The nursing process panel reflects the workflow of the nursing process. The Nursing Plan of Care panel shows the HIRS development of the Care Plan. The nursing terminology and codes in the following figures use the CCC.

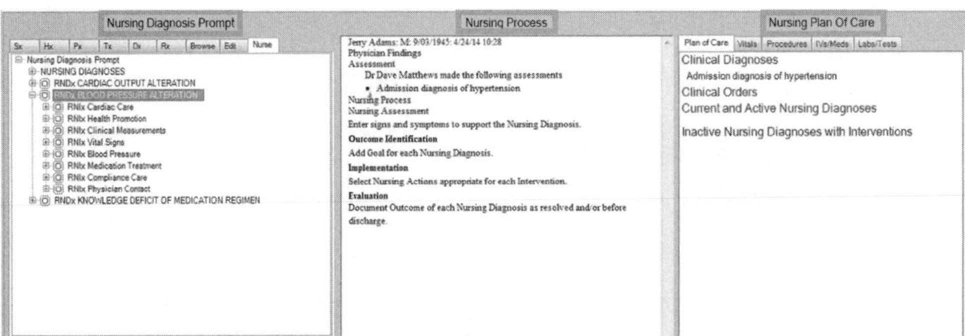

FIGURE 12.8 Example of Interactive Point-of-Care Nursing Plan of Care for hypertension using the nursing process and Intelligent PromptingTM in the MEDCIN® Engine (© 2014 Medicomp Systems).

The first step in the nursing process is to complete the patient **Assessment.** The assessment is shown in the next section. The second step of the nursing process is the selection of the appropriate **Nursing Diagnosis.** This is shown in Figure 12.9.

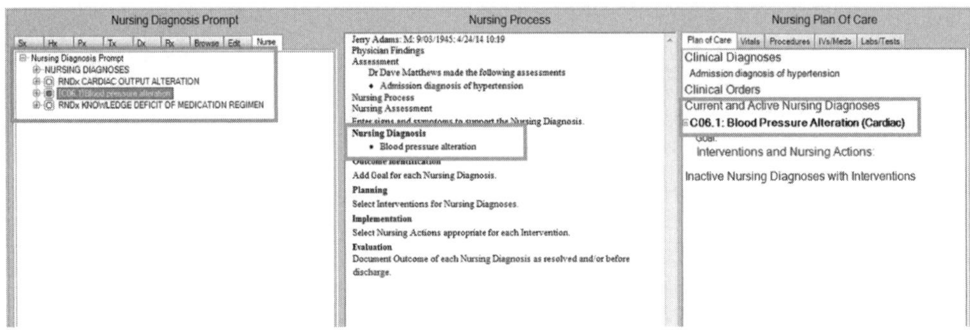

FIGURE 12.9 Selected **Nursing Diagnosis**: *Blood pressure alteration, C06.1* (© 2014 Medicomp Systems).

The next two figures reflect the selection of **Outcomes Identification** following the nursing process.

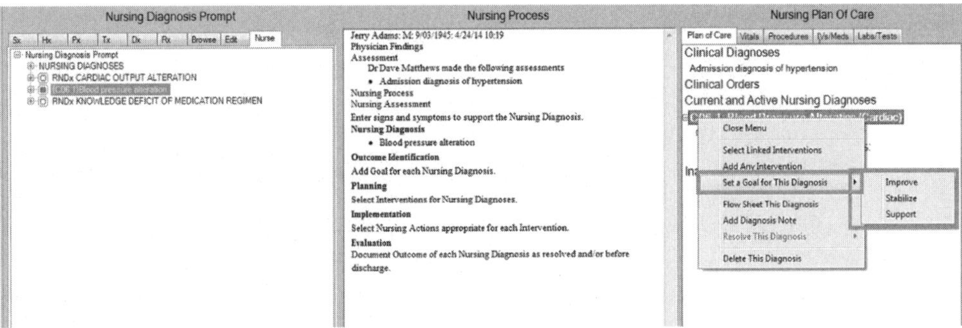

FIGURE 12.10A Selection of **Outcomes Identification** (Expected Outcome): *Improve (Qualifier .1) Blood pressure alteration* (© 2014 Medicomp Systems).

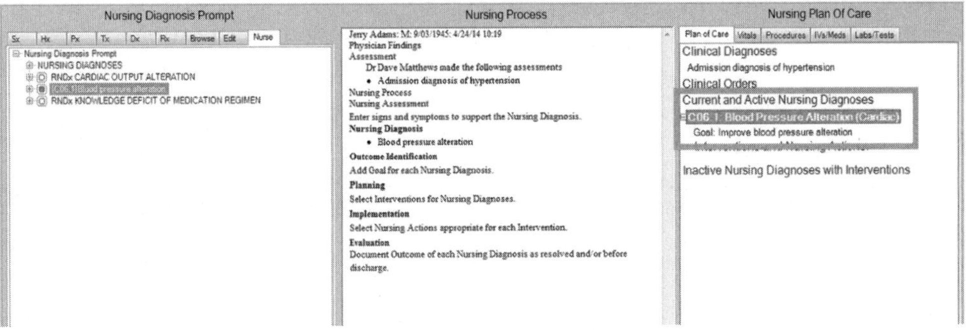

FIGURE 12.10B Outcomes Identification: Improve Blood Pressure Alteration, C06.1.1 (© 2014 Medicomp Systems).

The next two figures reflect the **Planning** step of the nursing process to meet goal of *Improve Blood Pressure Alteration.*

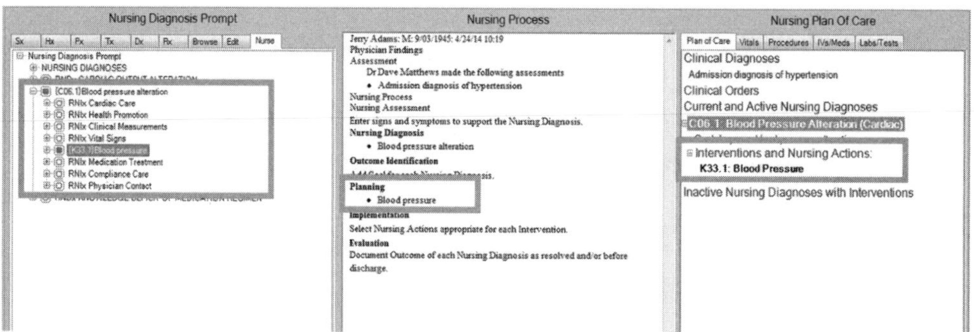

FIGURE 12.11A Planning (Interventions) using Nursing Intervention: Blood Pressure, K33.1 (© 2014 Medicomp Systems).

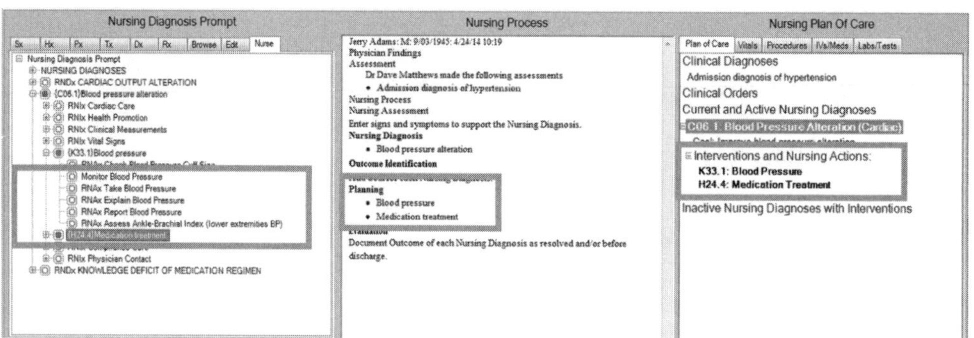

FIGURE 12.11B Planning (Interventions) using Nursing Intervention: Medication Treatment, H24.4 (© 2014 Medicomp Systems).

The next step in the nursing process is **Implementation** with the selection of appropriate nursing actions for each intervention. The nursing actions provide the evidence for clinical decision-making (Saba, 2007, p. 154). The nursing action for implementation of the Nursing Intervention, Blood Pressures is shown in Figure 12.12. To complete the Implementation, step appropriate actions were selected to support the Medication Treatment intervention.

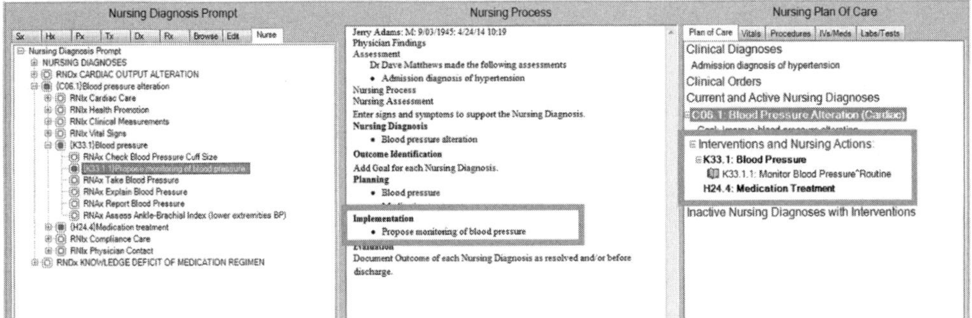

FIGURE 12.12 Implementation (CCC Action Types) such as Monitor Blood Pressure, K33.1.1 (© 2014 Medicomp Systems).

Figure 12.13 reflects the Nursing Plan of Care as developed to this point at the point-of-care based on nursing process using the CCC and MEDCIN®.

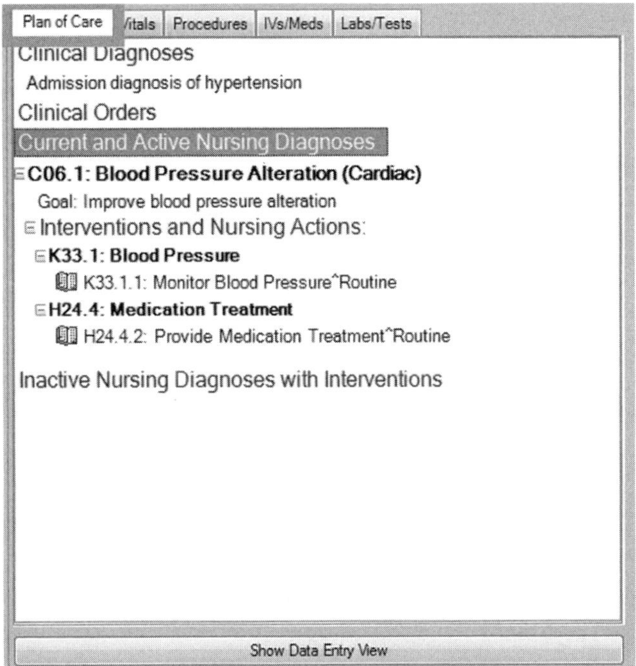

FIGURE 12.13 Sample patient-centered Nursing Plan of Care (© 2014 Medicomp Systems).

The last step of the nursing process is **Evaluation.** Figures 12.14a and 12.14b reflect the actual outcome after all nursing interventions and actions have been performed for a given Nursing Diagnosis. In the CCC, the actual outcomes are Improved, Stabilized, and Deteriorated (Supported).

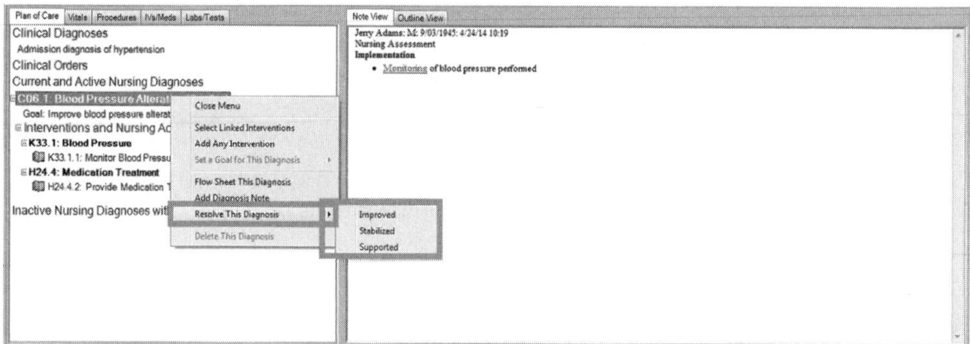

FIGURE 12.14A Choices for Evaluation (Actual Outcome) for Blood Pressure Alteration (Diagnosis) (© 2014 Medicomp Systems).

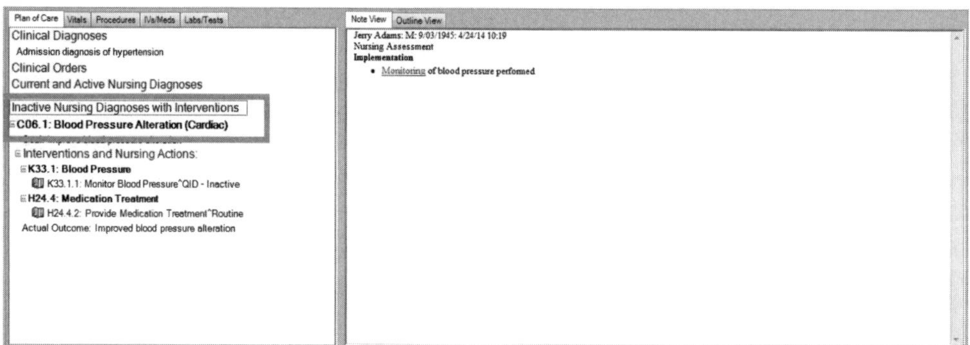

FIGURE 12.14B Nursing Plan of Care with Improved Actual Outcome selected (© 2014 Medicomp Systems).

In this application, when an Actual Outcome (Evaluation) has been assigned to a Nursing Diagnosis, the Diagnosis is placed in an inactive section.

The common language of the nursing process fosters the comparability of nursing data across patient populations and underscores that nursing and interprofessional care plans are needed to support continuous and efficient shared understanding of a patient's care history. The access to the patient's history by the healthcare team aids interprofessional communication and decision-making about the future care of patients (Keenan, Yakel, & Marriott, 2006). Considering that a health record system may have multiple purposes within an organization (such as fulfilling legal and accreditation documentation requirements, professional accountability, and financial billing), the primary function of nursing documentation—to communicate professional assessment about patients to other nurses and providers to ensure continuity and quality outcomes—may be overlooked; thus nursing, as a profession, misses a tremendous source of information about patient care outcomes and the evidence of nursing care effectiveness.

For nurses, patient care planning accompanies every stage of nursing care, beginning with the identification of a patient's problem as part of the nursing process. The acceleration of healthcare quality will require the ability to individualize a patient plan of care. The individual patient care planning process has been important to nursing for more than a century.

> "The diversity and size of the nursing profession make it difficult for us to communicate with each other, other health providers, and the public. It is imperative nurses share a common language for the purpose of fostering the comparability of nursing data across patient populations with the ultimate goal being the improvement of health care" (McCloskey & Bulechek, 1994, p. 56).

See Figures 12.15–12.20 for examples of a point-of-care nursing care plan prompted based on standard nursing terminology, the CCC, and patient-centered nursing assessments using MEDCIN® and Quippe™ (Medicomp Systems, 2014).

The nursing terminology in the following figures uses the CCC.

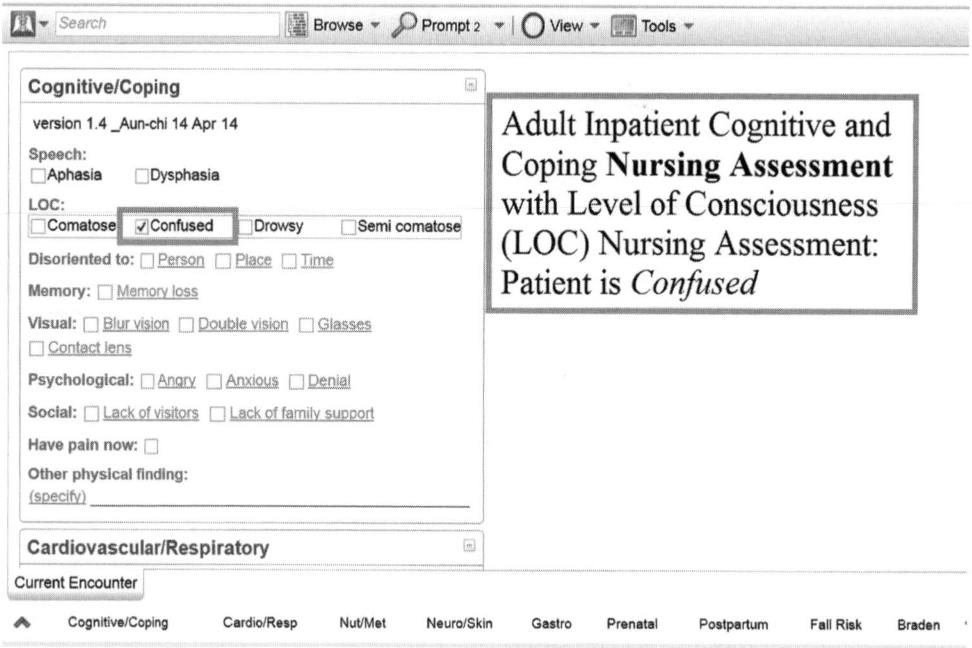

FIGURE 12.15 Example of point-of-care nursing care plan prompted based on standard nursing terminology and patient-centered nursing assessments using MEDCIN® and Quippe™ (© 2014 Medicomp Systems).

TIP

Quippe™ is a documentation tool deployed locally or over the Internet on both mobile and desktop devices powered by the MEDCIN Engine®.

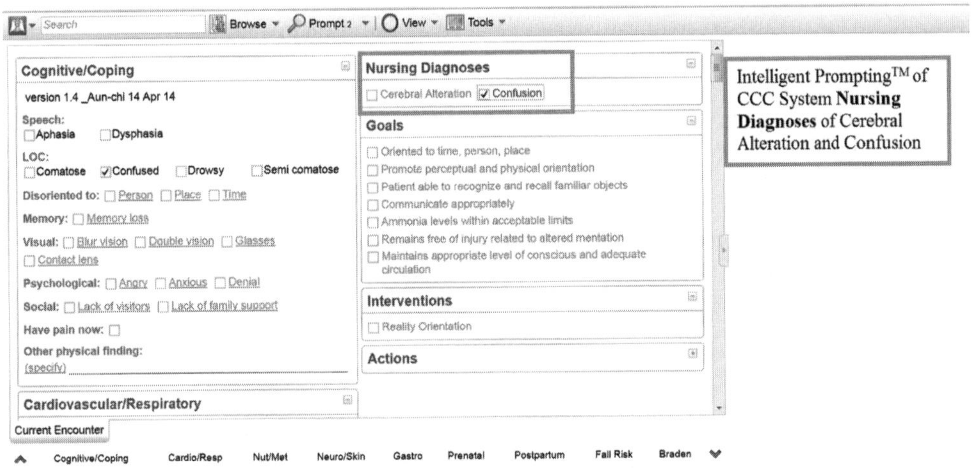

FIGURE 12.16 Nursing Diagnosis prompted based on Nursing Assessment documentation (© 2014 Medicomp Systems).

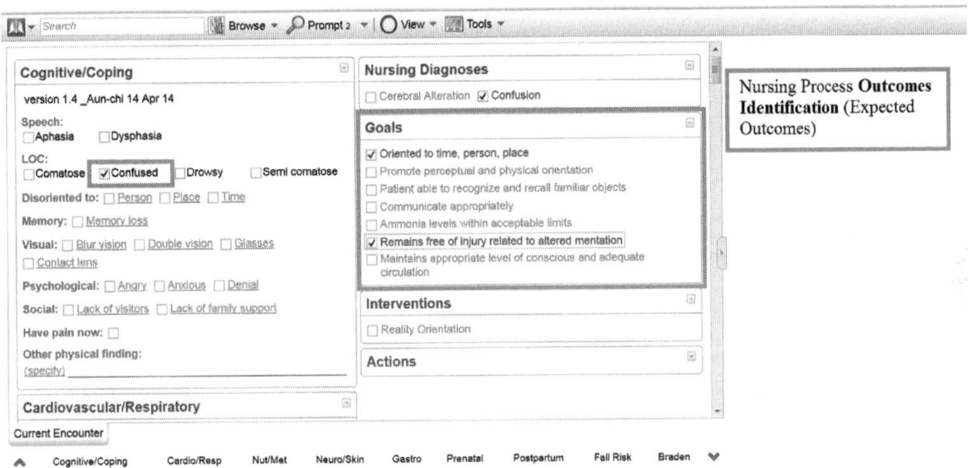

FIGURE 12.17 Prompted Outcomes Identification (© 2014 Medicomp Systems).

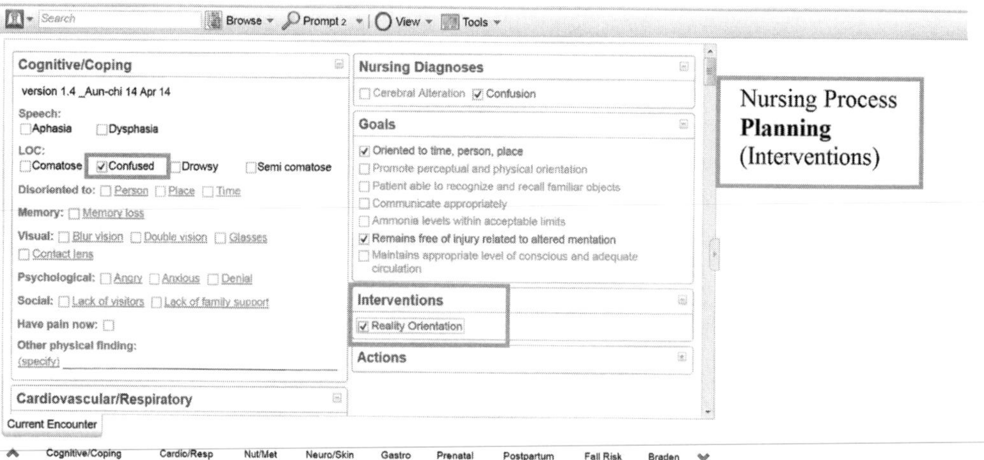

FIGURE 12.18 Prompted Planning (Intervention) (© 2014 Medicomp Systems).

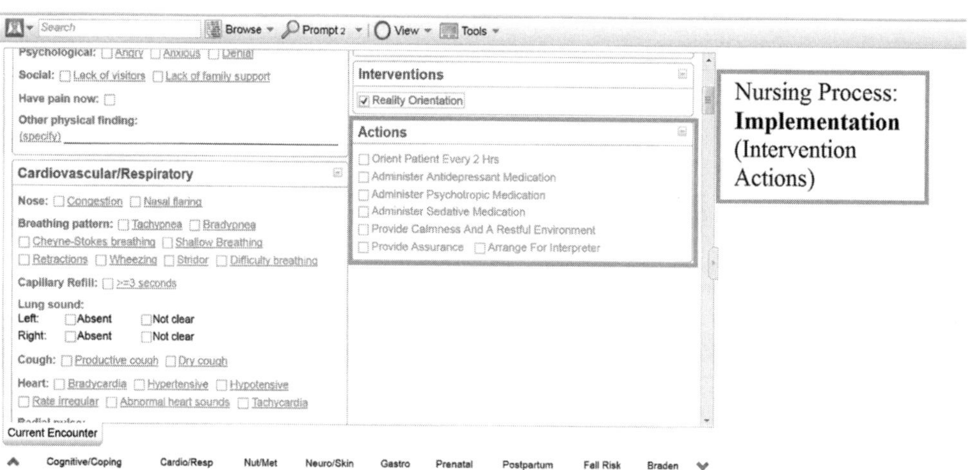

FIGURE 12.19 Prompted Implementation (Intervention Action Types) (© 2014 Medicomp Systems).

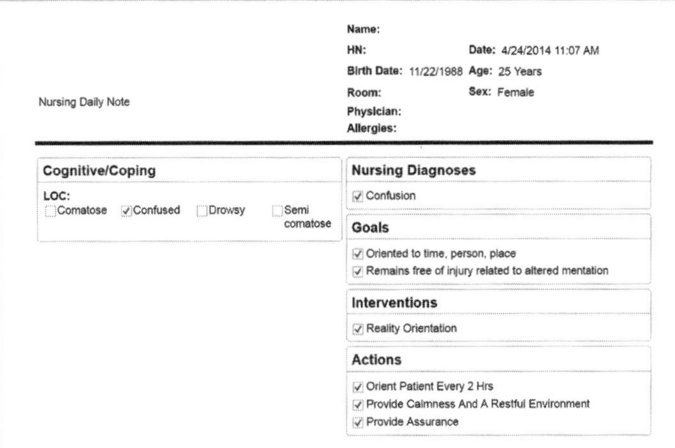

FIGURE 12.20 Sample Nursing Care Plan (© 2014 Medicomp Systems).

Future Directions

> "Two significant challenges have always faced nursing: (a) how to differentiate nursing's contributions to patient care from those of medicine; and (b) how to incorporate descriptions of nursing care into the health record in a manner that is commensurate with its importance to patients' welfare" (Thede & Schwiran, 2011, para. 1).

This chapter has discussed how to apply computer technology to nursing documentation by using standard terminology and the nursing process to achieve patient-centered, interprofessional care plans. Nurses who use nursing diagnoses need to define the patient assessment (signs and symptoms) of patient problems, provide the appropriate interventions and, finally, observe the patients' responses to the care process (Carpenito, 2000).

With the implementation of electronic nursing documentation systems using coded, standardized nursing language and the nursing process, nurse managers are able to query the electronic nursing documentation application about nursing workload, the actions required to provide care, and evaluate the outcomes of nursing care—the results of care—and examine what nursing actions improved care. We are confident the clinical documentation applications of the future that use standard nursing terminology and follow the nursing process will be sufficiently flexible to meet the professional documentation needs of nursing and allied health professionals in all clinical settings.

References

American Nurses Association (ANA). (2006, January 18). *Background on nursing practice information infrastructure.* In ANA Nursing World. Retrieved from http://ana.nursingworld.org/npii/about.htm

American Nurses Association (ANA). (2008). *Nursing Informatics: Scope and standards of practice.* Silver Spring, MD: Nursesbooks.org

American Nurses Association (ANA). (2010). *Nursing: Scope and standards of practice*, 2nd ed. Silver Spring, MD: Nursesbooks.org.

American Nurses Association (ANA). (2012, June 4). *ANA recognized terminologies that support nursing practice.* Retrieved from http://nursingworld.org/npii/terminologies.htm

Carpenito, L. J. (2000). *Nursing diagnosis: Application to clinical practice*, 8th ed. Philadelphia, PA: J. B. Lippincott.

Cimino, J. J. (1998). Desiderata for controlled medical vocabularies in the twenty-first century. *Methods of Information in Medicine, 37*(4-5), 394–403.

Cimino, J. J., Hripcsak, G., Johnson, S. B., & Clayton, P. D. (1989). Designing an introspective, multipurpose, controlled medical vocabulary. In L. C. Kingsland (Ed.). *Proceedings of the thirteenth annual symposium on computer applications in medical care.* New York, NY: IEEE Computer Society Press: 513–518.

Coenen, A. (2003). The International Classification for Nursing Practice (ICNP®) programme: Advancing a unifying framework for nursing. *OJIN: The Online Journal of Issues in Nursing.* Retrieved from www.nursingworld.org/MainMenuCategories/ANAMarketplace/ANAPeriodicals/OJIN/TableofContents/Volume82003/No2May2003/ArticlesPreviousTopics/TheInternationalClassificationforNursingPractice.aspx

Data. (n.d). In *Math is fun, using and handling data.* Retrieved from http://www.mathsisfun.com/data/data.html

Hardiker, N. R., Bakken, S., Casey, A., & Hoy, D. (2002). Formal nursing terminology systems: Means to an end. *Journal of Biomedical Informatics, 35*(5-6), 298–305.

Huber, D. G., Delaney, C., Crossley, J., Mehmert, M., & Ellerbe, S. (1992). A nursing management minimum data set: Significance and development. *Journal of Nursing Administration, 22*(7-8), 35–40.

Hunter, M. K., & Bickford, C. J. (2011). The practice specialty of nursing informatics. In V. K. Saba & K. A. McCormick (Eds.), *Essential of nursing informatics,* 5th ed. (pp. 171–189). New York, NY: McGraw Hill Medical.

ICNP. (2014). In World Health Organization, *Classification.* Retrieved from http://www.who.int/classifications/icd/adaptations/icnp/en/

IHTSDO. (n.d.). In SNOMED CT, *History of SNOMED CT.* Retrieved from http://www.ihtsdo.org/snomed-ct/history0/

IHTSDO. (2014). *SNOMED CT starter guide.* Retrieved from http://www.snomed.org/doc.

Institute of Medicine. (2001). *Crossing the quality chasm: A new health system for the 21st century.* Washington, DC: National Academies Press.

ISO. (n.d.). In ISO, *Standards.* Retrieved from http://www.iso.org/iso/home/standards.htm

Kane N. M. , & Siegrist, R. B. (2006). In L. Unruh & S. Hassmiller (2007). Legislative: Economics of nursing invitational conference addresses quality and payment issues in nursing care. *The Online Journal of Issues in Nursing, 13*(1), 5-9.

Keenan, G. M., Yakel, E., & Marriott, D. (2006, June). HANDS: A revitalized technology supported care planning method to improve nursing handoffs. Paper presented at the *9th International Congress on Nursing Informatics.* Seoul, Korea.

LOINC®. (1994-2014). In LOINC® from Regenstrief, *LOINC background.* Retrieved from http://loinc.org/background

Martin, K. S., & Scheet, N. J. (1992). *The Omaha System: Applications for community health nursing.* Philadelphia, PA: W. B. Saunders Company.

Matney, S., Bakken, S., & Huff, S. M. (2003). Representing nursing assessment in clinical information systems using the Logical Observation Identifiers Names and Codes database. *Journal of Biomedical Informatics, 36*(4-5), 287–293.

McCloskey, J. C., & Bulechek, G. M. (1994). Standardizing the language for nursing treatments: An overview of the issues. *Nursing Outlook, 42*(2), 56–63.

Medicomp Systems. (2013, February 19). In Media Center, Medicomp takes MEDCIN® global. Retrieved from http://www.medicomp.com/news/

Moen, A., Gregory, J., & Brennan, P. F. (2007). Cross cultural factors necessary to enable design of flexible consumer health informatics systems (CHIS). *International Journal of Medical Informatics, 76*(1), 168–173.

Park, H. T., Lu, D. F., Konicek, D., & Delaney, C. (2007). Nursing interventions classification in systematized nomenclature of medicine clinical terms: A cross-mapping validation. *CIN: Computers Informatics Nursing, 25*(4), 198–208. doi:10.1097/01.NCN.0000280590.35690.7d

Saba, V. K. (1992). The classification of home health care nursing diagnoses and interventions. *Caring, 10*(3), 50–57.

Saba, V. K. (2007). *Clinical Care Classification (CCC) System manual: A guide to nursing documentation.* New York, NY: Springer Publishing.

Saba, V. K. (2012). *Clinical Care Classification (CCC) System, version 2.5: User's guide.* New York, NY: Springer Publishing.

Schwiran, P., & Thede, L. (2012). Informatics: The standardized nursing terminologies: A national survey of nurses' experiences and attitudes – Survey II: Participants, familiarity and information sources. *OJIN: The Online Journal of Issues in Nursing, (17)*2. Retrieved from http://www.nursingworld.org/MainMenuCategories/ANAMarketplace/ANAPeriodicals/OJIN/Columns/Informatics/Standardized-Nursing-Terminologies-SURVEY-II.html; doi:10.3912/OJIN.Vol17No02InfoCol01

Smolij, K., & Dun, K. (2006). Patient health information management: Searching for the right model. *Perspectives in Health Information Management, 3,* 10–15.

Snyder, R., Weston, M. J., Fields, W., Rizos, A., & Tedeschi, C. (2006). Computerized provider order entry system field research: The impact of contextual factors on study implementation. *International Journal of Medical Informatics, 75,* 730–740.

Taylor, S. (2010). *Adult admission assessment care components* (unpublished manuscript).

Thede, L., & Schwiran, P. (2011). Informatics: The standardized nursing terminologies: A national survey of nurses' experiences and attitudes–Survey I. *OJIN: The Online Journal of Issues in Nursing, (16)*2. doi:10.3912/OJIN.Vol16No02InfoCol01. Retrieved from http://nursingworld.org/MainMenuCategories/ANAMarketplace/ANAPeriodicals/OJIN/Columns/Informatics/Standardized-Nursing-Terminologies.html

Thede, L. Q., & Sewell, J. P. (2010). *Informatics and nursing: Opportunities and challenges* (3rd ed.). Philadelphia, PA: Lippincott, Williams & Wilkins.

Turpin, P. (2005). Transitioning from paper to computerized documentation. *Gastroenterology Nursing, 6*(7), 61–62.

USA NMDS. (n.d.). In University of Minnesota School of Nursing, Minimum Data Sets. Retrieved from http://www.nursing.umn.edu/icnp/minimum-data-sets/

Werley, H. H., Devine, E., Zorn, C. R., Ryan, P., & Westra, B. L. (1991). The nursing minimum data set: Abstraction tool for standardized, comparable, essential data. *American Journal of Public Health, 81*(4), 421–426.

Whittenburg, L. (Ed.). (2013). *HIMSS dictionary of healthcare information technology terms, acronyms and organizations.* Chicago, IL: Healthcare Information and Management Systems Society.

Zielstorff, R. D. (1998). Characteristics of a good nursing nomenclature from an informatics perspective. *OJIN: The Online Journal of Issues in Nursing, 3*(2). Retrieved from http://www.nursingworld.org/MainMenuCategories/ANAMarketplace/ANAPeriodicals/OJIN/TableofContents/Vol31998/No2Sept1998/CharacteristicsofNomenclaturefromInformaticsPerspective.html

Recommended Reading

Rector, A. L. (1999). Clinical terminology: Why is it so hard? *Methods of Information in Medicine, 38*(4), 239–252.

Saba, V. K. (2002). Nursing classifications: Home Health Care Classification System (HHCC): An Overview, OJIN: The Online Journal of Issues in Nursing. Retrieved www.nursingworld.org/MainMenuCategories/ANAMarketplace/ANAPeriodicals/OJIN/TableofContents/Volume72002/No3Sept2002/ArticlesPreviousTopic/HHCCAnOverview.html

Saba, V. K., & Zuckerman, A. E. (1992). A new home health classification method. *Caring Magazine, 11*(9), 27–34.

Sicotte, C., Denis, J. L., & Lehoux, P. (1998). The computer based patient record: A strategic issue in process innovation. *Journal of Medical Systems, 22*(6), 431–443.

SNOMED CT. (n.d.). In NIH National Library of Medicine, Unified Medical Language System. Retrieved from http://www.nlm.nih.gov/research/umls/Snomed/snomed_main.html

Wooley, N. (1990). Nursing diagnosis: Exploring the factors which may influence the reasoning process. *Journal of Advanced Nursing, 15*, 10–117.

"To err is human, to cover up is unforgivable, and to fail to learn is inexcusable."

–Sir Liam Donaldson

Patient Safety and Healthcare IT

13

Patricia P. Sengstack, DNP, RN-BC, CPHIMS

OBJECTIVES

- Discuss challenges that have led to increased scrutiny of electronic health record (EHR) safety.
- Discuss the key areas of focus for healthcare IT safety work by the Office of the National Coordinator for Health IT.
- Identify resources and tools available for informatics specialists to use in the improvement of safety using healthcare IT.
- Describe the importance of a standard method for healthcare IT safety event reporting.

Every organization should ask itself two questions in regards to their electronic health record (EHR). First, is the EHR optimized to improve the safety of care delivery? In other words, have you taken advantage of the capabilities that an electronic record provides to improve patient safety that was just not possible with pen-and-paper records? And second, is the EHR safe to use? In other words, can you blame your EHR for errors or mistakes made in the healthcare setting? This second question has caused much discussion and even some controversy in recent years and will be the focus of this chapter on health information technology (IT) and patient safety.

Since the Institute of Medicine (IOM) report *To Err is Human* was published in 1999, patient safety has been on the healthcare agenda more than ever before (Kohn, Corrigan, & Donaldson, 1999). Those of us on the front lines of patient care may not have been as surprised as to the general public about the volume of errors reported in our healthcare organizations, because healthcare is complex, and care delivery is multifaceted and nonlinear, and can be a perfect set up for errors. If you consider the number of people, disciplines, and times a patient is "touched" literally and figuratively in some way during a healthcare encounter, it is a wonder that the reported errors are not higher. Enter the EHR. Will this be the answer to reduce medical errors and improve the quality and safety of care that we deliver to our patients?

Adoption of the EHR began back in the 1970s with relatively slow adoption until the signing of the Health Information Technology for Economic and Clinical Health (HITECH) Act in 2009 (Goolsby, 2002). The HITECH Act allocated more than $17 billion to stimulate the adoption of quality health IT systems or EHRs that demonstrate meaningful use as defined by the Office of the National Coordinator (ONC) for Health Information Technology (U.S. Department of Health & Human Services [HHS], 2009). As an agency of the Department of Health and Human Services (HHS), the ONC launched the Meaningful Use program that provided the impetus and structure for organizations to adopt EHRs in a meaningful way. In a 2013 report to Congress on the progress of the program, the ONC reported that between 2011 and 2012, the percentage of hospitals possessing certified EHR technology increased from 72% to 85% (ONC, 2013c).

Organizations have been installing these systems at a rapid pace as the much sought-after incentive dollars are captured. It should not come as a shock that implementation of these complex systems at such a fast pace would result in unintended consequences, many of which have the potential to impact patient safety. In this chapter, background information will be provided regarding the concept of healthcare IT and patient safety, along with U.S. federal government efforts to support technology to improve patient safety. More importantly, there will be a focus on resources, tools, and evaluative methods to apply to practice settings with the goal of improving the quality and safety of patient care using technology.

Background

Over the last several decades, the quest for a safer healthcare system has focused on technology as the solution. The resounding theme in the late 1990s and early 2000s was that the EHR would provide that safety net. In fact, there have been numerous publications supporting the concept that those EHRs that are implemented and configured well can improve the safety of our patients. These studies include randomized controlled trials, cohort studies, pre-/post-studies, and several systematic reviews. (Ammenwerth, Schnell-Inderst, Machan, & Sievert, 2008; Franklin, O'Grady, Donyai, Jacklin, & Barber, 2007; Kaushal, Shojania, & Bates, 2003; Reckmann, Westbrook, Koh, Lo, & Day, 2009; Shulman, Singer, Goldstone, & Bellingan, 2005). These articles conclude that EHRs with computerized provider order entry (CPOE) can result in improvements to patient safety, but also conclude that more research is needed and generalizability is limited.

As these EHR systems were introduced into the complex and chaotic world of healthcare, unintended consequences began to appear, some of which are adverse and result in harm to the patient. Reports and publications began to pepper the literature and the Internet with actual and potential errors that point to the EHR as the actual cause of errors. A study published by Koppel et al. in 2005 in the *Journal of the American Medical Association* reported that CPOE systems can actually facilitate medication errors. This article identified 22 types of medication error risks associated with the use of CPOE.

Other studies published indicating the error potential of EHRs include multiple retrospective and chart review studies, a retrospective pre-/post-study, case studies, and descriptive qualitative studies (Han et al., 2005; Horsky, Kuperman, & Patel, 2005; Walsh et al., 2006). In one qualitative study by Campbell, Sittig, Ash, Guappone, and Dykstra (2006), researchers attempted to identify the types of unintended consequences seen with the implementation of EHR systems with CPOE. One category, "Generation of New Kinds of Errors," indicated that new types of errors appear when EHRs with CPOE are implemented. Examples of items in this category include adjacency or juxtaposition errors when users select an item next to the intended choice; a wrong patient being selected; desensitization to alerts ("alert fatigue"); confusing order options; and system design issues with poor data organization and display. Users get frustrated or confused trying to find the right field to enter a particular data item and then end up entering orders on generic screens with free text fields, bypassing any rules and alerts configured—all potentially leading to medication errors (Campbell et al., 2006).

To reinforce, the literature on the potentially negative aspects of EHR safety concludes that more research is needed and that generalizability is limited.

Institute of Medicine – Health IT and Patient Safety Report

Noting increasing dissatisfaction in the usability and safety of EHRs, the ONC made a request to the Institute of Medicine (IOM) to assemble a panel of experts to assess the current state of health IT safety and provide recommendations for improvement. In November, 2011, the IOM published the report titled, "Health IT and Patient Safety: Building Safer Systems for Better Care" (IOM, 2011). This document provides a comprehensive description of the state of electronic health records in their quest to improve safety and offered 10 recommendations. A summarized version of these recommendations can be found in Table 13.1.

Table 13.1 IOM Recommendations for Improving Safety of Health IT

The Secretary of HHS should publish an action and surveillance plan within 12 months that includes a schedule for working with the private sector to assess the impact of health IT on patient safety and minimizing the risk of its implementation and use.
The Secretary of HHS should ensure insofar as possible that health IT vendors support the free exchange of information about health IT experiences and issues and not prohibit sharing of such information, including details (for example, screenshots of vendor EHRs) relating to patient safety.
The ONC should work with the private and public sectors to make comparative user experiences across vendors publicly available.
The Secretary of HHS should fund a new Health IT Safety Council to evaluate criteria for assessing and monitoring the safe use of health IT and the use of health IT to enhance safety. This council should operate within an existing voluntary consensus standards organization.
All health IT vendors should be required to publicly register and list their products with the ONC, initially beginning with EHRs certified for the Meaningful Use program.
The Secretary of HHS should specify the quality and risk management process requirements that health IT vendors must adopt, with a particular focus on human factors, safety culture, and usability.
The Secretary of HHS should establish a mechanism for both vendors and users to report health IT–related deaths, serious injuries, or unsafe conditions.
The Secretary of HHS should recommend that Congress establish an independent federal entity for investigating patient safety deaths, serious injuries, or potentially unsafe conditions associated with health IT. This entity should also monitor and analyze data and publicly report results of these activities.

The Secretary of HHS should monitor and publicly report on the progress of health IT safety annually, beginning in 2012. If progress toward safety and reliability is not sufficient as determined by the Secretary, the Secretary should direct FDA to exercise all available authorities to regulate EHRs, health information exchanges, and personal health records (PHRs).

The Secretary should immediately direct the Food and Drug Administration (FDA) to begin developing the necessary framework for regulation. Such a framework should be in place if and when the Secretary decides the state of health IT safety requires FDA regulation.

HHS, in collaboration with other research groups, should support cross-disciplinary research toward the use of health IT as part of a learning healthcare system. Products of this research should be used to inform the design, testing, and use of health IT.

The report reinforces the fact that sound evidence to clearly define the magnitude of the risk associated with EHRs is limited. IOM recognizes the current dissatisfaction with poor user interface design, poor workflow support, and complex data interfaces as being threats to patient safety. It is clear in this report that the need to develop strategies to standardize the reporting of health IT–related errors is needed. The problem cannot be measured or analyzed when error reporting structures are heterogeneous, not mandated, and often ignored.

There is also an emphasis on increasing the transparency of reporting from both vendors and system users as the industry learns and improves. It promotes a multifaceted approach and calls for vendor participation and IT user involvement, with governmental support and oversight (IOM, 2011). Understandably, one recommendation calls for further research to better understand many of the concepts surrounding the safe use of EHRs. Table 13.2 includes the recommended areas for further research. To ensure that follow-up was part of the ongoing plan, the IOM recommended that the ONC develop an action plan within 12 months of publication so that improvements would proceed in a strategic way.

Table 13.2 IOM Recommended Research Areas

Problem	*Solution Question*
Work organization	How can IT be designed to better support the clinical work activities of health professionals?
Information structure	How can health IT be used to create meaningful representations of clinical data and knowledge?
Pick-list	How can lists be presented so that their order and appearance make it easy to know what choices are available and easier to select the desired item?
Alarm/alert	How can the use of alerts be managed at the system level so that clinicians receive useful alerts?
Cooperative work	How can health IT be designed and configured to assist cooperative work?
Accountability and reimbursement	Can health IT be configured to encourage recording of high-quality clinical observations rather than just the accumulation of clinically meaningless filler?
Availability	What is the real impact of system outages? How often does this occur? How can the effects be determined?
Interoperability at the user level	Is it possible to make health IT interoperable at the user level so that clinicians moving from one facility to another do not have to learn a new way of doing things each time?

ONCs Safety Plan

In response to the IOM report, the ONC published the *Health IT Patient Safety Action & Surveillance Plan* in July, 2013 (ONC, 2013a), which reiterated the challenge of determining whether health IT can be identified as the true cause of medical errors given the limitations on the recent research. With so many unknowns and the need to clearly define health IT–related errors, a call to action is stressed. The *ONC Action and Surveillance Plan* addresses the need to focus on learning and the assessment of the current state prior to moving toward a quick solution. It calls for strong leadership at all levels to continue to take on the task of realizing the safety potential of these systems with a goal of inspiring confidence and trust in health IT.

The ONC Action and Surveillance Plan revolves around three key areas—Learning, Improving, and Leading—with two main objectives: (1) Use health IT to make care safer, and (2) continuously improve the safety of health IT (ONC, 2013a). Recognizing the limited body of evidence in this area, the ONC learning focus aims to increase the quantity and quality of data and knowledge about health IT safety. The establishment of processes and mechanisms that facilitate reporting among users and vendors of health IT is recommended, along with strengthening the use of state and national Patient Safety Organizations (PSOs) to help collect and report on these issues. PSOs have emerged as part of the Patient Safety and Quality Improvement Act of 2005. As of this writing, the Agency for Healthcare Research and Quality (AHRQ) lists 77 PSOs in 29 states. These evolving organizations will help in the collection of data on patient safety and submit nonidentified data to the AHRQ Network of Patient Safety Databases (ONC, 2013a).

Additionally, it is recognized that not only do we need standard terminologies to report health IT related errors, but we also need processes to report them centrally and a method to aggregate and analyze the data. The goal is to make it easy for clinicians to report patient safety events to PSOs using standard terminologies such as the AHRQ Common Formats that are reviewed later in the chapter. The ONC proposes to support PSOs in their work to collect, aggregate, and analyze the data related to health IT safety.

In addition to learning more about health IT and patient safety, the ONC plans to focus on improvement efforts. Capitalizing on the potential of health IT and its ability to support safe care—like that never possible with the hard copy chart—is clearly the mission of this work. The objective is to develop resources and evidence-based corrective actions to improve health IT safety and patient safety. To support the establishment of priorities in health IT safety initiatives, the ONC will align with the National Quality Strategy, the Meaningful Use program as part of the HITECH Act, and the Centers for Medicare and Medicaid Services Partnership for Patients initiative. Through priorities established by these organizations, ONC safety work will focus on:

- Adverse drug events
- Catheter-associated urinary tract infections

- Central line–associated blood stream infections
- Readmissions
- Ventilator-associated pneumonia
- Pressure ulcers
- Surgical site infections
- Obstetrical adverse events
- Venous thromboembolism
- Injuries from falls and immobility

Using health IT to improve in these areas will help drive the patient safety effort. The plan additionally intends to continue the work of the Meaningful Use program that supports and encourages safe and meaningful use of health IT. This effort includes configuring EHRs with CPOE to reduce medication errors using decision-support tools, such as allergy alerting, dose range checking, improving reconciliation of medications across care settings, and many other methods to assist in error reduction (ONC, 2013a).

To support this work over the next several years, ONC recognizes the need for strong leadership. Several strategies address the direction that needs to be supported to make these efforts successful. In addition to providing methods to engage all key stakeholders, ONC is planning to develop a strategy and recommend an appropriate, risk-based regulatory framework for health IT. This framework includes working collaboratively with other federal agencies, such as the U.S. Food and Drug Administration (FDA) and the Federal Communications Commission (FCC) (FDA, 2013).Through efforts coordinated by ONC, HHS will monitor the Health IT Safety Program and strive toward the goal of patients and providers having confidence in the safety of health IT (ONC, 2013a).

Health IT Safety Tools and Resources

Resources for organizations to use when configuring, assessing, and evaluating the safety of their clinical systems have been emerging over the last several years. They provide excellent tools for informaticists with varying levels of expertise in charge of developing organizational health IT safety strategies. These tools include:

- AHRQ web-based *Guide to Reducing Unintended Consequences in Electronic Health Records*
- AHRQ Common Formats for reporting adverse events
- AHRQ Hazard Manager
- Institute for Safe Medication Practices *Guidelines for Standard Order Sets*
- Safety Assurance Factors for EHR Resilience (SAFER) Guides
- ECRI Institute "How to Identify and Address Unsafe Conditions Associated with Health IT"
- The CPOE Design Recommendations Checklist
- The Pick-list Checklist

AHRQ Guide to Reducing Unintended Consequences of Electronic Health Records

The AHRQ *Guide to Reducing Unintended Consequences of Electronic Health Records* is a web-based tool designed to help organizations identify, anticipate, mitigate, and address problems that can occur when implementing and using an EHR. The guide addresses both future and current EHR users with practical knowledge as well as recommendations for safety assessments. Within the links on the website, there are resources that guide new and experienced EHR adopters through the identification and remediation of the unintended consequences that can surface when using an electronic record. It provides information on how to survive a system downtime and includes a copy-and-paste toolkit as organizations struggle to address the complexities of this functionality. Case studies are provided on safety-related topics along with remediation solutions to several challenges in health IT (Jones et al., 2011), and can be accessed via the ONC website:

http://www.healthit.gov/unintended-consequences/

QUESTIONS

How does your organization identify unintended consequences or errors related to the use of EHRs?

After looking through the *AHRQ Guide to Reducing Unintended Consequences of Electronic Health Records,* what tools or resources would you find the most helpful in your organizations journey to improve safety using technology?

Do you have a method for the end users of your system to report any potentially unsafe conditions or practices when using the EHR?

AHRQ Common Formats

With the increasing adoption of health IT, AHRQ has increased efforts to study and provide resources to help organizations make improvements to care delivery using technology. One area of focus for AHRQ has been the development of Common Formats for reporting patient safety events. The AHRQ vision, along with that of the ONC, is that the reporting of health IT safety issues will occur not just at the organizational level but at the national level as well. In using the Common Formats for reporting, it is hoped that standardized aggregate data will provide valuable analysis and trending that can lead to more focused efforts and significant improvements in patient safety. In line with the saying that we have all become familiar with, "If you can't measure it, you can't improve it," AHRQ hopes that organizations will adopt these formats as they collect, analyze, and report health IT–related errors. Interestingly though, the Common Formats themselves, along with resources and tools for implementation, are not found on the AHRQ website. They are found on the PSO Privacy Protection Center (PSOPPC) website (AHRQ, 2013):

https://psoppc.org/web/patientsafety/commonformats

To collect data using the AHRQ Common Formats (Hospital Version 1.2 – April 2012), a report has been developed and is offered via the PSOPPC website. This specific Patient Safety Event Report is titled, "Device or Medical/Surgical Supply, Including Health Information Technology (HIT)." There are 26 questions to respond to in this report, each with multi-select lists to identify at a more granular level the exact error and its potential cause. Although this report is not mandated for use by organizations, it is hoped that adoption will increase, or that the terms will be integrated into current tools used to capture adverse events and near-miss situations. A screenshot of some questions from this report is shown in Figure 13.1 (AHRQ, 2013).

21. Which of the following best characterizes the type of HIT device related to the event or unsafe condition?
CHECK ONE:

a. ☐ Administrative/billing or practice management system

> **22. Which component of the administrative/billing system?**
> CHECK ONE:
>
> a. ☐ Master patient index
> b. ☐ Registration/appointment scheduling system
> c. ☐ Coding/billing system
> d. ☐ Unknown
> e. ☐ Other: PLEASE SPECIFY ______

b. ☐ Automated dispensing system

c. ☐ Electronic health record (EHR) or component of EHR

> **23. Which type or component of the EHR?** CHECK ONE:
>
> a. ☐ Computerized provider order entry (CPOE) system
> b. ☐ Pharmacy system
> c. ☐ Electronic medication administration record (e-MAR)
> d. ☐ Clinical documentation system (e.g., progress notes)
> e. ☐ Clinical decision support (CDS) system
> f. ☐ Unknown
> g. ☐ Other: PLEASE SPECIFY ______

d. ☐ Human interface device (e.g., keyboard, mouse, touchscreen, speech recognition system, monitor/display, printer)

e. ☐ Laboratory information system (LIS), including microbiology and pathology systems

f. ☐ Radiology/diagnostic imaging system, including picture archiving and communications system (PACS)

g. ☐ Other: PLEASE SPECIFY ______

FIGURE 13.1 AHRQ Common Formats: PSO Privacy Protection Center.

AHRQ Hazard Manager

In 2011, AHRQ completed beta testing of another tool called the Health IT Hazard Manager. This tool has undergone extensive testing, and gives health IT developers and researchers a method of capturing and managing error event data using web-based software. It includes areas to document near miss-errors and actual errors with an ultimate goal of providing essential improvement information as well as data transmission to PSOs. With widespread use, healthcare organizations, vendors, policymakers, and researchers could request access to view de-identified, aggregate reports of hazard attributes (Walker, Hassol, Bradshaw, & Rezaee, 2012). The terms used in the Hazard Manager are mapped to those in the Common Formats, so data can be aggregated and analyzed. Although the Hazard Manager tool itself has not yet been released for public use, the research surrounding its development is available in a formal report for those interested in health IT safety and its reporting, which can be found at

http://healthit.ahrq.gov/sites/default/files/docs/citation/HealthITHazardManagerFinalReport.pdf

QUESTIONS

How does your organization report health IT safety–related events?

Are you using a standard terminology, such as AHRQs Common Formats, for reporting health IT–related safety events?

Do you have a plan in place to address any health IT–related safety events?

Do you submit your health IT safety events to a PSO?

Have you contacted your PSO to discuss reports and data available for analysis, trending, and benchmarking?

Institute for Safe Medication Practices

Another organization committed to patient safety is the Institute for Safe Medication Practices (ISMP), which has been in existence for more than 30 years and is devoted entirely to medication error prevention and safe medication use. The ISMP mission is to lead efforts to improve the medication use process, and to that end, has published multiple guidelines and tips for the designers of EHRs as they configure medication orders and order sets. A five-page checklist for order sets containing medications helps organizations evaluate the safety of their CPOE systems (ISMP, 2010).

The ISMP *Guidelines for Standard Order Sets* (www.ismp.org/tools/guidelines/standardordersets.pdf) includes recommendations for screen/user interface lay out, use of symbols and abbreviations, and order set content. The following examples are adapted from ISMP's *Guidelines for Standard Order Sets:*

> Use separate lines/entries for each medication order so that multiple orders do not appear on one line or within a single entry.
>
> Avoid listing products with look-alike names near each other.

> List the most common or preferred drug, strength, and dose first, if multiple drugs, strengths, and doses are available from which to choose.
>
> Provide adequate space between the medication name and dose (for example, *propranolol 20 mg*, not *propranolol20 mg*, which may look like *120 mg*), and between the numerical dose and unit of measure (for example, *3 units*, not *3Units*, which can look like *30units*).
>
> Adhere to a consistent facility template regarding placement and format of prompts for documenting the date and time of the order, including how the date (month, day, year) and time (for example, a 24-hour clock) should be documented/displayed.
>
> Include leading zeroes (for example, *0.1 mg*) when expressing medication doses (or other numerical values, as appropriate).
>
> Include commas when expressing whole numbers greater than 999 (for example, *1,000 units*; *1,000 mg*).
>
> Exclude trailing zeroes for example, *1.0 mg*) when expressing medication doses (or other numerical values, as appropriate).
>
> Exclude error-prone abbreviations (for example, *U* for units, *QD* for daily, *ml* instead of *mL*), including those on the organization's Do Not Use list.

ISMP also has a robust voluntary error-reporting program: the Medication Errors Reporting Program (MERP). In this system, practitioners can report any errors related to medication use. The goal for this program is to learn about errors occurring nationwide, understand their origins, and share lessons learned with the healthcare and health IT community. Each year, ISMP receives hundreds of error reports from healthcare professionals. Additionally, ISMP is certified as a Patient Safety Organization by the AHRQ (ISMP, 2014).

You can find the ISMP *List of Error-Prone Abbreviations, Symbols, and Dose Designations* at

www.ismp.org/Tools/errorproneabbreviations.pdf

QUESTIONS

Does someone in your pharmacy department report medication errors related to health IT to MERP?

When your organization's configuration team develops medication orders and order sets containing medications, do they use a standard set of guidelines, such as the ISMP guide?

Does your organization have processes in place that include a multidisciplinary approach to the development of order sets, including pharmacists?

SAFER Guides

The SAFER (Safety Assurance Factors for EHR Resilience) Guides were developed under the sponsorship of the ONC to enable healthcare organizations to conduct self-assessments of EHR safety in a variety of areas and to help identify recommended practices to optimize the safety and safe use of EHRs. These guides are based on available evidence and are intended to be useful for all EHR users, developers, PSOs, and others who are concerned with optimizing the safe use of health IT. They consist of nine guides organized into three categories: foundational guides, infrastructure guides, and clinical process guides.

Each guide contains a listing of recommended practices. See Table 13.3 for the categories and high-level descriptions of the nine recommendation guides. These recommended practices are then broken down further into rationale, including published evidence, suggested sources of input for reviewing the practice, and examples of potentially useful practices or scenarios. The two foundational guides are recommended as a good starting point for organizations as they represent key and critical functions of EHR safety.

Table 13.3 Categories and High-Level Descriptions of SAFER Recommendation Guides

Foundational Guides	***Description***
High Priority Practices	Identifies "high risk" and "high priority" recommended safety practices intended to optimize the safety and safe use of EHRs
Organizational Responsibilities	Identifies individual and organizational responsibilities (activities, processes, and tasks) intended to optimize the safety and safe use of EHRs
Infrastructure Guides	***Description***
Contingency Planning	Identifies recommended safety practices associated with planned or unplanned EHR unavailability—instances in which clinicians or other end users cannot access all or part of the EHR
System Configuratioin	Identifies recommended safety practices associated with the way EHR hardware and software are set up ("configured")
System Interfaces	Identifies recommended safety practices intended to optimize the safety and safe use of system-to-system interfaces between EHR-related software applications
Clinical Process Guides	***Description***
Patient Identification	Identifies recommended safety practices associated with the reliable identification of patients in the EHR
Computerized Provider Order Entry with Decision Support	Identifies recommended safety practices associated with CPOE and clinical decision support (CDS)
Test Results Reporting and Follow up	Identifies recommended safety practices intended to optimize the safety and safe use of processes and EHR technology for the electronic communication and management of diagnostic test results
Clinician Communication	Identifies recommended safety practices associated with communication between clinicians and is intended to optimize the safety and safe use of EHRs

Examples of these important practices include:

- Data and application configurations are backed up and hardware systems are redundant.
- EHR downtime and reactivation policies and procedures are complete, available, and reviewed regularly.
- Hardware and software modifications and system-system interfaces are tested (pre–/post–go-live) to ensure data are not lost or incorrectly entered, displayed, or transmitted within or between EHR system components
- Information required to accurately identify the patient is clearly displayed on screens and printouts.
- The status of orders can be tracked in the system.
- EHR–related patient safety hazards are reported to all responsible parties, and steps are taken to address them.

An emphasis is placed on the need to review and analyze these recommendations with all key stakeholders at the table. A multidisciplinary approach with IT staff, clinicians, risk managers, administrators, and other appropriate team members is believed to be the key to the success in using these guides (ONC, 2013b). These guides are available at

http://healthit.gov/safer/safer-guides

QUESTIONS

What tools does your organization use to assess the safety of its EHR?

How often does your organization review its policies and procedures related to system downtime?

What key safety metrics are you using to monitor safe use of your EHR?

ECRI Institute

Another organization focused on patient safety is the ECRI Institute, which is a federally certified PSO. This nonprofit organization has 45 years of experience focused on scientific research to discover the effectiveness of medical procedures, devices, drugs, and processes.

In 2012, ECRI conducted an evaluation of health IT–related events and unsafe conditions to better understand technology's impact on healthcare delivery, publishing "ECRI Institute PSO's Deep Dive: Health Information Technology." This report included more than 170 health IT–related events reported by 36 healthcare organizations over a 9-week period. The events included numerous health IT–related events, such as wrong patient data entries, users ignoring alerts, and gaps in reporting critical test results due to poor system interoperability. The five most frequently identified health IT–related problems identified are shown in Table 13.4 (ECRI Institute, 2013).

Table 13.4 ECRI Top Safety Issues from Health IT Events

Issue	*Example*
System Interface Issues	These problems arise if there are failures with the system interfaces, often resulting in missed orders for medications and various other types of tests.
System/Software Configuration	Issues were also associated with the configuration of a system's hardware and software.
Software Function	A health IT system's software failed to function as intended.
Wrong Data Input	The most common problem encountered with the human-computer interface in ECRI Institute PSO's analysis occurred when a computer user entered incorrect data about the patient, such as weight, drug allergies, or an identification number.
Wrong Record Retrieved	Another common problem at the human-computer interface occurred when the wrong record was retrieved by the computer user, often resulting in a medication order for an incorrect patient.

This report was followed by a white paper titled "Anticipating Unintended Consequences of Health Information Technology and Health Information Exchange: How to Identify and Address Unsafe Conditions Associated with Health IT." In this report, several examples of commonly encountered health IT–related incidents are shared. Examples include users ignoring or overriding an alert; test results sent to the wrong provider, causing a delay in action; text entries not shared due to poorly designed interfaces between systems; and an item from an outside source scanned into the wrong patient record.

The report further explored these phenomena of health IT and patient safety, and strongly advocated for using standardized reporting methods that funnel up to PSOs. Issues to be addressed by healthcare managers are listed that provide a foundation for a solid health IT safety program, including a checklist of questions that a manager should ask while health IT safety is evaluated. Questions include topics of how adverse events are reported; whether a standard terminology is used in the reporting; what processes are in place for follow up after an incident; policies/procedures in place for system corrective action; and the existence of a budget to support health IT safety activities.

These questions can be used as part of a toolkit when developing an organizational health IT safety plan (Wallace, Zimmer, Possanza, Giannini, & Solomon, 2013):

- Are health IT system users instructed on using the organization's patient safety adverse event reporting system to report events, near-misses, and hazardous conditions involving health IT?
- Do patient safety, risk, and/or quality staff have a process in place to forward any event reports raising health IT issues to the IT department for resolution?
- Does a representative from the IT department, in addition to other appropriate stakeholders, participate in all follow-up systems analyses of health IT–related events?
- Are the findings from the event analysis reported to appropriate departments and individuals within the organization?
- Does the organization have a process to identify health IT–related events that will be reported to external organizations or entities (for example, ECRI Institute, PSOs, Institute for Safe Medication Practices, The Joint Commission)?

CPOE Design Checklist and the Pick-list Checklist

The CPOE Design Checklist and the Pick-list Checklist address health IT safety and provide methods to evaluate current EHRs and EHRs under development. Their intent is to be easy to use for both the novice and expert informaticist, and they are appropriate to use at any phase of the EHR lifecycle. Items contained in each of these checklists are based on the current literature and represent a concise, consolidated tool with which to evaluate EHR configuration proven to reduce errors.

CPOE Design Checklist

The CPOE Design Checklist is a 46-item list and provides a tool that can be used during software selection, design, or evaluation. It can be used at any point in time—not just at the time of initial configuration. Each list item list was pulled from published peer-reviewed journals that indicated that they either improved the safety of EHR use or resulted in an error because it was not configured properly. The items in the list fall into four categories: *clinical decision support, order form configuration, human factors configuration,* and *workflow process configuration* (Sengstack, 2010). Examples of some of the checklist items are included in Table 13.5. Organizations can evaluate their CPOE systems and determine their gaps in configuration and work toward improvement.

Table 13.5 CPOE Design Recommendations

Clinical Decision Support

Display alert when an allergy has been documented or an allergy to another drug in same category is documented.

Provide alert of potential allergy at time of order entry, not order submission.

Display alert when the same medication is ordered and when separate doses of the same medication are to be given within a "closely spaced time."

Display alert when order specifying a route of administration that is not appropriate for the ordered medication (for example, antifungal topical cream ordered with route of IV).

Create an alert informing users ordering potassium when there has not been a serum potassium value recorded in the past 12 hours or if the most recent potassium value is greater than 4.0.

continues

Table 13.5 CPOE Design Recommendations *(continued)*

Order Form Configuration

All ordering screens should be designed in a similar fashion. Fields for drug, dose, route, frequency, and so on should be in the same place on all screens.

Do not use field labels that require a negative answer for a positive response: for example, *Is IV contrast contraindicated?*

Human Factors Configuration

Use alternate line colors between patients to help visual separation of names.

Workflow Process Configuration

Provide a way to alert caregivers to new orders.

Pick-list Checklist

One of the ten recommendations mentioned in the IOM report, "Health IT and Patient Safety: Building Safer Systems for Better Care" emphasizes the need to conduct more research in the area of health information technology and patient safety (IOM, 2011). The IOM specifically stated that there should be more research in the area of the "pick-list" (drop-down list) problem.

A review of the literature, including documentation from our nation's top agencies for developing usability standards, finds relatively little information on how to properly configure a pick-list in an EHR. No research studies have been conducted to date on the pick-list itself. It is surprisingly easy to choose the wrong item from a pick-list/drop-down list. The ability to identify an adjacency or juxtaposition error is difficult, making this potential error even more troublesome.

This 11-item Pick-list Checklist can be used by all levels of informatics specialists to assess current configuration based on the best evidence available. An easy-to-use checklist such as this has multiple benefits and represents a starting point for informatics specialists to evaluate and improve the systems that care providers rely on to deliver safe patient care. The items contained within this checklist can be found in Table 13.6 along with their rationale (Sengstack, 2013).

Each of the items listed in The Pick-list Checklist seem to be common sense, but taken collectively, they have the potential to strengthen the quality and safety that clinical systems were meant to deliver.

Table 13.6 Pick-list Checklist

Checklist Item	*Rationale*
Use alternate line colors between patients to help visual separation of names and any list that spans across the screen horizontally.	Keep rows separated visually in order to reduce wrong patient choice.
Do not put patient lists in alphabetical order.	This places similar patient names next to each other, making it easier to choose the incorrect patient.
Number of items in drop-down list should be manageable. Keep list to 12 items or less.	Lists that are too long make it difficult to view all the choices at once and require scrolling down to see unviewed items.
If using more than 12 items, group the most commonly used items at the top.	Provides increased chance that desired item is viewable near the top of the list, without scrolling.
Do not put similar terms on top of one another in drop-down lists.	If list items are close together and similar in name, there is an increased risk of clicking on the wrong item.
Use 1.5 lines of spacing between items (not single-line spacing).	Increased space between each item fosters better readability.
Avoid using abbreviations in drop-down lists.	Having similar abbreviation choices atop each other in a drop-down list for medication route can create errors: for example, terms such as *IV* and *IP*.
By default, there should not be an item pre-selected when opening the list.	A pre-selected item may not always be the desired choice. Over-reliance on assuming that the default is the right choice can lead to errors.

continues

Table 13.6 Pick-list Checklist *(continued)*

Do not truncate items on a pick-list.	The truncated information may be critical to the choice.
Use a font size of at least 12 point (pt).	Anything smaller than 12pt font can be challenging to read, leading to more mistakes and finger fumbles
Provide the ability to search from medication lists that use "Tall Man" letters	Tall Man letters help to differentiate similar looking medications: for example, *NIFEdipine* versus. *niCARdipine*, or *predniSONE* versus *prednisoLONE*.

QUESTIONS

When developing new orders for your EHR with CPOE, does your organization use a standard template to ensure placement of fields are consistent across all orders?

When an order requires knowledge of a specific laboratory result, are order forms configured to display the most recent lab values on the ordering screens (with associated date and time the blood was drawn)?

How is a nurse alerted when a new order has been entered into the EHR for his/her patient?

Are any of your patient lists in alphabetical order?

Are any of your pick-lists truncated so that the entire item does not completely display?

Future Directions

Evaluating the safety of our electronic systems in healthcare is in its infancy. The rush has been to adopt these systems, and now the emphasis needs to be on using them to their full extent in order to capture their power and address the safety needs of our patients. Not only do we need to ensure that we configured them in the safest way possible, but we need to work in partnership with vendors, PSO organizations, federal entities, risk managers, and organizational safety teams to continue to make improvements. At a foundational level, the future emphasis needs to be on making these systems easier and safer to use. There should never be an incident in which the way a system has been configured can be pointed to as the cause of a patient error.

Using the tools covered in this chapter should drive significant improvements toward this goal of continuously improving the safety of health IT. Additionally, patient engagement will continue to increase in the future. We should enlist our patient partners in reviewing data contained within the EHR and have them report any errors so they can be corrected prior to any adverse consequence occurring. Our patients and our system end users are untapped safety resources when it comes to making improvements to the EHR. Consider how your organization can include them in EHR use and safety.

As improvements continue, the future must focus on the use of health IT to make care safer. To put it simply, the future must focus on strategies to use the electronic record in ways that users of the paper-based system could never imagine. We need to take advantage of the potential and address better, easier methods to get evidence-based knowledge into the hands of practitioners to improve decision-making. We need to better evaluate our current alerts, warnings, and reminders to see whether they are working, and continue to tweak them until they are meaningful and we can confidently state that safety has improved as a result. A clear future direction will be to contribute to the health IT safety body of knowledge by conducting outcome evaluations of our systems and disseminating the information throughout our industry.

We will also see in the near future the involvement of the FDA in the evaluation of clinical information systems including EHRs. In July of 2012, the U.S. Congress enacted the Food and Drug Administration Safety and Innovation Act (FDASIA). Section 618 of FDASIA instructs the Secretary of HHS, acting through the FDA Commissioner and in collaboration with ONC and the FCC, to issue a report on a proposed strategy that includes recommendations on an appropriate risk-based regulatory framework for health IT. The intent is for the framework to promote innovation, protect patient safety, and avoid regulatory duplication. As of this writing, the proposed report is being reviewed by the ONC Health IT Policy Committee, with input from the public, and will incorporate what the agencies learn about risk, safety, and opportunity for innovative technologies to support improved health and safety outcomes. The agencies will consider how to make it easier for innovators to understand the regulatory landscape, ways to minimize regulatory burden, and how to design an oversight approach that supports innovations and patient safety (FDA, 2013).

Conclusion

The culture that we should adopt is one that thinks nationally but acts locally. Our federal government and professional organizations cannot improve health IT safety without the expertise of informatics specialists. It will take each organization working in partnership with the government, health IT vendors, and PSOs to drive improvements in patient safety using health IT. The tools, knowledge, and resources offered in this chapter can help lay the foundation for a strong health IT strategic plan that can assist organizations as they strive to capture the full potential of their systems. In summary, healthcare organizations need to ensure the safety of their health IT systems. A committed team of stakeholders must become involved and increase transparency as we learn and share safety lessons from the implementation and use of health IT. The EHR is fast becoming the standard in healthcare today, and thus it is imperative that organizations commit time, energy, and funding to ensure that these clinical systems are integral to reaching their error-reduction goals.

References

Agency for Healthcare Research and Quality (AHRQ). (2013). AHRQ Common Formats: PSO Privacy Protection Center website. Retrieved from https://www.psoppc.org/c/document_library/get_file?uuid=75912503-7bd1-4e99-a678-5dbb70008e95&groupId=10218

Ammenwerth, E., Schnell-Inderst, P., Machan, C., & Sievert U. (2008). The effect of electronic prescribing on medication errors and adverse drug events: A systematic review. Journal of the American Medical Informatics Association, *15*(5), 585–600.

Campbell, E. M., Sittig, D. F., Ash, J. S., Guappone, K. P., & Dykstra, R. H. (2006). Types of unintended consequences related to computerized provider order entry. Journal of the American Medical Informatics Association, *13*, 547–556.

ECRI Institute. (2013, February 6). ECRI institute PSO uncovers health information technology-related events in deep dive analysis. Retrieved from https://www.ecri.org/Press/Pages/Health-Information-Technology-HIT-Deep-Dive.aspx

Franklin, B. D., O'Grady, K., Donyai, P., Jacklin, G., & Barber, N. (2007). The impact of a closed-loop electronic prescribing and administration system on prescribing errors, administration errors and staff time: A before and after study. Quality and Safety of Health Care, *16*(4), 279–284.

Goolsby, K. (2002). CPOE odyssey: The story of evolving the world's first computerized physician order entry system and implications for today's CPOE decision makers. Retrieved from www.outsourcing-information-technology.com/cpoe.html

Han, Y., Carcilla, J. , Venkataraman, D., Clark, R., Watson, S., Nguyen, T., . . . Orr, R. (2005). Unexpected increased mortality after implementation of commercially sold computerized physician order entry system. *Pediatrics, 116*(6), 1506–1512.

Horsky, J., Kuperman, G. J., & Patel, V. L. (2005). Comprehensive analysis of a medication dosing error related to CPOE. *Journal of the American Medical Informatics Association, 12*(4), 377–382.

Institute for Safe Medication Practices (ISMP). (2010). *Guidelines for standard order sets.* Retrieved from http://www.ismp.org/newsletters/acutecare/articles/20100311.asp

Institute for Safe Medication Practices (ISMP). (2014). *The National Medication Errors Reporting Program (ISMP MERP).* Retrieved from https://www.ismp.org/orderforms/reporterrortoismp.asp.2014

Institute of Medicine (IOM). (2011). *Health IT and patient safety: Building safer systems for better care.* Washington, DC: National Academies Press. Retrieved from http://www.iom.edu/Reports/2011/Health-IT-and-Patient-Safety-Building-Safer-Systems-for-Better-Care.aspx

Jones, S. S., Koppel, R., Ridgely, M. S., Palen, T. E., Wu, S., & Harrison, M. I. (2011). *Guide to reducing unintended consequences of Electronic Health Records.* Prepared by RAND Corporation under Contract No. HHSA290200600017I, Task Order #5. Rockville, MD: Agency for Healthcare Research and Quality (AHRQ).

Kaushal, R., Shojania, K. G., & Bates, D. W. (2003). Effects of computerized physician order entry and clinical decision support systems on medication safety. Archives of Internal Medicine, *163*(12), 1409–1416.

Kohn, L.T., Corrigan, J. M., & Donaldson, M. S. (Eds.). (1999). *To err is human: Building a safer health system.* Washington, DC: National Academies Press.

Koppel, R., Metley, J. P., Cohen, A., Abaluck, B., Localia, A. R., Dimmel, S. E., & Strom, B. L. (2005). Role of computerized physician order entry systems in facilitating medication errors. Journal of the American Medical Association, *5*(293), 1197–1203.

Office of the National Coordinator for Health Information Technology (ONC). (2013a). Health information technology patient safety action & surveillance plan. Retrieved from http://www.healthit.gov/sites/default/files/safety_plan_master.pdf

Office of the National Coordinator for Health Information Technology (ONC). (2013b). Safety Assurance Factors for EHR Resilience: SAFER guides. Retrieved from http://www.healthit.gov/policy-researchers-implementers/safer

Office of the National Coordinator for Health Information Technology (ONC). (2013c). *Update on the adoption of health information technology and related efforts to facilitate the electronic use and exchange of health information: A report to Congress.* Retrieved from http://www.healthit.gov/sites/default/files/rtc_adoption_of_healthit_and_relatedefforts.pdf

Reckmann, M. H., Westbrook, J. I., Koh, Y., Lo, C., & Day, R. O. (2009). Does computerized provider order entry reduce prescribing errors for hospital inpatients? A systematic review. Journal of the American Medical Informatics Association, *16*(5), 613–622.

Sengstack, P. (2010). CPOE configuration to reduce medication errors: A literature review on the safety of CPOE systems and design recommendations. *Journal of Healthcare Information Management*, *24*(4), 26–34.

Sengstack, P. (2013). The pick-list checklist: Reducing adjacency errors in health information technology. *Journal of Health Information Management, 27*(2), 68–71.

Shulman, R., Singer, M., Goldstone, J., & Bellingan, G. (2005). Medication errors: A prospective cohort study of hand written and computerised physician order entry in the intensive care unit. Critical Care, *9*, R516–R521.

U.S. Department of Health & Human Services (HHS). (2009). Health IT legislation and regulations. Retrieved from http://www.healthit.gov/policy-researchers-implementers/hitech-act

U.S. Food and Drug Administration (FDA). (2013). Food and Drug Administration Safety and Innovation Act (FDASIA). Retrieved from http://www.fda.gov/regulatoryinformation/legislation/federalfooddrugancosmeticactfdcact/significantamendmentstothefdcact/fdasia/ucm20027187.htm

Walker, J. M., Hassol, A., Bradshaw, B., & Rezaee, M. E. (2012). AHRQ Hazard Manager. AHRQ Publication No. 12-0058-EF May 2012, Retrieved from http://www.ahrq.gov/news/events/conference/2011/walker-hassol/index.html

Wallace, C., Zimmer, K. P., Possanza, L., Giannini, R., & Solomon, R. (2013). ECRI Institute. *Anticipating unintended consequences of health information technology and health information exchange: How to identify and address unsafe conditions associated with health IT.* Retrieved from http://www.healthit.gov/sites/default/files/How_to_Identify_and_Address_Unsafe_Conditions_Associated_with_Health_IT.pdf

Walsh, K. E., Adams, W. G., Bauchner, H., Vinci, R. J., Chessare, J. B., Cooper, M. R., … Landrigan, C. P. (2006). Medication errors related to computerized order entry for children. Pediatrics, *118*(5), 1872–1879.

"When patients participate more actively in the process of medical care, we can create a new healthcare system with higher quality services, better outcomes, and happier, healthier patients. We must make this the new gold standard of healthcare quality and the ultimate goal of all our improvement efforts: Not better hospitals. Not better physician practices. Not more sophisticated electronic medical systems. Happier, healthier patients."

–Dr. Charles Safran (Ferguson, 2007)

Patient Engagement in Healthcare IT

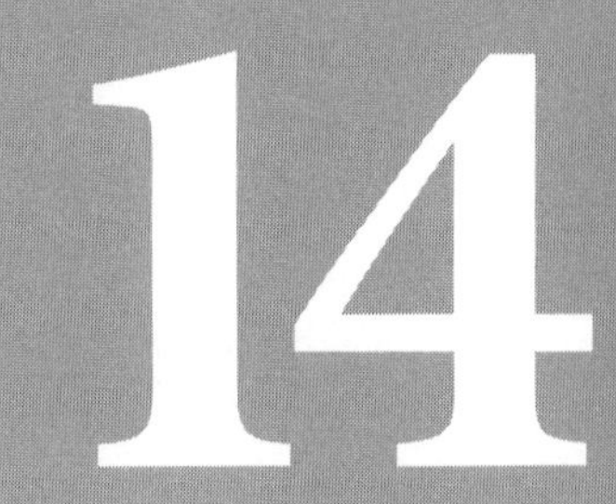

Daniel Gracie, DNP, RN-BC
Melissa Barthold, MSN, RN-BC, CPHIMS, FHIMSS

OBJECTIVES

- Identify how technology can influence the engagement of patients in their own healthcare.
- Evaluate new technologies and their potential impact in the healthcare arena.
- Describe how a provider can assess levels of patient engagement.

Mentioned in the 1999 groundbreaking publication, "To Err is Human," by the Institute of Medicine (IOM) and as a national priority of the National Quality Forum in 2008, patient engagement has become a cornerstone of modern healthcare. As technology and our environment evolve, our healthcare, communication practice, and expectations evolve.

During this process, we reevaluate and challenge once-accepted practices. Over the past 20 years, technology and healthcare have changed how the patient is viewed, changed both provider and patient expectations, and completely altered how patients share in the decision-making process of their care plan. Patient engagement has been referred to as the "next blockbuster drug," the "holy grail" of healthcare, and as a key to achieve the "Triple Aim" in healthcare of improved outcomes, better care, and decreased costs (James, 2013; Kish, 2012; Wilkins, 2012).

TIP

Read more about the Triple Aim in Chapter 17.

We like to think that we have engaged our patients in their healthcare. However, until recently, that engagement was lacking a key element: namely, data sharing. With recent advancements in communication and healthcare technology, along with legislative incentives, patients are now assuming an increasingly greater partnership role in their healthcare team.

Pew Research has found that 87% of adults use the Internet, and 78% have reported going online for health-related information in 2014 (Pew Research Center, 2014). The ultimate goal of this evolution is to create a better healthcare system centered on providing quality care that is efficient and inclusive of the patient.

We often think of "patient engagement" as simply including patients in every facet of their healthcare. Although this term sounds simple, it has been used synonymously in the literature with other terms—such as *patient activation* or as a part of *patient-centered care*—making its usage unclear. Although these terms all work toward the same goal, they have varied meanings and roles in the active process of patient engagement. Table 14.1 lists some of the common definitions for patient engagement found in the literature.

Table 14.1 Common Definitions for Patient Engagement

Author	*Definition of Patient Engagement*
Coulter (2012, p. 10)	"[W]orking together to promote and support active patient and public involvement in health and healthcare and to strengthen their influence on healthcare decisions, at both the individual and collective levels."
Center for Advancing Health (2010, p. 2)	"Actions individuals must take to obtain the greatest benefit from the healthcare services available to them."
Rob Lambert (2013, para. 15)	"Engagement is about interaction, listening, and learning in relationship to another person. Engagement is not a strategy, it is care."

Author	*Definition of Patient Engagement*
Donna Cryer (Polta, 2012, para. 14)	"Properly done, patient engagement in action looks like shared responsibility between patients (and their families if applicable), health care practitioners (the entire team: surgeons, physicians, nurses), and health care administrators (providers of the infrastructure and payment models) to co-develop pathways to optimal individual, community and population health. Patient engagement brought to life means involving patients and caregivers in every step of the process, providing training or financial support if necessary."

Carman et al. (2013) have proposed an updated framework that provides a fluid model, focusing on the various forms of patient engagement. They looked at the patient provider engagement relationship as it has evolved on a continuum through levels in the healthcare system that spans from the consultation to partnership phase. They characterized patient engagement in their continuum by "...how much information flows between the patient and provider, how active a role the patient has in care decisions, and how involved the patient or patient organization becomes in health organization decisions and policy making" (Carman et al., 2013, p. 224).

At the higher end of their framework is a state in which the provider and patient are engaged and share responsibility in the care plan. This state is characterized by a bidirectional flow of data that takes into consideration the preferences and wishes of the individual. This would seem to mirror the ideal state that we commonly think of as "patient engagement." At the opposite end of the continuum, the situation is different in that patients take on more of an unequal relationship wherein they are given decisions on their care, with minimal input on their preferences or wishes. The authors pointed out that the higher end of the continuum is not always the goal or ideal position: rather, it changes with the patient and their preferences. Regardless of the definition used, it is undeniable that technology is enabling patients to become engaged in their care by providing a conduit to share and find information. Educating patients leads to more involved patients and improves healthcare outcomes. Patients can make better decisions, work more closely with their providers, improve patient-provider communication, and can ask more questions and evaluate their providers (Robert Wood Johnson Foundtion, 2014).

Patients who have not looked at their medical records in the past are now asking for copies of that record. Healthcare providers need to be aware of this change in patient engagement, as well as be aware that regulations require that the patient's request be fulfilled. Providers, who have had discussions as to whether the patient was entitled to read his/her chart, now have no choice: A patient can review his chart at any time. Although providers might have been concerned that patients would worry about information in the chart that they did not understand, studies show that this change may improve doctor-patient communication (Ross & Lin, 2003). With patients improving medication adherence, as well as possibly improving patient safety with patients catching errors in their records, the "open notes" movement is continuing, and with legislation, will grow more (Walker, Darer, Elmore, & Delbanco, 2014).

This chapter will discuss patient engagement, what it is and is not, how providers can support it, how technology can add to that engagement, as well as the value to the patient—improved health status—to be truly engaged in their own healthcare.

Assessing Patient Engagement

Patients are taking advantage of the opportunity to review their medical records. According to a study by Walker et al. (2014), four out of five patients had read their notes, and the majority stated they had better recall and understanding of their plans of care—and that they were more in control of their healthcare. Ralston et al. (2014) looked at patients with HIV who used web-based shared medical records. As more patients become aware of the regulations requiring that they have access to their records, it seems likely that more patients will access those records. Additional studies are in progress to evaluate what changes may occur when the patients read their records.

Provider Driving Forces

As email and the Internet became commonplace in the late twentieth century, some early adopter patients and providers began using Internet technology to communicate and monitor their progress. Although communication across the Internet was often public and insecure, it did not stop patients from seeking support from other patients who shared their disease or condition. They found that simply talking to another person—one who really understood—helped. The shared understanding came from shared conditions, becoming virtual support groups.

As a part of the American Recovery and Reinvestment Act (ARRA) of 2009, the United States federal government made available financial incentives to assist providers and organizations in the adoption of electronic health records (EHRs). These systems were required to meet set guidelines and demonstrate that the systems were being used meaningfully and to improve patient outcomes. Patient engagement was a key part of this Meaningful Use incentive program, and the criteria set forth by the Office of the National Coordinator for Health Information Technology (ONC) is highlighted in Table 14.2. Although this legislation provides incentives initially, the incentive program switches after a few years to reimbursement penalties for those not meeting the Meaningful Use criteria.

Table 14.2 Meaningful Use of Healthcare IT

STAGE 1	
Eligible Hospital	***Metric***
Objective Measure Core 11: Provide patients with an electronic copy of their health information (including diagnostic test results, problem list, medication lists, medication allergies, discharge summary, procedures) upon request.	More than 50% of all patients of the inpatient or emergency departments (ED) of the eligible hospital or critical access hospital (CAH) (place of service (POS) 21 or 23) who request an electronic copy of their health information are provided it within three business days.
Objective Measure Core 12: Provide patients with an electronic copy of their discharge instructions at time of discharge, upon request.	More than 50% of all patients discharged from an eligible hospital or CAH's inpatient or ED (POS 21 or 23) and who request an electronic copy of their discharge instructions are provided it.
Eligible Provider	***Metric***
Objective Measure Core 12: Provide patients with an electronic copy of their health information (including diagnostic test results, problem list, medication lists, medication allergies) upon request.	More than 50% of all patients who request an electronic copy of their health information are provided it within three business days.

continues

Table 14.2 Meaningful Use of Healthcare IT *(continued)*

Eligible Provider	*Metric*
Objective Measure Core 13: Provide clinical summaries for patients for each office visit.	Clinical summaries provided to patients for more than 50% of all office visits within three business days.
Objective Measure Menu 5: Provide patients with timely electronic access to their health information (including lab results, problem list, medication lists, and allergies) within four business days of the information being available to the EP.	At least 10% of all unique patients seen by the EP (Eligible Provider) are provided in a timely manner (available to the patient within four business days of being updated in the certified EHR technology). This electronic access to their health information is made available to the patient, with the content subject to the EP's discretion to withhold certain information.
STAGE 2	
Eligible Hospital	*Metric*
Objective Measure Core 6: Provide patients the ability to view online, download, and transmit information about a hospital admission.	(1) More than 50% of all unique patients discharged from the inpatient or ED of the eligible hospital or CAH (POS 21 or 23) during the EHR reporting period have their information available online within 36 hours of discharge. (2) More than 5% of all patients (or their authorized representatives) who are discharged from the inpatient or ED (POS 21 or 23) of an eligible hospital or CAH view, download or transmit to a third party their information during the EHR reporting period.

Eligible Provider	*Metric*
Objective Measure Core 7: Provide patients the ability to view online, download, and transmit their health information within four business days of the information being available to the EP.	(1) More than 50% of all unique patients seen by the EP during the EHR reporting period are provided timely (available to the patient within four business days after the information is available to the EP) online access to their health information. (2) More than 5% of all unique patients seen by the EP during the EHR reporting period (or their authorized representatives) view, download, or transmit to a third party their health information.
Objective Measure Core 8: Provide clinical summaries for patients for each office visit.	Clinical summaries provided to patients or patient-authorized representatives within one business day for more than 50% of office visits.
Objective Measure Core 17: Use secure electronic messaging to communicate with patients on relevant health information.	A secure message was sent using the electronic messaging function of certified electronic health record technology (CEHRT) by more than 5% of unique patients (or their authorized representatives) seen by the EP during the EHR reporting period.

STAGE 3 MEANINGFUL USE

Not released as of this writing. However, it is expected that the requirements of Stage 3 will focus on patient access to self-management tools; access to comprehensive patient data through robust, secure, patient-centered health information exchange; and improving population health.

Excerpted from http://cms.gov/Regulations-and-Guidance/Legislation/EHRIncentivePrograms/Downloads/Hosp_CAH_MU-toc.pdf

Health Consumer Driving Forces

Technology is changing our lives and allowing us to perform tasks that once required a professional. Take, for example, performing a real estate listings search, completing a bank or stock transaction from home, or searching multiple airlines to make travel arrangements. Healthcare is following a similar trend. Because of these advances, consumers are increasingly relying on technology to provide real-time access to help them find and organize information.

Additionally, the hardware relied on by patients has become "smaller" and more mobile with wireless Internet access. Smartphones have the same computing ability as an entire room full of servers did 20 years ago. Applications ("apps") are becoming the norm in our everyday lives. These apps easily perform the tasks that not long ago required specialized hardware or software, making these tasks much easier to address now. The standard response to improving any task is, "There's an app for that!" From editing photos, recording events on a group calendar, creating a shopping list, managing your checkbook, paying a bill from your bank account or sending an email to your healthcare provider, there are apps created to handle this work. More apps are being created every day.

In a 2014 survey, the Pew Research Center found that 90% of adults own a wireless phone, and 58% use a smart phone (Skiba, 2014). The increased speeds—both cellular and broadband—are supporting the increased use of smartphones and devices. And with users carrying them at all times, finding healthcare–related applications is growing easier by the day.

This virtual communication shift has spurred new ways for patients to find support, resources, and data previously not available to them. As people turn to the Internet for information, they are also discovering individuals with similar health conditions to support connection.

Patient portals are specialized, secure websites created to allow patients 24/7 access to their health information anywhere there is Internet access. Some portals are 'home-grown' to permit access for patients; some portals are part of a large electronic health record, and some are part of the provider's office. The portal provides selected information to patients, from x-ray results from recent lab tests, discharge summaries and instructions, medication listings, appointment scheduling, and usually a secure method to communicate with a provider (HealthIT.gov, 2014).

Although portals were created about ten years ago, their functionality was limited, because there was (usually) no EHR to connect to. And without the lab results, scheduling abilities, etc., portals had limited value to patients. Some patient portals have intricately designed web interfaces, but many still rely on email-based listserv (automated email lists services), to provide information and then facilitate connection with others. Some portals, such as Microsoft's HealthVault, are designed as personal health records, but have the ability to connect to some EHRs, making them much more like a portal.

Note

A *listserv* is an automated service that uses a 'listserv' email address. Users subscribe to the list. An email sent to the list goes to all subscribers and replies go to all subscribers, too. A webpage is very different in that it is a location on the Internet accessed by typing in the webpage address.

The following websites offer patient portals:

- **PatientsLikeMe (www.patientslikeme.com):** Offers a forum to blog about their experience, connect with others afflicted by similar conditions, and also track their personal health.
- **CaringBridge (www.caringbridge.org):** Offers a blog service for patients and families to help communicate and provide updates to their support network.
- **CarePages (www.carepages.com):** Provides health information and blogging capabilities for patients to learn more about their condition and also communicate with their support network.
- **ACOR.org (www.acor.org/):** A listserv that has been around since the early days (1996) of the Internet that offers 142 cancer support networks.
- **Reviewing Personal Health Records (www.myphr.com/StartaPHR/what_is_a_phr.aspx):** This website, originally developed for seniors, explains how to evaluate an EHR.

Applying the Technology: Some Tools and Growing Evidence

Technology provides support for patient engagement. It provides better information access for clinicians and for their patients. For the clinician, it can provide information at the point of care. For the patient, it can provide information when needed, and support and inform decision-making.

To ensure that technology does help the patient, the patient's level of health literacy must be assessed. *Health literacy* is the ability of the patient to receive and understand provided health information, from clinicians' instructions to disease-specific information. According to Berkman, Sheridan, Donahue, Halpren, and Crotty (2011), there is a connection between the patient's health literacy and their better health outcomes. The converse is also true. Patients with low literacy are hospitalized more often; use more specific healthcare services, including increased hospitalizations; and their preventive healthcare, such as influenza immunization and mammograms, is lower. Low health literacy also leads to lower health status and higher mortality rates. According to Berkman, there is evidence showing that techniques to increase patient engagement are effective, and providers who encourage patient engagement will be assisting in improving the patient's health outcomes (Berkman et al., 2011).

Whatever can be done that supports the patient's attempt to increase health literacy will support that patient's improving health outcomes (Dentzer, 2013; Hibbard, Mahoney, Stock, & Tusler, 2007).

Being able to navigate the Internet is not an indicator of health literacy. Providing educational material in electronic as well as paper format is enhanced when that material is delivered by a clinician (Coulter, 2012). Supporting health literacy supports improved care.

Several tools are available to assess health literacy:

Rapid Estimate of Adult Literacy in Medicine (REALM): This tool has been available since 1991. It can be used to determine a patient's reading ability in primary care, patient education, and medical research (Davis et al., 1991). It is available from the Agency for Healthcare Research and Quality (AHRQ), and you can find a Spanish tool available on the AHRQ website at http://www.ahrq.gov/professionals/quality-patient-safety/quality-resources/tools/literacy/sahlsa.pdf as well.

Shortened Test of Functional Health Literacy in Adults (S-TOFHLA): This tool was evaluated in patients, most of whom were older than age 65. This test is a timed administration, which had a negative effect on the test scores (Robinson et al., 2011), so it may not be a true indicator of literacy for seniors or someone reading in a second language. Strategies to improve health literacy are available at:

Quick Guide to Health Literacy

http://www.health.gov/communication/literacy/quickguide/decision.htm

National Institutes of Health

http://www.nih.gov/clearcommunication/healthliteracy.htm

Social Media, Healthcare, and Patient Engagement

Social media has a potential to improve patient engagement. Sites such as PatientsLikeMe have demonstrated that patients are interested in using the Internet to get involved with others. However, the quality of information, as well as ensuring that the information is up to date, has not been standardized from an industry perspective. Health information can change quickly. Because there are no regulations or rules governing healthcare websites, or directives as to who can set up a website or the accuracy of any information posted therein, a web page can provide whatever information the authors want to provide, accurate or not.

At times, social media networks that are not primarily healthcare focused still have discussion on or information about healthcare. Facebook, Twitter, LinkedIn, and Instagram can all have discussions or posts about a healthcare issue. In 2009, Erin Turner saw a schedule posted for an online chat with a Mayo Clinic surgeon, who had cured the wrist pain of Jason Werth, an outfielder for a major league baseball team. She logged into that chat and heard that a split tear in a ligament often goes undiagnosed. She drove across the country to meet the surgeon about the cause of the wrist pain she had experienced for the past 5 years. She did have the same split tear and had curative surgery 5 weeks later. She considers herself cured by 'Mayo and YouTube' (Mayo Clinic, 2010).

There is little research regarding how patients use the information they obtain on these sites, as well as how these sites may increase either healthy behaviors or the patients' decision-making abilities (Househ, Borycki, & Kushniruk, 2013). There is a possibility of erroneous material being circulated via social media because the information—from videos and text information—is created by patients, usually with little clinical oversight. In additional, many of these sites have little to no policies on privacy and security of patient-entered information (Househ et al., 2013). Evaluation tools are available to assist healthcare providers and patients, though, in determining the accuracy and safety of a healthcare website. The Health On the Net Foundation site (http://www.hon.ch/) is a good starting point. Vargas (2013) provides additional information on assessing healthcare websites.

Albeit with no promise of improved outcomes, there is the possibility that social media will support patients' involvement in their own care. Although cancer survivors use the Internet less frequently than other patients with chronic diseases, once there, they use it for more health-related information than others do (Chou, Liu, Post, & Hesse, 2011; Househ et al., 2013).

Supporting the use of social media in healthcare is increasingly prevalent. Healthcare institutions are expected to, at the least, have a Facebook page, a Twitter feed, and an Internet presence. Patients use social media and will look for their provider and their hospital on Facebook. Providers should use social media to promote their institution and to provide improved information to patients. According to Kevin Pho, the founder and author of a well-known medical blog, "[H]ealth professionals need a strong social media presence to establish themselves as reputable sources as well as to properly point patients toward legitimate sites to be used as secondary sources" (Kotenko, 2013). Patients need to think of their providers as good sources for Internet information as well as a source for face-to-face information.

The American Academy of Orthopedic Surgeons has developed a social media primer for surgeons (Soyer, 2012). Additional information, including brochures and white papers directed specifically toward nurses, is available from the National Council of State Boards of Nursing (National Council, 2011). Barry and Hardiker (2012) discussed the use of social media by nurses and described how to keep it safe and professional. In their article,

Schmidt, Sims-Giddons, and Booth (2012) presented the importance of incorporating the education of nursing students in the ethical use of social media and other technologies in course work in colleges of nursing. They reminded educators that this technological education is equally as important as teaching students how to change dressings and administer medications. Weaver, Lindsay, and Gitelman (2012) emphasized the importance of nurses assuming a leadership role in the use of social media technology in healthcare, both to support patient care and to support nursing.

As another hardware device in use, the devices in the patients' rooms—from heart monitors, blood oxygenation monitors, or pumps for intravenous fluids—can do more than provide television access, Internet access, and other entertainment. Patient devices at the bedside often look like small televisions, and can indeed serve as a television—but they can also display patient information, from data such as pulse rates or blood pressure to reports on different studies. In the use of these bedside patient devices, an article by Caligtan, Carroll, Hurley, Gersh-Zaremski, and Dykes (2012) showed that both patients and providers were able to identify the necessary information that should be available on those devices.

Although there was agreement between patients and staff on much of the information that should be available on the devices, there was concern among the clinicians about giving the patients access to too much information. For example, patients want to see their current laboratory results, x-ray reports, echo reports, ECG reviews, as well as most other reports. This knowledge can support patient engagement in their healthcare. Outpatients ranked access to information very high, and studies have shown that inpatients want more information about their disease processes and ordered testing and great involvement in their healthcare (Caligtan et al., 2012). Although clinicians were concerned that too much information may be given to patients who will not completely understand the information, negative effects from providing information to patients has not been seen (Caligtan et al., 2012; Darkins et al., 2008).

Blue Button: Announced by President Obama in 2010, the Blue Button Initiative has proven popular among veterans and consumers as a way to download their healthcare information and become more informed about their health. The program, initially available as a part of the Department of Veterans Affairs My Health*e*Vet portal (https://www.myhealth.va.gov/index.html), was launched as a program to the public and private electronic medical record vendors by the United States Department of Health and Human Services through the Office of the National Coordinator and the HealthIT.gov website.

The Blue Button initiative focuses on making information—such as current medication history, active problem list, allergies, medical and procedure history, lab test results, immunizations, and other vital information—into a portable document that can help patients learn more about their medical history or transition between providers.

Open Notes: Initially started as part of a Robert Wood Johnson Foundation–funded study in 2010, the Open Notes project sought to open key parts of patient medical records that were previously readily available only to their provider. The study has evolved and now is a national program that gives patients the same view to their healthcare visit notes that their providers see. This monumental study found that "[W]hen patients have access to their doctors' notes, they feel more in control of their health care, better understand their medical issues, and report they are more likely to take their medications as prescribed" (Delbanco et al., 2012; Robert Wood Johnson Foundation, n.d.).

The Future Is Now: Patient-Provided Data

Healthcare is being challenged today from many sides. Patients would prefer to stay home—and third-party payers prefer that they stay home. Providing the necessary assessments while the patient is in the community setting is spurring innovation and use of different methods and new devices.

Telemedicine is providing an increase in technology to patients in all parts of the United States. Current devices use cellular or broadband circuits to transmit data obtained, using specific devices, to a telehealth center where it is reviewed by clinicians. For example, patients with congestive heart failure (CHF) have their heart rate, weight, oxygen level, and blood pressure monitored using these wireless devices. In essence, the process is that a patient uses wireless devices to obtain the data, and then the data is automatically sent to the central monitoring device in the patient's home. That central device then uploads data to the telehealth center, using either cellular or broadband connectivity. The devices are easy to use; even patients who are not "techie'" have little trouble using them because the data transmission is automatic (Darkins et al., 2008).

Figure 14.1 shows a heathcare provider demonstrating how to use a health-monitoring device.

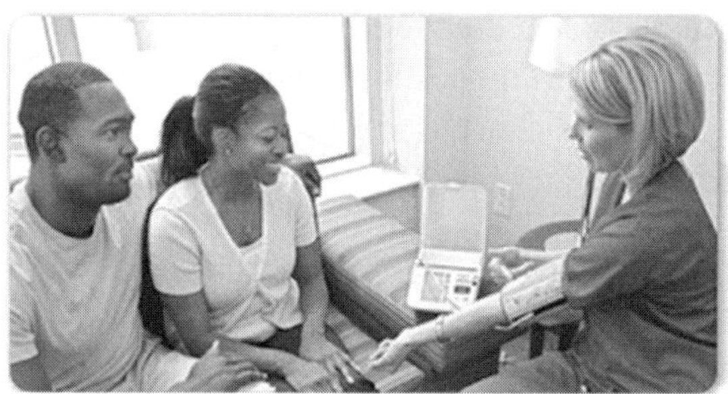
Home monitoring can
record your improvements.

FIGURE 14.1 Health-monitoring device.

If the clinician reviewing the data is concerned about the patient's status, the nurse can contact the patient for further information and interventions. Almost any patient data is available to be monitored, from heart rates to blood sugar test results. All these devices can automatically send data to a provider's office or a telehealth center, where expert nurses can review the information or use decision support software to assist in evaluating the data. Telehealth centers are maintained around the clock and usually staffed with nurses or monitor technicians. Some of these centers are part of a university system, such as the Arizona Telehealth Center (The University of Arizona, 2014); some centers are companies that provide telehealth monitoring services (Cardiocom, 2014).

The evidence clearly supports the use of telehealth technologies for those with chronic diseases. An abridged Cochrane review by Inglis, Clark, McAllister, Stewart, and Cleland (2011) stated that home telehealth monitoring should be the standard of care for patients with CHF. They also noted that an additional benefit of telemonitoring was that "[T]he patient is less likely to be a passive recipient of services from health professionals and becomes more actively involved in their care" (Inglis et al., 2011, p. 1037). The Veterans Administration has been using home monitoring for chronic diseases for some years, resulting in decreased mortality and morbidity, decreased admissions and readmissions, decreased use of resources, and increased quality of life (Darkins et al., 2008).

Hardware and Software

Much of the hardware making possible the transmission of patient-provided data already exists. Eric Topol, the Gary and Mary West Endowed Chair of Innovative Medicine and Professor of Genomics at the Scripps Research Institute, supports this new technology;

from a 12-lead ECG available with a small smartphone add-on to an application that permits the provider to view physiological monitoring devices from an intensive care unit remotely on a tablet (Topol, 2012). Topol stated that technology is reshaping healthcare and supports empowering patients. He insists that "[I]t's the patients' data" (Reed & Topol, 2012).

Topol is convinced that empowered patients are going to drive the adoption of mobile healthcare technology and that those patients will convince the change-resistant physician to adopt new mobile applications. There is currently no reimbursement for a provider who evaluates the ECG sent wirelessly from a patient's mobile device. Added to the financial concern, there is the possibility of legal implications and perhaps the provider receiving a large amount of data, directly from the patient. The avalanche of data from patients—continuous blood sugars, heart rates, blood pressures—is all information that is not available, and certainly not continuously available now. Providers do not have any processes set up to handle—and use—all this patient-generated data (Dolan, 2014b; Reed & Topol, 2012).

To increase the treatment options to rural patients, InvisionHeart (http://signup.invisionheart.com/) in Nashville, Tennessee has developed both hardware and the software to run the hardware that will allow first responders to obtain, store, and then transmit ECGs to providers in real-time from remote areas (Blum, 2014).

Wearable Devices

The first wearable tech was used in the 1960s by Thorp, the self-appointed inventor of wearable technology. In 1994, a wrist computer was invented by Matias and Ruicci, although today's devices are smaller. Today's wearable tech communicates with a designated computer selected by the user, uploading data to it. Approximately 13 million wearable devices shipped in 2013; it is expected that by 2018, that number will increase to 130 million (Gross, 2014). Many of the devices on the market as of this writing are used in the sports arena to monitor biometric information and support improvement of the athlete.

One of the largest U.S. electronics retailers, Best Buy (www.bestbuy.com), has more than 10 different devices (and the associated software) available for the tech-conscious. This equipment will track activities, especially sports activities, performance, calories burned, and multisport tracking, including speed and location. A sports enthusiast can monitor data from workouts and then analyze that data with a goal of improving performances.

These devices can be used for health tracking. These wearable devices monitor a person's activity level, sleep, steps, or body fat, and then transmit data wirelessly to each person's smartphone, tablet, or computer for further monitoring and analysis. Some companies are incorporating more of the possible healthcare use into their hardware and software and tracking heart rate, weight, and blood pressure. They are being made by different companies, from Microsoft (www.microsoft.com) and Samsung (www.samsung.com/us/mobile/wearable-tech/all-products?filter=gear-fit) to Fitbit (www.fitbit.com/) and Bose (www.bose.com). They include step counters, stairs step counters, and assessment of sleep quality (www.bestbuy.com).

The Scripps Translational Science Institute (STSI) has started a trial of three wearable devices that will monitor (dependent on the patient's condition) blood sugar, blood pressure, or heart rate/rhythm. The goal of the study is to evaluate the possibility of using this type of mobile health to lower healthcare costs and resource use (Comstock, 2013). Additionally, STSI has begun a pilot with two companies on their sensor that detects lung cancer (Dolan, 2014c). After trials at STSI, with results published by E. Topol, Aetna (insurance company) has agreed to reimburse for the use of the iRhythm ZIO patch (Dolan, 2014a) to monitor certain cardiac problems that the patch can detect better than a Holtor monitor can.

As of this writing, the design of these wearable monitors can be awkward, but to address that lack, Intel has sponsored a wearable design contest, with prizes of $1.25 million dollars. The wrist has been considered the best location for these devices, but designers of wearable devices are looking for different body locations (Wood, 2014). The Shine, the newest monitor, can be worn as a pendant or a bracelet, not confined to the wrist, although that greater flexibility costs more than other monitoring devices:

> http://www.fastcoexist.com/1680863/the-shine-a-self-tracking-device-that-youd-wear-even-if-it-didnt-do-anything

Wearable devices need to improve, in style and function, to meet the demands of today's techie folks. Qrest Devices (http://mimobaby.com/mimo/), as a change from the current audible baby monitor, is producing an infant monitor with sensors built into a "*onesie*" (one-piece garment) for the youngest babies. The monitor uploads data on the infant's heart rate, temperature, and breathing to the parents' smartphones for analysis by the parents, who can also discuss the information with their healthcare provider. The Mimo Baby Monitor will be available in stores for those parents that want to (and have the funds) to buy one at $199 for the starter model. The onesie will have to be replaced when it is outgrown (a set of two onsies costs $29.99 and is available in size 0 to 12 months). This is not a designated medical device, but is a consumer purchase.

Apple is close to releasing a wearable wristband watch, the iWatch, and this device will permit the user's input. It is anticipated that the device will allow reading of messages as well as collecting and permitting the management of biometric data and is due for release in late fall, 2014 (Sullivan, 2014).

PulsePoint

There's an app for that—PulsePoint. This hardware/software combination was developed to address the more than 350,000 cardiac arrests that occur yearly outside the hospital. According to the American Heart Association, most patients who arrest away from immediate help die (American Heart Association, 2013). Many cities across the United States have implemented this application, which comprises software that is installed at the community's fire department and the mobile application available from the PulsePoint website (http://www.pulsepoint.org/) or on websites for Mac or Android systems and downloaded to volunteers' smartphones.

People who volunteer to be notified about 911 calls from people needing CPR can download the mobile software. When a 911 call is received, in addition to notifying the usual emergency staff, PulsePoint sends out a page to their smartphones to CPR–trained community members (volunteers) and off-duty emergency staff within walking distance (configurable, but usually one-quarter of a mile) of the stricken person. The application tells the volunteer where the person is and provides a map to the location and to the location of the automatic external defibrillator (AED) closest to the patient.

Often, these PulsePoint volunteers arrive much faster than the official emergency vehicles and staff and are able to provide initial CPR. Typically, three to eight people are notified by the system: It is completely dependent on the location of the patient and the location of the volunteers. The numbers of daily activations of the application are viewable in real-time on Twitter at @1000livesaday.

The application has been installed in more than 600 different communities, from Los Angeles to Cleveland. However, implementing the software is expensive ($25,000), with additional monies needed for marketing to publicize it in the community (Aleccia, 2014).

Even so, adoption of PulsePoint is an example of the height of patient engagement, where patients are helped by community residents who are so engaged into the community that they volunteer to install the software and be available in case a person needs help. Patient engagement extends to helping others, as well as becoming engaged in one's own healthcare.

Google Glass and CHaRM™

Google Glass and CHaRM™ provide a heads-up display (HUD) to the wearer or viewer. A *heads-up display* permits the wearer to see a video display straight ahead on a screen, so that the head is not moved and the wearer can still see ahead. The data that is included in the display is configurable, from the ED physician's view of the EHR to a display screen for the surgeon in the OR.

Google Glass is being trialed in many situations, including being worn by providers. The glasses can display the patient's EHR, lab results, and any radiology or cardiology results in a hands-free format. Google is estimating that more than 6.5 million units will be sold by 2016. The glasses can take pictures that are automatically added to the patient's EHR, as well as ensure improved billing by taping procedures for later coder review (Diana, 2014).

CHaRM™ is a heads-up display for the operating room. Although it is not worn, it is completely configurable, with windows displaying a body image with the surgical site indicated, an image gallery, the patient's name and medical record number, any allergies, the list of staff in the room, and any other information the users think is necessary. The users can devise different checklist screens and change them at different points in the surgery. The screen's displayed content is controlled by the end users' voices (Combs, 2014).

And because many of the devices are being created for monitoring sports, it is not a far leap to have those devices monitoring healthcare information. Although not all these items are commercially available (Google Glass is available for purchase and CHaRM™ is still in late research), all are in production, with estimated release dates of 2014 to 2016. An article in *Scientific American* discusses the many different possibilities for wearable technology, saying that futurists predict that most people will be wearing four to six different devices in the near future (Westervelt & Climate Confidential, 2014). Not all the devices will have healthcare implications, but many can.

Regarding a very patient-orientated device, David Evans reported, “This concept is evolving to be even more personal, and not just for the benefit of the wearer. Expectant mothers will wear electronic ‘tattoos’—smart sensing stickers that can monitor fetal heart rate and brain waves, detect early signs of labor, and even notify the doctor directly when it is time to go to the hospital” (Evans, 2013). The device has a predicted launch in 2014.

To ensure that wearable healthcare technology is useful—and used—providers have to be able to accept and analyze any data electronically delivered to them, which most cannot do now. According to Scher (2014), wearable technology for consumers does not have to demonstrate efficacy, but it will need payer participation as well as involving the caregivers in the data collection and analysis.

As of this writing, no applications are available that can interface with any EHR that can accept and store data from these wearable technologies. The HealthIT.gov website has several articles about patient-generated data and its importance and has published several guides to the incorporation of this patient data into the electronic record. The Office of the National Coordinator published “Issue Brief: Patient Generated Health Data and Health IT,” which details the issues involved in incorporating this important information into the patient’s record. There is caution about regulation of the data format, given that it is thought that regulation may well slow down the data’s inclusion in the EHR. Rob McCray, President and CEO of the Wireless-Life Sciences Alliance, has insisted that the incorporation of patient-generated data is absolutely essential to healthcare (Deering, 2013). Although the importance is recognized, little progress has been made in that data incorporation. Currently, many patient portals do not permit any editing by the patient. Even if the patient is capable and articulate, patient data is entered into the record only by healthcare providers—even if that person is a clerk.

The application of wearable technology in healthcare, especially in areas that really require hands-free access, is growing (Diana, 2014). And that growth is increasing the possibility of point-of-care data delivery and improving patient care with better access to patient information.

Conclusion

Technology will continue to change our lives and open up more data and communication options for our patients. In the future, patients will be able to securely communicate with their care team, use telehealth technologies, research reviews and publicly reported outcomes for providers and facilities, view and upload information from consumer devices to their medical record, and seek out virtual support groups and education, all from their homes. As patients become engaged and empowered with their data and online forums, we expect to see better health outcomes, increased efficiency of our health systems, and higher levels of patient satisfaction. This makes it increasingly imperative that as nurses, we stay up to date on current trends and technologies so that we can have a better understanding of how our patients seek information and communicate and foster positive, caring relationships.

References

Aleccia, J. (2014, June 3). Heart attack rescue? There's an app for that. *NBC News.* Retrieved from http://www.nbcnews.com/health/health-news/heart-attack-rescue-theres-app-n121911

American Heart Association. (2013). Cardiac arrest statistics. [Data file]. Retrieved from http://www.heart.org/HEARTORG/General/Cardiac-Arrest-Statistics_UCM_448311_Article.jsp

Barry, J., & Hardiker, N. R. (2012). Advancing nursing practice through social media. *OJIN: The Online Journal of Issues in Nursing, 17*(3). Retrieved from http://www.medscape.com/viewarticle/780048_3

Berkman, N. D., Sheridan, S. L., Donahue, K. E., Halpren, D. J., & Crotty, K. (2011). Low health literacy and health outcomes: An updated systematic review. *Annals of Internal Medicine, 155*(2), 97–107.

Blum, S. (2014, June 4). InvisionHeart's portable EKG device attracts $1.9 million in Series A round. *MedCity News.* Retrieved from http://medcitynews.com/2014/06/invisionhearts-portable-ekg-device-attracts-1-9-million-series-round/?utm_source=MedCity+News+Subscribers&utm_campaign=2e0025d176-RSS_Medical+Devices&utm_medium=email&utm_term=0_c05cce483a-2e0025d176-67041049

Caligtan, C. A., Carroll, D. L., Hurley, A. C., Gersh-Zaremski, R., & Dykes, P. C. (2012). Bedside information technology to support patient-centered care. *International Journal of Medical Informatics, 81*(7), 442–451. Retrieved from http://dx.doi.org/10.1016/j.ijmedinf.2011.12.005

Cardiocom. (2014). Nurse call center. Retrieved from http://www.cardiocom.com/nurse_call_center.asp

Carman, K. L., Dardess, P., Maurer, M., Sofaer, S., Adams, K., Bechtel, C., & Sweeney, J. (2013). Patient and family engagement: A framework for understanding the elements and developing interventions and policies. *Health Affairs, 32*(2), 223–231.

Center for Advancing Health. (2010). A new definition of patient engagement: What is engagement and why is it important? Retrieved from http://www.cfah.org/file/CFAH_Engagement_Behavior_Framework_current.pdf

Chou, W. Y., Liu, B., Post, S., & Hesse, B. (2011). Health-related Internet use among cancer survivors: Data from the Health Information National Trends Survey, 2003–2008. *Journal of Cancer Survivors, 5*(3), 263–270. Retrieved from http://dx.doi.org/10.1007/s11764-011-0179-5

Combs, V. (2014, June 27). Heads up displays for surgeons moves closer to launch. *MedCity News*. Retrieved from http://medcitynews.com/2014/06/parallax/

Comstock, J. (2013, August 7). More details emerge on Scripps Wire for Health trial. *MobiHealthNews*. Retrieved from http://mobihealthnews.com/24513/more-details-emerge-on-scripps-wired-for-health-trial/

Coulter, A. (2012). Patient engagement: What works? *Journal of Ambulatory Care Management*, *35*(2), 80–89. Retrieved from http://dx.doi.org/10.1097/JAC.0b013e318249e0fd

Davis, T. C., Crounch, M. A., Long, S. W., Jackson, R. H., Bates, P., George, R. B., & Bairnsfather, L. E. (1991). Rapid assessment of literacy levels of adult primary care patients. *Family Medicine, 23*(6), 433–435.

Darkins, A., Ryan, P., Kobb, R., Foster, L., Edmonson, E., Wakefield, B., & Lancaster, A. (2008). Care coordination/home telehealth: The systematic implementation of health informatics, home telehealth, and disease management to support the care of veteran patients with chronic conditions. *Telemedicine and e-Health, (14)*10, 1118–1126. Retrieved from http://dx.doi/org/10.1089/tmj.2008.0021

Deering, M. (2013, December). Patient-generated health data and health IT. [Issue Brief]. Retrieved from http://www.healthit.gov/sites/default/files/pghd_brief_final122013.pdf

Delbanco, T., Walker, J., Bell, S. K., Darer, J. D., Elmore J. G., Farag, N., … Leveille, S. G. (2012). Inviting patients to read their doctors' notes: A quasi-experimental study and a look ahead. *Annals of Internal Medicine, 157*(7), 461–470.

Dentzer, S. (2013, February). Rx for the "blockbuster drug" of patient engagement. *Health Affairs*, *32*(2), 202. Retrieved from http://dx.doi.org/10.1377/hlthaff.2013.0037

Diana, A. (2014, June 18). Google Glass gains momentum in healthcare. *Information Week*. Retrieved from http://www.informationweek.com/healthcare/mobile-and-wireless/google-glass-gains-momentum-in-healthcare/d/d-id/1278648

Dolan, B. (2014a, January 31). Aetna now reimburses for iRhythm's ZIO Patch. *MobiHealthNews*. Retrieved from http://mobihealthnews.com/29484/aetna-now-reimburses-for-irhythms-zio-patch/

Dolan, B. (2014b, March 21). In depth: Providers' inevitable acceptance of patient-generated health data. *MobiHealthNews*. Retrieved from http://mobihealthnews.com/31268/in-depth-providers-inevitable-acceptance-of-patient-generated-health-data/

Dolan, B. (2014c, February 11). Scripps to test NASA-developed, smartphone enabled lung cancer sensor. *MobiHealthNews*. Retrieved from http://mobihealthnews.com/29840/scripps-to-test-nasa-developed-smartphone-enabled-lung-cancer-sensor/

Evans, D. (2013). The future of wearable technology: Smaller, cheaper, faster and truly personal computing. Retrieved from http://www.linkedin.com/today/post/article/20131024145405-122323-the-future-of-wearable-technology-smaller-cheaper-faster-and-truly-personal-computing

Ferguson, T. (2007). e-Patients how they can help us heal health care. Retrieved from http://e-patients.net/e-Patients_White_Paper.pdf

Gross, D. (2014, January 9). Is wearable technology the fad or the future? [Web log post]. Retrieved from http://www.thedailybeast.com/articles/2014/01/09/is-wearable-technology-a-fad-or-the-future.html

HealthIT.gov. (2014). What is a patient portal? Retrieved from http://www.healthit.gov/providers-professionals/faqs/what-patient-portal

Hibbard, J., Mahoney, E., Stock, R., & Tusler, M. (2007). Do increases in patient activation result in improved self-management behaviors? *Health Services Research, 42*(4), 1443–1463.

Househ, M., Borycki, E., & Kushniruk, A. (2013). Empowering patients through social media: The benefits and challenges. *Health Informatics Journal, 20*(1), 50–58. Retrieved from http://dx.doi.org/10.1177/1460458213476969

Inglis, S. C., Clark, R. A., McAllister, F. A., Stewart, S., & Cleland, J. G. (2011). Which components of heart failure programmes are effective? A systematic review and meta-analysis of the outcomes of structured telephone support or telemonitoring as the primary component of chronic heart failure management in 8323 patients: Abridged Cochrane Review. *European Journal of Heart Failure, 13*(9), 1028–1040. Retrieved from http://dx.doi.org/10.1093/eurjhf/hfr039

James, J. (2013, February). Health policy brief: Patient engagement. *Health Affairs,* pp. 1–6

Kish, L. (2012, August 28). The blockbuster drug of the century: An engaged patient. Retrieved from http://www.hl7standards.com/blog/2012/08/28/drug-of-the-century/

Kotenko, J. (2013, April 18). The doctor will see you now: How the Internet and social media are changing healthcare. Retrieved from http://www.digitaltrends.com/social-media/the-internet-and-healthcare/#!2q2R6

Lamberts, R. (2013, May 2). This is what patient engagement really is [Web log post]. Retrieved from http://www.kevinmd.com/blog/2013/05/patient-engagement.html

Mayo Clinic. (2010). Referred to Mayo Clinic by Twitter and YouTube. Retrieved from http://sharing.mayoclinic.org/discussion/referred-to-mayo-clinic-by-twitter-and-youtube/

National Council of State Boards of Nursing. (2011). A nurse's guide to the use of social media. [White Paper]. Retrieved from https://www.ncsbn.org/Social_Media.pdf

Pew Research Center. (2014). Health fact sheet. Retrieved from http://www.pewinternet.org/fact-sheets/health-fact-sheet/

Polta, A. (2012, March 30). Defining patient engagement [Web log post]. Retrieved from http://healthbeat.areavoices.com/2012/03/30/defining-patient-engagement/

Ralston, J. D., Silverberg, M. J., Grothaus, L., Leyden, W. A., Ross, T., Stewart, C., . . . Carzasty, S. (2014). Use of web-based shared medical records among patients with HIV. *American Journal of Managed Care, 4*(19), e114–e124.

Reed, J. C., & Topol, E. J. (2012, April 13). Medscape one-on-one: Reed Topol on the creative destruction of medicine [Video file]. Retrieved from http://www.medscape.com/viewarticle/761951#2

Robert Wood Johnson Foundation. (n.d.). Grants. Retrieved from http://www.rwjf.org/en/grants/grantees/OpenNotes.html

Robert Wood Johnson Foundation. (2014). New era of patient engagement. Website of Robert Wood Johnson Foundation. Retrieved from http://www.rwjf.org/en/about-rwjf/newsroom/features-and-articles/empowering-patients.html

Robinson, S., Moser, D., Pelter, M, Nesbitt, T., Paul, S., & Dracup, K. (2011). Assessing health literacy in heart failure patients. *Journal of Cardiac Failure, 17*(11), 887–892. Retrieved from http://dx.doi.org/10.1016/j.cardfail.2011.06.651

Ross, S. E., & Lin, C.-T. (2003). The effects of promoting patient access to medical records: A review. *Journal of the American Medical Informatics Association, 10*(2), 129–138. Retrieved from http://dx.doi.org/10.1197/jamia.M1147

Scher, D. (2014, June 3). Five differences between consumer and patient sensor technologies. *Medcity News.* Retrieved from http://www.medcitynews.com

Schmidt, T. L., Sims-Giddons, S. S., & Booth, R. G. (2012). Social media use in nursing education. *OJIN: The Online Journal of Issues in Nursing, 17*(3). Retrieved from http://www.medscape.com/viewarticle/780051_9

Skiba, D. (2014). The connected age: Mobile apps and consumer engagement. *Nursing Education Perspectives, 3*(35), 199–201. Retrieved from http://dx.doi.org/10.5480/1536-5026-35.3.199

Soyer, A. (Ed.). (2012). Social media in healthcare: A primer for orthopaedic surgeons. [White Paper] Retrieved from http://www3.aaos.org/member/prac_manag/Social_Media_Healthcare_Primer.pdf

Sullivan, M. (2014). "Industry sources" say Apple's anticipated health wearable will be on wrists by fall. *MedCity News.* Retrieved from http://medcitynews.com/2014/06/industry-sources-say-apples-anticipated-health-wearable-coming-fall/

Topol, E. J. (2012, June 5). The creative destruction of medicine: Topol on 5 devices physicians need to know about. [Video file]. Retrieved from http://www.medscape.com/viewarticle/765017?src=mp&spon=25

The University of Arizona. (2014). Arizona Telehealth Program. Retrieved from http://telemedicine.arizona.edu/about-us/home

Vargas, K. (2013). Evaluating health websites. Retrieved from http://nnlm.gov/outreach/consumer/evalsite.html

Walker, J., Darer, J. D., Elmore, J. G., & Delbanco, T. (2014). The road toward fully transparent medical records. *The New England Journal of Medicine, 370*(1), 6–8. Retrieved from http://dx.doi.org/0.1056/NEJMp1310132

Weaver, B., Lindsay, B., & Gitelman, B. (2012). Communication technology and social media: Opportunities and implications for healthcare systems. *OJIN: The Online Journal of Issues in Nursing, 17*(3). Retrieved from http://www.medscape.com/viewarticle/780049_4

Westervelt, A., & Climate Confidential. (2014, May 29). Wearable tech helps you live in the moment. *Scientific American.* Retrieved from https://www.scientificamerican.com/article/wearable-tech-helps-you-live-in-the-moment/

Wilkins, S. (2012, January 27). Patient engagement is the holy grail of health care [Web log post]. Retrieved from http://www.kevinmd.com/blog/2012/01/patient-engagement-holy-grail-health-care.html

Wood, M. (2014, March 5). No longer clashing, wearable tech embraces fashion. *The New York Times.* Retrieved from http://www.nytimes.com

"Do not wait for leaders; do it alone, person to person."

–Mother Teresa

Informatics in Non-Acute Care Settings

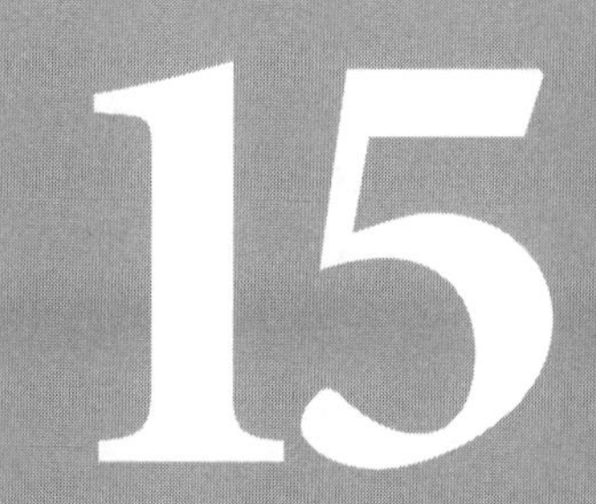

Maria Arellano, MS, RN
Rick Gagnon, RN, FNP

OBJECTIVES

- Discuss various non-acute settings and their challenges for informaticists.
- Review obstacles to adoption of health information technology within non-acute settings.
- Understand the health IT industry's priorities for action with long-term post-acute care settings.

Much of the attention surrounding health information technology (IT) focuses on the acute care setting; however, the healthcare industry serves a population that predominantly needs ongoing, chronic care. Patients requiring chronic care make up a significant percentage of the healthcare costs today, seeking care in many of the non-acute care settings discussed in this chapter. According to the Centers for Disease Control (2009), about 133 million Americans—nearly 1 in 2 adults—live with at least one chronic illness, and more than 75% of healthcare costs are due to chronic conditions. Many of these adults living with chronic conditions are Medicare beneficiaries, and significant gaps exist in care coordination within the traditional Medicare fee-for-service (FFS) payment structure. These gaps occur because of fragmented care, poor communication among providers in a variety of settings, and the lack of financial incentives to coordinate care (MedPac, 2012).

Payment reform driving the shift to paying for quality versus FFS will require all healthcare providers to have a fundamental change in mindset, culture, and attitude about volume and practice to eliminate redundant or unnecessary care and drive patients into the lowest possible cost setting in which quality care can be delivered. Managing a population's health across the entire continuum of care, keeping patients healthy through preventive and primary care services and out of acute care facilities whenever possible is the ultimate goal (York, Kaufman, & Grube, 2013).

If true healthcare reform is to be achieved, all settings where patients receive care must be connected and coordinated. One of the key requirements for the success of healthcare reform requires that the silos that exist across the healthcare settings be abolished. These silos lead to fragmented and redundant care that very frequently lowers the quality and increases the cost of care. Interoperability of health information technology, along with clinical informatics, plays a significant role in the removal of these silos and continues to show promise to revolutionize the way care is provided in all areas (Brailer, 2005).

The usage of Long-Term and Post-Acute Care (LTPAC) services is expected to grow rapidly as the population of the United States ages. LTPAC settings can range from complex care in long-term acute care hospitals (LTACH), inpatient rehabilitation facilities (IRF), or skilled nursing facilities (SNF) to simple supportive services in a community from assisted living facilities and home-based care. Patients receiving services from LTPAC providers typically are more complex, with multiple comorbidities resulting in frequent transitions between these settings. The frequent transitions of these patients require the sharing of relevant data in a timely fashion in order to successfully coordinate care. To achieve this goal, providers in all settings must have the systems to support information capture, use, and exchange. The Office of the National Coordinator for Health Information Technology (ONC) states that as adoption of electronic health records (EHRs) and health information exchange (HIE) by eligible professionals and hospitals increases, the need to understand and support EHR and HIE adoption across the LTPAC community is heightened (2012b).

The clinical informaticist in each of these non-acute settings plays an important role in advancing improvements in healthcare quality and cost. Some of these settings, however, may not have the same level of maturity in the informatics role compared with the acute care setting. The functions and roles that the informaticist performs in the non-acute settings are very similar to their counterparts in acute care and are consistent with those set forth by the American Nurses Association *Nursing Informatics: Scope and Standards of Practice* (2008). These informaticists are primarily serving in the following functional areas:

- Leadership, administration, management
- Compliance and integrity management
- Coordination, facilitation, and integration
- Development

Health Information Technology in Non-Acute Settings

Even though nursing and medical standards of practice exist that are consistent across all settings, each setting is challenged by its unique workflow, business models, and regulations that require assistance from operational experts to guide selection, design, implementation, and optimization of tools and technology. This section will provide an overview of each setting and discuss key issues and challenges that the informaticist must understand for successful adoption of health IT.

Ambulatory Care

Ambulatory care is characterized by healthcare settings that provide treatment and services that can be delivered to the patient safely as an outpatient and also include independent office-based settings or clinics with single or multiple specialties, dental clinics, dialysis centers, infusion therapy centers, hospital outpatient departments and surgical centers, and clinics owned and operated by hospitals or government entities. The Medicare/Medicaid EHR incentive program included many of the ambulatory care setting providers—such as physicians, dentists, and nurse practitioners—as eligible providers to receive the incentives to adopt EHR systems.

Since the passage of the Health Information Technology for Economic and Clinical Health (HITECH) Act in 2009, physician adoption of EHR technology has increased substantially. In 2012, 72% of office-based physicians had adopted any EHR system, which was up 48% since 2009; and 66% of physicians intended to participate or intended to apply for the Medicare or Medicaid incentive program (Hsiao & Hing, 2012). This steady growth in physician adoption of EHR technology to meet Meaningful Use objectives aims to improve quality, safety, and efficiency. According to the ONC (2012), some of the key capabilities adopted so far by physicians include:

- E-prescribing (73%), more than doubled since 2009
- Electronic medication lists (68%)
- Drug interaction checks (67%)
- Providing patients with clinical summaries after each visit (56%)
- Secure messaging with patients increased in 1 year (40%)

According to Xierali, Phillips, Green, Bazemore, and Puffer (2013), EHR adoption varies significantly along primary care practice settings. Family physicians in health maintenance organizations, government, and faculty settings were more likely to adopt EHRs than physicians in solo practices, small partnerships, and other settings. Rural physicians are only slightly behind their urban peers in EHR adoption. Some of the obstacles to EHR adoption cited include lack of capital and support resources for system implementation and maintenance.

And despite the steady growth in adoption for primary care providers, adoption rates in the non–primary care specialists; physicians older than age 55; and physicians in small, physician-owned practices are lower, according to Decker, Jamoom, and Sisk (2012). Decker et al. believed that in order to achieve nationwide adoption for all provider types, federal policies should focus on encouraging adoption among non–primary care specialists, addressing persistent gaps in the use of electronic record systems by practice size, physician age, and ownership status.

For some ambulatory care providers, the availability of affordable resources or informatics support for all phases of adoption may be limited, especially in the independently owned offices and clinics. Frequently, these providers must use costly consultant services for vendor selection, system design, implementation, and training. To address this issue, the Federal HITECH Act authorized the creation and funding of health information technology Regional Extension Centers (RECs) to accelerate the adoption of EHRs. RECs offer free or low-cost technical assistance and guidance by helping providers navigate the EHR adoption process from vendor selection and workflow analysis to implementation and meaningful use attestation.

The ONC–established goal for the RECs is to bring 100,000 primary care providers to Meaningful Use of EHRs as defined by the Centers for Medicare and Medicaid Services (CMS) within 2 years. As of January 2014, the ONC (on the Health IT Dashboard) reports achieving 85% of the original goal through the RECs' efforts. As of this writing, more than 147,000 providers are enrolled with an REC for support and guidance, which accounts for 41% of primary care providers (PCPs) nationwide and 51% of rural PCPs. RECs are clearly demonstrating their success, with 85% of REC–enrolled providers "live" on an EHR compared with 62% live on an EHR in the general provider population.

Informaticists supporting the ambulatory care setting must fully understand the clinical documentation requirements and practice management needs of the ambulatory care provider. Every practice has its individual needs and preferences based on its specialty, but there are some common issues that apply to most practices, such as patient registration, scheduling, and billing. Additional knowledge and skill set requirements that the informaticist must possess for the ambulatory setting include:

- Meaningful Use requirements and timelines for EHR incentives
- Federal, state, and local regulatory requirements for ambulatory care/physician practices
- Tight integration of billing with clinical workflows in order to help with compliance with CMS billing and provide supportive documentation for services billed
- Support of code sets used in practice including Current Procedural Terminology (CPT) codes, Healthcare Common Procedure Coding System (HCPCS), and International Classification of Diseases (ICD) 9 and 10
- Physician Quality Reporting System (PQRS) to satisfactorily report data on quality measures for covered Physician Fee Schedule (PFS) services furnished to Medicare Part B FFS beneficiaries
- Person-centered medical homes (PCMH)

Skilled Nursing and Long-Term Care Facilities

Care provided in an SNF is evolving rapidly, due in part to changing regulations and reimbursement models as well as the increase in complexity of these patients with multiple comorbidities. Patients in the SNF setting can receive short-term rehabilitative care before returning to their prior living situation or long-term care (LTC), depending upon their healthcare needs and available resources. National data on the adoption of health information technology in skilled nursing centers and long-term care facilities is not available, but the ONC reports that it is believed to be lagging behind the acute care hospitals. One key reason for the lack of adoption may be that these providers are currently not eligible for the Medicare and Medicaid EHR incentive programs. According to an ONC Issue Brief released in 2013, some of the main challenges that affect LTPAC health IT adoption and use include:

- Differences in clinical processes and information needs
- Lack of staff, leadership, and organizational skills and capacity to acquire, implement, and use technology
- Lack of awareness of and need for interoperable health information exchange solutions
- Lack of access to capital for IT expenditures

Although these providers have electronic systems, they are generally focused on creating and transmitting the *Minimum Data Set (MDS),* which is a federally required assessment tool used for care planning, payment, and quality reporting (ONC, 2013). Many of these facilities maintain patient medical records in both paper and electronic formats, which could lead to fragmented documentation and ineffective communication among the interdisciplinary team.

Similar to the ambulatory care setting, the informaticist supporting skilled nursing and long-term care facilities must have a strong working knowledge of the clinical and business operations. Workflows and needs may vary based on facility size, payer mix, acuity of the patients, and geographic location. SNFs and LTC facilities are highly regulated, and these regulations must be supported within the financial and clinical applications. One of the key requirements in this setting is the support of the MDS and the full Resident Assessment Instrument (RAI) process. The MDS has both clinical and financial implications for the facility and must be tightly integrated throughout the application to ensure accurate assessment and care planning as well as appropriate reimbursement.

Additional knowledge and skill set requirements that the informaticist must possess for the SNF/LTC facility setting include:

- Quality Measures and public reporting on Nursing Home Compare
- Quality Assessment Process Improvement (QAPI)
- Quality Indicator Survey process (QIS)
- Clinical documentation standards for LTC facilities (Medicare/Medicaid/Managed Care)
- Compliance
- Transitions of care and care coordination with health information exchange

Nursing Home Compare

Nursing Home Compare is a CMS website that allows consumers to compare information about nursing homes. It contains quality of care information on every Medicare and Medicaid–certified nursing home in the country, including over 15,000 nationwide. For more information, visit the following website

> www.medicare.gov/nursinghomecompare/About/What-Is-NHC.html

QAPI – Quality Assurance Performance Improvement

Section 6102(c) of the Affordable Care Act requires CMS to establish regulations in Quality Assurance and Performance Improvement (QAPI) and provide technical assistance to nursing homes to help them develop best practices to comply with the forthcoming regulations. CMS has developed a program of technical assistance that includes tools, resources, and training materials to help nursing homes implement QAPI and establish best practices to continuously improve the care and services delivered in each nursing home. Information on the Nursing Home Quality Initiatives can be viewed here

> www.cms.gov/Medicare/Provider-Enrollment-and-Certification/QAPI/Downloads/Aligning_QAPI_FAQ.pdf

QIS – Quality Indicator Survey

The QIS is a two-staged computer assisted survey process used by surveyors to systematically review specific nursing home requirements and objectively investigate any regulatory areas that are triggered. The process is used by selected State Survey Agencies and CMS to determine if Medicare and Medicaid–certified nursing homes meet the federal requirements. Information on the QIS process can be found at the following URL

www.cms.gov/Medicare/Provider-Enrollment-and-Certification/SurveyCertificationGenInfo/Downloads/QIS-Brochure.pdf

Home Healthcare

Home care encompasses several types of care that can be safely provided in the patient's home: certified home care after discharge from an acute care hospital stay, hospice and palliative care, and nonmedical private duty home care. Much like the other LTPAC settings, the home care environment is changing rapidly and is moving toward the use of more automation, increased adoption of EHRs, and the need for comprehensive information management despite not being eligible for incentives to adopt EHRs. Home care is very different from hospital and ambulatory settings and can be an effective way of successfully transitioning patients from hospital to home and of managing their chronic illness. According to the Centers for Medicare and Medicaid Services, more than three million Medicare beneficiaries discharged from the hospital receive nearly 104 million home care visits annually (2010).

According to Resnick and Alwan (2007), approximately 29% of the 10,000 home care agencies in the United States report having implemented point-of-care EHR, and 21% of home care agencies use telemedicine. Among home health agencies using telemedicine, more than 90% used telephone monitoring, and about two-thirds used nonvideo monitoring. Despite concerns about acceptance, there is evidence to suggest that 75% of older people would consent to use telehealth and telemedicine applications that would help diagnose and/or monitor their health conditions in the comfort of their own home. The motivation to accept these technologies was based on the value that older people place on staying in their own homes and remaining as independent as possible (Barrett, 2008).

Medicare, Medicaid, and many private insurance plans pay for certain types of home care provided by Medicare-certified agencies based on medical necessity. Medicare-certified home health agencies (HHA) assess the patient's condition by using the Outcome and Assessment Information Set (OASIS) instrument (a federally mandated assessment form) and initiate the required care. HHAs have been completing and submitting the OASIS tool electronically since 1999; and similar to the MDS, it drives the interdisciplinary care plan and reimbursement and is the basis for the quality measures reported on Home Health Compare. The OASIS tool is required for all agencies that received Medicare and Medicaid funding. Hospice and palliative care agencies are required to complete the Hospice Item Set (HIS) and submit it electronically to CMS. The *HIS* is a data collection tool and one component of the *Hospice Quality Reporting Program (HQRP),* which collects data on seven hospice quality measures.

The National Association for Home Care & Hospice (NAHC) claims that agencies providing nonmedical home care are not as highly regulated as the other types of home care and are not required to submit any assessment data; therefore, the adoption of technology is much lower and may be limited to only the financial aspects of the business (2013). In the past, these providers have not been involved with the other settings. However, as we look at strategies to prevent hospital readmissions, there is great potential for these private-duty home care providers to assist with successful care at home.

The home healthcare aspect of post-acute care also offers tremendous opportunities for the clinical informatics professional because it presents a set of challenges not seen in brick-and-mortar institutions. Clinicians in home care have clinical practice workflows and issues not experienced in other settings, and they take place in a disconnected state in an unfamiliar home environment. The interdisciplinary team assigned to the patient must work closely while it plans and delivers the care; however, ongoing team communication is challenged by offline documentation that may not be readily available until the data has been synchronized on the network. Each team member visits the patient in the home at different times, and the visits are intermittent from one to three days per week, so collaboration is usually conducted over the phone (Sockolow, Adelsberger, & Bowles, 2011).

Equipment needs in home care may also differ from other settings. Mobile devices, such as laptops, must be evaluated on factors such as durability, weight, ease of use in a mobile environment, as well as their capacity to run appropriate home care information technology applications.

Security and privacy are important in all settings, but home care poses additional threats because devices could be lost or stolen when clinicians travel from the patient's home back to the agency office. Patient records could also be compromised if the clinician uses a public (nonsecure) Wi-Fi connection to complete documentation in between visits.

Additional knowledge and skill set requirements that the informaticist must possess for the home care setting include:

- State and federal regulations governing home care
- Documentation standards for home care and payers
- OASIS-C (current version) and HIS mandated by CMS
- Quality measures reported on Home Health Compare
- Hospice Quality Reporting Program
- Home care compliance programs and documentation to support claims
- Survey and certification processes for home care and hospice

Telehealth

The Health Resources and Services Administration (HRSA, 2014) defines telehealth as:

> "[T]he use of electronic information and telecommunications technologies to support long-distance clinical health care, patient and professional health-related education, public health and health administration."

Telehealth technologies are constantly evolving but primarily include videoconferencing, the Internet, store-and-forward imaging (find more on this topic later herein), streaming media, and terrestrial and wireless communications. Telehealth is often confused with telemedicine, and the two terms are sometimes used interchangeably. Telehealth differs from telemedicine because *telehealth* refers to a broader scope of remote healthcare services. *Telemedicine* involves only remote clinical services. Telehealth can involve more than just clinical services, including remote nonclinical services such as provider training, administrative meetings, and continuing medical education (HRSA, 2014).

Telehealth is not necessarily concerned about new healthcare services but simply provides a new way to deliver existing healthcare services. One of the key advantages of telehealth is allowing patients to remain in their communities while being seen by a healthcare provider at a remote site. Patients benefit greatly from the savings of time and money as well as reducing the time that patients are away from work. It also plays a more important role as we move away from the traditional FFS system and toward new models of care, including Accountable Care Organizations (ACO), patient-centered medical homes (PCMHs), and other strategies that focus on outcomes. Telehealth technologies are becoming more widely available in the marketplace, are much easier to use and implement, and are becoming much more affordable (Missouri Telehealth Network, 2014).

There are many examples of innovative ways that telehealth is being used to improve care within all healthcare settings. Simple technologies, such as videoconferencing equipment, provide patients with a live, real-time interaction with a specialist—across town or across country—that feels like they are in the same room. The physician is able to conduct an evaluation of the patient that includes questioning about history and current symptoms and also using electronic diagnostic equipment and other peripheral cameras to provide the visual examination.

For example, in teledermatology, a high-resolution camera or a digital camera is used for the dermatologist to see a close-up view of the patient's wound or skin condition. Remote monitoring equipment used in home healthcare allows a nurse to monitor a patient's adherence to medications or vital sign and weight readings. Family caregivers can be alerted to potential issues that may need intervention to prevent complications or hospital admissions. Telepsychiatry is also being explored within skilled nursing facilities located in communities where psychiatrists and other mental health providers are limited. By visually connecting with a provider early to evaluate the patient in the skilled nursing facility, these technologies show a great deal of promise to aid in the reduction of unnecessary hospital readmissions.

Store-and-forward imaging is another technology used in telehealth that allows x-rays, CT scans, MRI images, and digital and other images to be transmitted from the patient site to a physician located at a remote healthcare facility. In the case of teleradiology, images are sent to a radiologist to be read, and the results are transmitted back to the patient site, which could be ambulatory, acute, care or long-term post-acute care (HRSA, 2014; Missouri Telehealth Network, 2014).

One of the most comprehensive studies in telehealth was conducted at the Veterans Administration (VA). In 2003, the VA introduced home telehealth services to help patients with chronic conditions stay at home successfully rather than moving into an assisted living setting or other care setting. The program used technologies including videophones, digital cameras (for telewound care and teledermatology), and vital sign monitors. By 2007, the program had realized significant cost savings after enrolling 30,000 patients and achieving a 19% reduction in hospital visits. The VA model empowered patients and encouraged self-management by incorporating healthcare into daily routines. Additional telehealth programs developed at the VA have also demonstrated positive outcomes because of regular phone contact with a nurse in managing chronic conditions, such as diabetes, depression, and hypertension (Darkins et al., 2008).

Reimbursement for services using telehealth is variable among private and government payers. Medicare reimburses for certain telehealth services based on the location of the services. Coverage may be available if the originating site is in a Health Professional Shortage Area (HPSA) or in a county that is outside any metropolitan statistical area (MSA). The originating site must be a medical facility and not the patient's home. Under Medicaid, telemedicine is considered a cost-effective alternative compared with the more traditional face-to-face way of providing medical care that states can choose to cover under Medicaid (HRSA, 2014). According to the American Telemedicine Association (2014), 20 states and the District of Columbia require that private insurers cover telehealth in the same way as they cover in-person services. Many other insurers cover at least some telehealth service, and more states have expressed interest in expanding their telehealth coverage as well. As more evidence becomes available on the efficacy of telehealth and telemedicine, more payers are expected to expand their coverage of these services.

The informaticist working in the telehealth arena faces challenges that many other settings do not pose. The requisite knowledge and skill set for each provider setting is needed, as well as knowledge of the patient as an end user as well. According to the ANA *Nursing Informatics: Scope and Standards of Practice* (2008), the informaticist must consider the consumer's needs so that key health information is presented in a format to ensure understanding. Assessment of key considerations—including culture, language, and literacy levels—should be completed prior to implementing any technology. Additional knowledge and skill set requirements the informaticist must possess for the delivery of telehealth services include:

- Assessment of appropriateness of telehealth for the patient's ability and status
- Evaluation of equipment options
- Infection control and cleaning of equipment
- Information safety/security
- Technology infrastructure/interoperability and connectivity
- Financial impact to practice/patient
- Licensure and credentialing
- Reimbursement
- Evaluation of outcomes

Long-Term Acute Care Hospitals and Inpatient Rehabilitation Facilities

Long-term acute care hospitals (LTACHs) provide extended medical and rehabilitative care to clinically complex patients that need hospital-level care for an extended period of time.

For Medicare reimbursement purposes, patients generally have an average inpatient length of stay (LOS) greater than 25 days. LTACHs have recently implemented the Continuity Assessment Record and Evaluation (CARE) Data Set for submission to CMS which will be the basis for the LTACH quality measures.

Inpatient rehabilitation facilities (IRFs) provide intensive rehabilitation programs to patients who are able to tolerate 3 hours of intense rehabilitation services per day. IRFs can be free-standing rehabilitation hospitals or rehabilitation units within acute care hospitals. These facilities are paid under the IRF Prospective Payment System (PPS) and must submit the IRF-PAI (patient assessment instrument) similar to the aforementioned MDS and OASIS.

Although these facilities may be part of an acute care hospital and operate more like an acute care setting, they are worth mentioning because they are included in the post-acute care sector of healthcare and also do not qualify (as of this writing) for the EHR incentives. The adoption of EHR for these two settings is dramatically lower than the acute care setting. Wolf, Harvell, andJha (2012) found that only 6% of LTACHs and 4% of IRFs had any type of EHR system, and only 2% of LTACHs were using a comprehensive system that had functionality robust enough to have an impact on quality and efficiency.

CMS has established the LTACH and IRF Quality Reporting Program, with payment adjustments if facilities do not comply. Facilities must report quality measures in order to avoid a 2% reduction to their annual payment update. CMS believes that performance on these quality measures will be improved through better coordinated patient care and facilitated via EHR data collection and reporting. These quality reporting programs supplement the preexisting CMS LTPAC quality reporting programs for hospice, home health, and SNFs. The informatics professional can take a leadership role in the development and management of processes and workflows to streamline the collection and submission of the required data and ongoing management of the quality measures.

LTPAC Provider Recommendations to the ONC

In May 2012, the ONC organized a roundtable of LTPAC providers to better understand the information needs of these providers, as well as obstacles to health information exchange. The roundtable participants included representatives from LTPAC providers, professional associations, system vendors, consumer advocates, and representatives from related U.S. federal programs and committees. The roundtable discussions supported two main objectives to ensure:

- LTPAC provider needs for EHRs and HIE services are well understood, and to facilitate the availability of products in the marketplace that meet those needs.
- LTPAC providers know what EHR system features and functions to look for, and to adopt systems that support transitions of care (TOC), care coordination, and related HIE functions.

Table 15.1 highlights the key recommendations provided to the ONC (ONC, 2012a) from the roundtable participants.

Table 15.1 ONC LTPAC Roundtable Participants Recommendations

General Recommendations	Current Activities
Topic: Advancing LTPAC adoption of Health IT	
Consider policy levers for driving change in addition to Meaningful Use and EHR Certification Criteria.	
Develop and administer a survey to more fully understand LTPAC HIT adoption.	
Stage 3 MU Recommendations	**Current Activities**
Topic: Transitions of Care: Patient-centered view of care	
Frame healthcare IT needs around care teams, including patients, families, and caregivers, and have a patient-centered view versus a provider-centric one.	Longitudinal Care Coordination (LCC) Work Group is addressing.
Consider healthcare IT impact on communication among specific team members across the continuum.	
Topic: Transitions of Care: Standards to support HIE	
Consider a broader range of TOC data elements and use cases in Stage 3 MU to support LTPAC.	LCC Transitions of Care Standards Work Group (SWG) is identifying standards.
Support care coordination among the care team and across care settings. At transition, transmit a core set of data and a care plan to all members of the care team in the receiver's preferred transmission method (even if not electronic).	
Acknowledge data received in a reasonable time frame and actionable. Recommend a time stamp to automate acknowledgement of receipt.	

continues

Table 15.1 ONC LTPAC Roundtable Participants Recommendations *(continued)*

Topic: Care Plans: Integrated Care Plans Across Settings	
Move toward vision of a dynamic, longitudinal care plan that can be shared among care team members, including providers, patients, families, and caregivers and exchanged across care settings. Come to consensus around the definition of a care plan, the components of a care plan and their definitions, and standards related to care planning needed across the spectrum of care, including inpatient, outpatient, and LTPAC settings. • Include patient-defined goals, problems, and interventions to support patient-centered care plans. • Include a time stamp with care plans to inform providers about when the plans were last updated. • Identify care team members and related information, such as name, role, and contact information. • Reconcile care plan and patient goals at each care transition.	LCC Care Planning SWG is addressing.
Topic: Patient Assessments	
Support the capture and exchange of patient assessment content, including cognitive status, functional status, and pressure ulcer content, to support care coordination, delivery, and planning.	LCC Patient Assessment SWG is identifying standards and considering.
Topic: Quality Measures	
Support a new MU quality measure related to skin integrity and pressure ulcers.	

Topic Advance Directives
Consider inclusion of advance directive content, including patient preferences and goals.
Consider adoption of a document schema to support exchange.

LTPAC Industry-Led Initiatives and Priorities for Action

In 2005, the LTPAC Health Information Technology (IT) Collaborative was formed to advance health IT issues through coordinated efforts of its members. The Collaborative hosts an annual LTPAC Health IT Summit and publishes of a LTPAC HIT Road Map. The 2012–2014 LTPAC Health IT Road Map is the fourth Road Map published by the Collaborative to provide guidance to provider organizations, policy-makers, vendors, payers, and other stakeholders.

The Collaborative has identified five priority areas for action for the 2012–2014 Road Map for LTPAC stakeholders:

- **Care Coordination:** LTPAC must be a leading participant and enabler of customer-centered longitudinal care planning and coordination across providers and contexts.
- **Quality:** LTPAC must leverage technology to support transparent, accountable delivery, measurement, and improvement of quality of care, services, and outcomes as experienced by consumers both within and across care settings.
- **Business Imperative:** LTPAC must leverage technology to generate innovative, efficient business and service strategies and models that will assure it a leading role in the future of health and wellness delivery.
- **Consumer-centered:** LTPAC's unique opportunity lies in its ability to leverage technology to build on its legacy of longitudinal person-centered care and services through effective integration of care and hospitality paradigms.
- **Workforce Acceleration:** LTPAC must re-equip, re-empower, and re-educate its workforce to effectively leverage technologies as part of care and hospitality service delivery to create great customer relationships, experiences, and outcomes.

2012–2014 LTPAC Health IT Road Map can be viewed in its entirety by downloading it from

http://www.ltpachealthit.org/content/2012-2014-roadmap-hit-ltpac

This collaborative effort and roadmap have guided many LTPAC providers in their efforts to develop their infrastructure for healthcare IT and effectively select and implement technologies to enhance the quality of care. It is not until recently that the ONC and CMS have started offering the LTPAC communities some guidance on how health IT should be adopted. EHR vendors supporting LTPAC providers are not required to be certified; however, several vendors have sought out the 2011 or 2014 certification used in the inpatient and ambulatory settings. These vendors have received the modular certification given that some of the criteria do not apply to their setting.

Recently, the ONC released the Proposed Voluntary Electronic Health Record (EHR) Certification Criteria for Long-Term and Post-Acute Care and Behavioral Health and offered a comment period for stakeholders. There are fewer certification criteria than on the acute and ambulatory care EHR side, and they are more relevant to these providers.

The organizing principles for these recommendations for all providers include:

- Support of transitions of care
- Privacy and security
- Data segmentation/consent management

The full document can be accessed at

http://www.healthit.gov/buzz-blog/federal-advisory-committees/seeking-feedback-voluntary-ehr-certification-behavioral-health-longterm-postacute-care-settings/

It is important to point out that significant work has been accomplished by many LTPAC providers even in the absence of government financial incentives or guidance. As more attention is given to these providers by the ONC, and the full effects of healthcare reform are realized, their participation in health information exchange will be critical to their success. There are tremendous opportunities for the informatics professional to support the providers in these non-acute care settings, and with emphasis on the workforce development, these opportunities are expected to grow. Advancing the adoption of certified EHRs for LTPAC providers supports the implementation of the nationwide health IT infrastructure, ensures that EHR systems meet national standards for data exchange, and contributes to the provision of high quality, well-coordinated care for the nation's most vulnerable patients.

References

American Nurses Association (ANA). (2008). *Nursing informatics: Scope and standards of practice,* (2nd ed.). Silver Spring, MD: Nursesbooks.org.

American Telemedicine Association. (2014). Telemedicine frequently asked questions. Retrieved from http://www.americantelemed.org/about-telemedicine/faqs#.U-408E10zIU

Barrett L. L. (2008). *Healthy @ home.* AARP Knowledge Management Report. Retrieved from http://assets.aarp.org/rgcenter/il/healthy_home.pdf

Brailer, D. J. (2005, January 19). Interoperability: The key to the future health care system. *Health Affairs* [Web log post]. Retrieved from http://content.healthaffairs.org/cgi/content/full/hlthaff.w5.19/DC1

Centers for Disease Control (CDC). (2009). *Chronic disease: The power to prevent, the call to control: At-a-glance.* Retrieved from http://www.cdc.gov/chronicdisease/resources/publications/aag/pdf/chronic.pdf

Centers for Medicare and Medicaid Services (CMS). (2010). Home health quality initiative. Overview webpage. Retrieved from http://www.cms.gov/HomeHealthQualityInits/

Darkins, A., Ryan, P., Kobb, R., Foster, L., Edmonson, E., Wakefield, B., & Lancaster, A. E. (2008). Care coordination/home telehealth: The systematic implementation of health informatics, home telehealth and home management to support the care of veteran patients with chronic conditions. *Telemedicine and e-Health, 14*(10), 1118–1126.

Decker, S. L., Jamoom, E. W., & Sisk, J. E. (2012). Physicians in nonprimary care and small practices and those age 55 and older lag in adopting electronic health record systems. *Health Affairs, 31*(5), 1108–1114.

Health Resources and Services Administration (HRSA). (2014). Rural health IT toolbox: Telehealth. Retrieved from www.hrsa.gov/healthit/toolbox/RuralHealthITtoolbox/Telehealth/index.html

Hsiao, C. J., & Hing, E. (2012). *Use and characteristics of electronic health record systems among office-based physician practices: United States, 2001–2012.* NCHS Data Brief Number 111. Hyattsville, MD: National Center for Health Statistics.

MedPac. (2012). *Care coordination in fee-for-service Medicare. Report to Congress: Medicare and the health care delivery system.* Washington, DC: Medicare Payment Advisory Commission.

Missouri Telehealth Network. (2014). What is telehealth? Retrieved from http://medicine.missouri.edu/telehealth/general.html

National Association of Home Care & Hospice. (2013). CMS provides hospice item set update. Retrieved from http://www.nahc.org/NAHCReport/nr131024_2/

Office of the National Coordinator for Health Information Technology (ONC). (2012a). Long-Term and Post-Acute Care (LTPAC) Roundtable Summary Report of Findings. Retrieved from http://www.healthit.gov/sites/default/files/pdf/LTPACroundtablesummary.pdf

Office of the National Coordinator for Health Information Technology (ONC). (2012b). *Physician adoption of electronic health record technology to meet Meaningful Use objectives: 2009-2012 Health IT Dashboard.* Retrieved from http://dashboard.healthit.gov/rec/

Office of the National Coordinator for Health Information Technology (ONC). (2013). Health IT in long-term and post-acute care [Issue Brief]. Retrieved from http://www.healthit.gov/sites/default/files/pdf/HIT_LTPAC_IssueBrief031513.pdf

Resnick, H. E., & Alwan, M. (2010). Use of health information technology in home health and hospice agencies: United States, 2007. *Journal of the American Medical Informatics Association,* 17(4), 389–395.

Sockolow, P. S., Adelsberger, M. C., & Bowles, K. H. (2011). Identifying certification criteria for home care EHR Meaningful Use. *American Medical Informatics Association annual symposium proceedings, 1,* 1280–1289.

Wolf, L., Harvell, J., & Jha, A. (2012). Hospitals ineligible for federal Meaningful-Use incentives have dismally low rates of adoption of electronic health records. *Health Affairs, 31*(3), 505–513.

Xierali, I. M., Phillips, R. L., Green, L. A., Bazemore, A. W., & Puffer, J. C. (2013). Factors influencing family physician adoption of electronic health records (EHRs). *Journal of the American Board of Family Medicine, 26*(4), 388–393. Retrieved from http://www.jabfm.org

York, R., Kaufman, K., & Grube, M. (2013, March 8). decline in utilization rates signals a change in the inpatient business model. *Health Affairs* [Web log post]. Retrieved from www.healthaffairs.org

"In order to succeed, you have to look at everything from your own unique perspective. When you think, you have to think in your own creative way—not accepting everything that's already out there... ."

–Jacob Barnett, 2012

Healthcare Analytics

16

Charles M. Boicey, MS, RN-BC, PMP, CLNC, CPHIMS

Healthcare analytics serves the clinical, quality, operational, and research needs of our organizations. The field of healthcare analytics is advancing exponentially due to new and emerging technologies; these exponential advances make it difficult for the clinical informaticist to stay current. This chapter surveys healthcare analytics, covering the following topics: data visualization, predictive analytics, and Big Data. The deepest dive is on the visualization of healthcare data, the importance of which cannot be overstated. We can build the best predictive algorithms, make important data discoveries, and build the most efficient decision-support systems—but if we do not visualize the data in a manner in which the viewer can immediately understand it, then we have failed.

OBJECTIVES

- Discuss the science of sight and its application to healthcare analytics.
- Describe various methods of effective healthcare data visualization.
- Discuss the introduction of infographics and Big Data technologies to healthcare.
- Identify appropriate data sources for population management.
- Discuss the various educational opportunities available to clinical informaticists to successfully deploy healthcare analytic solutions.

Assessing Healthcare Analytics

Healthcare analytics can best be described as an evolutionary process. As technology evolves, so too must the clinical informaticist's role and skill set evolve. This also holds true for healthcare organizations. In most cases, this process is organic, but due to necessity, this process has been expedited in many healthcare organizations (Boicey, 2014). As shown in Figure 16.1, there are four stages to this evolution. To better help understand the stages, go through them by looking at the workflow of a department we are all familiar with: Quality.

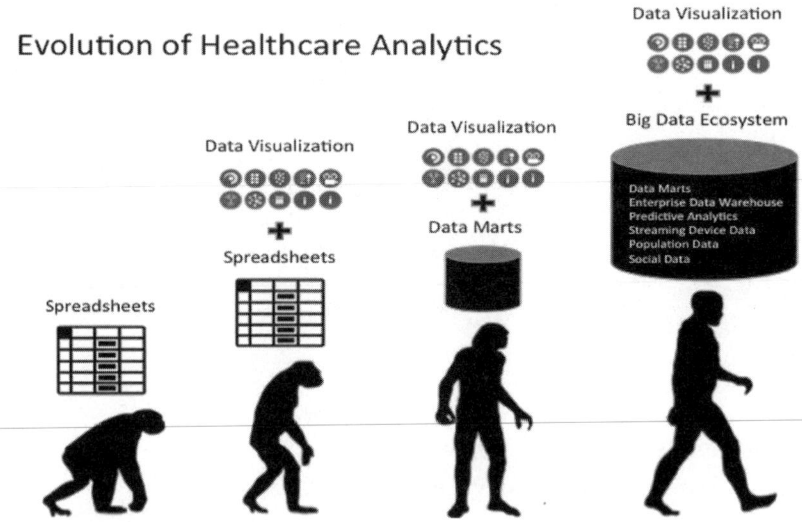

FIGURE 16.1 Healthcare analytics evolution (Boicey, 2014).

The first stage is the use of spreadsheets to collect and analyze quality data. At this stage, quality data is accumulated in spreadsheets via manual abstraction of quality data from such sources as paper documentation, electronic health records (EHRs), and other healthcare systems. The folks in Quality spend 25 or so days on data collection and analysis and have little time to produce data visualizations in the form of reports that are then emailed, posted in SharePoint, or distributed at departmental meetings. After analysis of the quality data is complete, 30 days have passed, leaving very little time for quality improvement projects as the cycle now repeats itself.

In stage 2, we introduce a data visualization application to the spreadsheet. This one addition to the technology stack reaps many benefits. First, by using a data visualization application to build quality dashboards, we now have a means for members of the healthcare organization to view and interact with the quality dashboards. Second, the work of creating visualizations each month is eliminated because after the quality visualizations are built within the application, there is no need to do this work again. This can eliminate one or two days of work for a quality analyst.

In stage 3, we add a data mart to the mix. In our Quality example, this would be a quality data mart. The advantage here is that we are now using data coming directly from the EHR and other healthcare systems, thus decreasing the workload of abstraction.

Additionally, as the data is fed to the data mart daily, we now have dashboards that are much more current.

In stage 4, we see the introduction of a Big Data ecosystem comprising real-time EHR feeds as well as data from other healthcare systems, devices in the hospital and at home, social media, open data, health information exchange (HIE), and population management systems (PMS). Abstraction for our quality peers is minimal: We now have real-time alerts around quality—and best of all, our Quality peers now have time for quality improvement projects.

A *data mart* is a subset of data oriented to a particular service line or organizational unit such as Quality or Surgery.

Big Data

Although not new, the term Big Data is becoming more prevalent in healthcare and will be with us for the future. For healthcare, Big Data comprises the accumulation of healthcare-related data from various sources, combined with new technologies that allow for the transformation of data to information, to knowledge, and ultimately to wisdom.

Best Practices, Applications, and Resources for the Application of Healthcare Analytics

"Data visualization is the use of visual representations to explore, make sense of, and communicate data." –*Stephen Few (2009)*

As healthcare transitions from a pay-for-service model to a pay-for-value model, applying best practices of healthcare analytics is crucial for success. Proper visualization of data is an essential skill for the informaticist to learn to turn data into useful information. To properly visualize data, we must first understand how data visualizations are interpreted.

Science of Sight

Vision is our dominant sense and is tightly coupled with the process of thought. In his book *Thinking, Fast and Slow,* Daniel Kahneman (2011) presents two distinct processes of the brain:

- System 1 represents the automatic and intuitive thinking process.
- System 2 represents the thinking process that requires effort and attention.

For the purpose of visualizing healthcare data from Quality and Operations, you want to ensure that your visualizations invoke System 1 processes. You do not want viewers spending time trying to figure out what the data is representing. You want them to understand immediately. Figure 16.2 represents the presentation of data that requires a System 2 response. Tabular data and data poorly represented in a pie chart causes the viewer to rely heavily on thinking and very little on intuition, thus causing confusion and an out-of-balance state. Conversely, in Figure 16.3, the data is represented so that the viewer can understand the patient waiting time data at a glance.

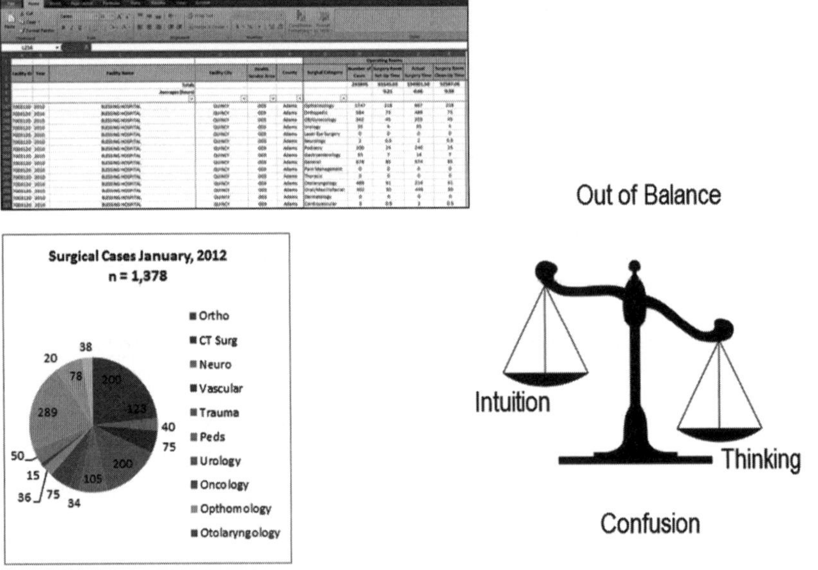

FIGURE 16.2 Out-of-balance state.

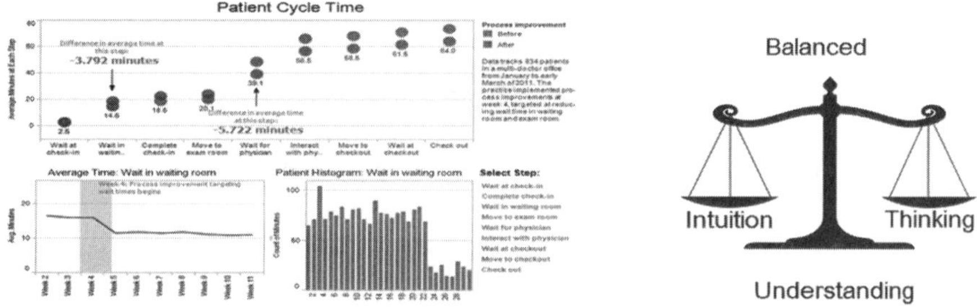

FIGURE 16.3 Balanced state.

Figure 16.4 shows another example of tabular data compared with that same data but shown as a line graph. In this example, we can see that the central line infection rate is improving in this nursing unit. The viewer of this visualization does not have to think but can see the improvements. Consider which technique allows you to understand the trend with the least amount of effort in the quickest amount of time.

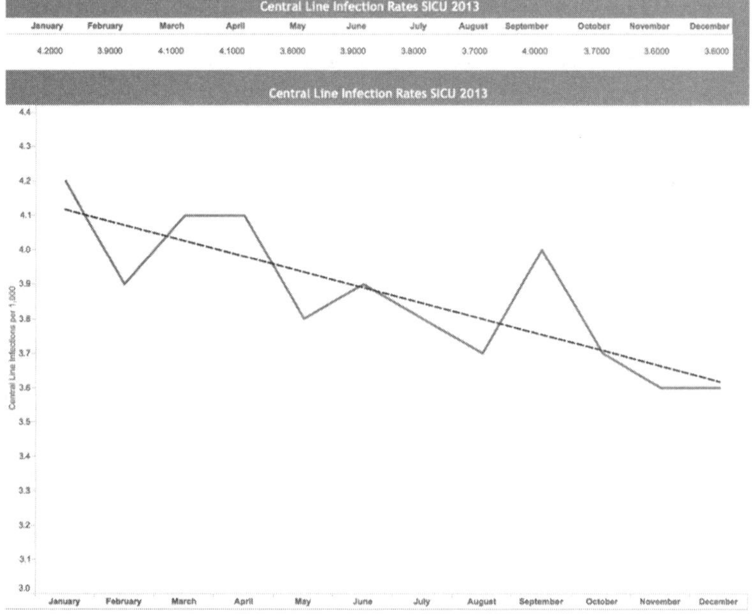

Central Line Infection Rates SICU 2013

January	February	March	April	May	June	July	August	September	October	November	December
4.2000	3.9000	4.1000	4.1000	3.8000	3.9000	3.8000	3.7000	4.0000	3.7000	3.6000	3.6000

FIGURE 16.4 Line graph of central line infection data.

Pie charts can get you into as much trouble as tabular data—and here is why. People tend to throw in too many variables and end up with a chart like that shown in Figure 16.5. Too many variables combined with a color code for each variable is confusing.

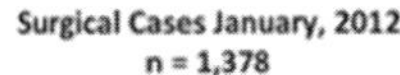

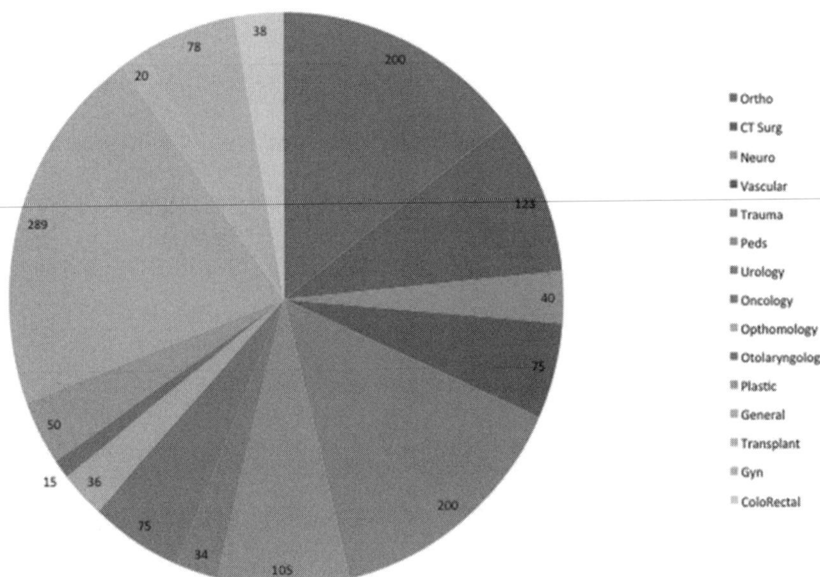

FIGURE 16.5 Pie chart confusion.

Also, as you look at the pie chart, you will likely catch your gaze going back and forth between the chart and the legend. The white space breaks your concentration and affects your short-term memory, causing you to repeatedly go back and forth between the pie chart and the legend. Last but not least, if you do not pay attention, you could possibly end up with a percentage pie chart that makes little sense, as illustrated in Figure 16.6.

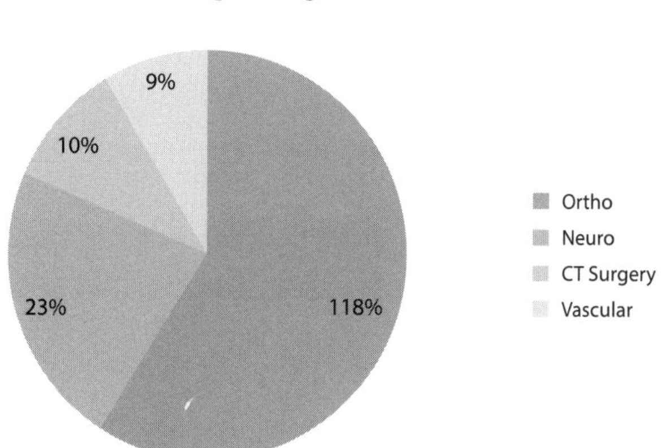

FIGURE 16.6 Pie chart percentages gone awry.

Color plays a very important role in visual perception. As much as 10% of the population has some form of color blindness (Xie et al., 2014); data broken down by ethnicity from a recent study in children is shown in Figure 16.7. It is best practice to consider the use of a colorblind-friendly palette. A colorblind healthcare executive could perceive a dashboard that uses green, red, and yellow as all green, so proceed with caution. Data visualization applications now include a colorblind-friendly palette, so use it.

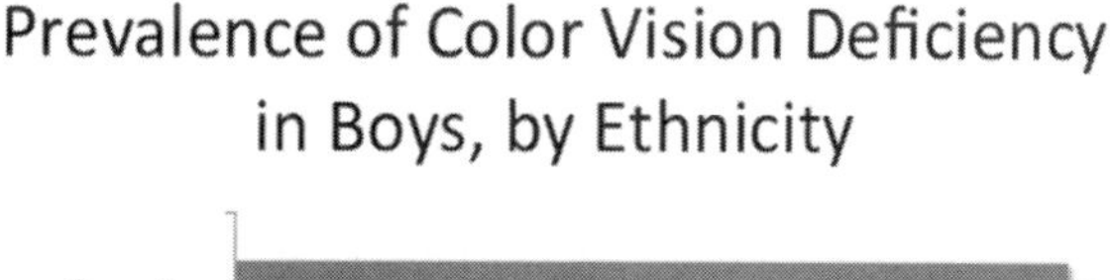

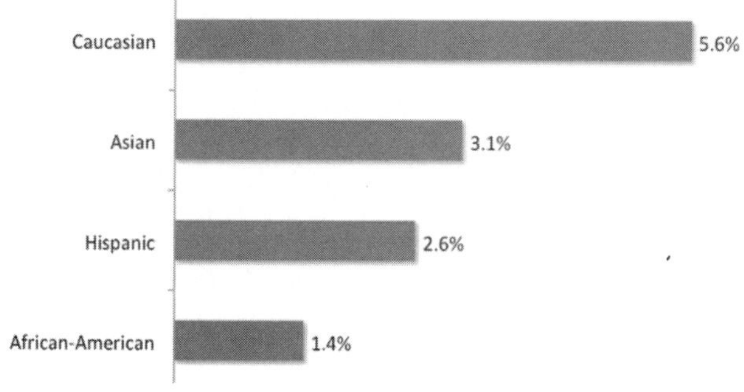

FIGURE 16.7 Breakdown of color deficiencies by ethnicity (Xie et al., 2014).

For further understanding of color blindness and how other visual processing disorders play a role in the interpretation of data, see the following references:

- **Change Blindness:** www.gocognitive.net/demo/change-blindness
- **How the Color Blind See the World:** www.color-blindness.com/coblis-color-blindness-simulator/
- **Visual Perception Videos:** www.dansimons.com/videos.html
- **Visual Processing Disorders:** www.ncld.org/types-learning-disabilities/adhd-related-issues/visual-processing-disorders/visual-processing-disorders-by-age-group

Data Visualization Techniques

Most of the healthcare data you will visualize is quantitative data. For best results representing that data, pay close attention and use attributes that yield the most precise understanding. Reviewing the attributes shown in Figure 16.8, you can see that the length of a line is very precise in that the longer the line the greater the value. Two-D position is also very precise, with higher equating to greater, and a lower placement lesser. Not as precise is using width and size as attributes, with wider equating to greater, and bigger being better.

Precision of Quantitative Perception	Attribute	Example	Description
Very precise	Length	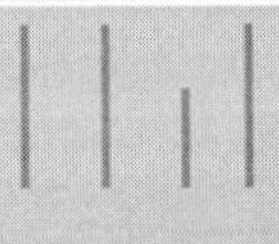	Longer = greater
	2-D Position	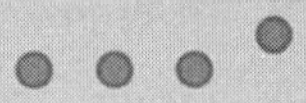	Higher or farther to the right = greater
Not very precise	Width	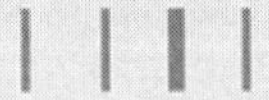	Wider = greater
	Size	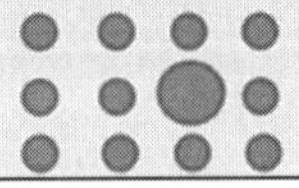	Bigger is greater

FIGURE 16.8 Precision of quantitative perception.

Other attributes that are even less precise include:

- Shape
- Curvature
- Color
- Hue
- Color Intensity
- Direction of Motion

For further study of the various visualization techniques, please visit the following references. Included in the references are my favorite data visualization expert's websites, Stephen Few (Perceptual Edge) and Edward Tufte (Edward Tufte).

- **Introduction to Data Visualization:** http://guides.library.duke.edu/vis_types
- **Perceptual Edge:** http://www.perceptualedge.com/
- **Periodic Table of Visualization Methods:** http://www.visual-literacy.org/periodic_table/periodic_table.html
- **A Tour through the Visualization Zoo:** http://queue.acm.org/detail.cfm?id=1805128
- **Data Driven Documents:** http://d3js.org/
- **The Work of Edward Tufte and Graphics Press:** http://www.edwardtufte.com

I find the best way to become proficient at data visualization is to study the effective visualizations of others. The following are commercially available data visualization tools that offer a trial of their product with a full feature set. Download one or more of these products, and try out various visualization techniques.

- **Alteryx:** www.alteryx.com
- **Birst:** www.birst.com
- **Birt:** www.actuate.com

- **MicroStrategy:** www.microstrategy.com
- **Pentaho:** www.pentaho.com
- **QlikView:** www.qlik.com
- **TIBCO Spotfire:** http://spotfire.tibco.com
- **Tableau:** www.tableausoftware.com

Data Visualization for Clinical Practice

The outcome of the visual perception experiments conducted by Feldman-Stewart, Kocovski, McConnell, Brundage, and Mackillop (2000) concluded that clinical decision support data should be presented in a manner that first evokes a System 1 response—quick and intuitive—and then further data presentation should evoke a System 2 response, which provides data for a more in-depth analysis. For example, when a patient enters an early sepsis pathway, an icon or image is presented to the clinician, and clicking or touching that image brings up the supporting visualization of the pertinent data from which the clinician can make an informed therapeutic decision.

Infographics

Infographics comprise the graphic representation of information which the viewer instantly connects with and understands. When done well, infographics synchronize the visualization with our visual perception capabilities.

The two most iconic and often-referenced infographics did not originate in our century but came to be in the 1850s and 1860s. First is Charles Minard's depiction of Napoleon's ill-fated 1812–1813 march to Moscow and back. As you can see in Figure 16.9, Minard successfully "mashes up" four variables; geography, direction of the march, dwindling army size, and temperature. Not to be outdone, Florence Nightingale created a remarkable visualization of the causes of soldier mortality during the Crimean War that she called a "Rose Diagram," which we now refer to as a "circular histogram." Yes, Florence gave us the circular histogram. In Figure 16.10, Florence cleverly visualized the causes of mortality over a period of time.

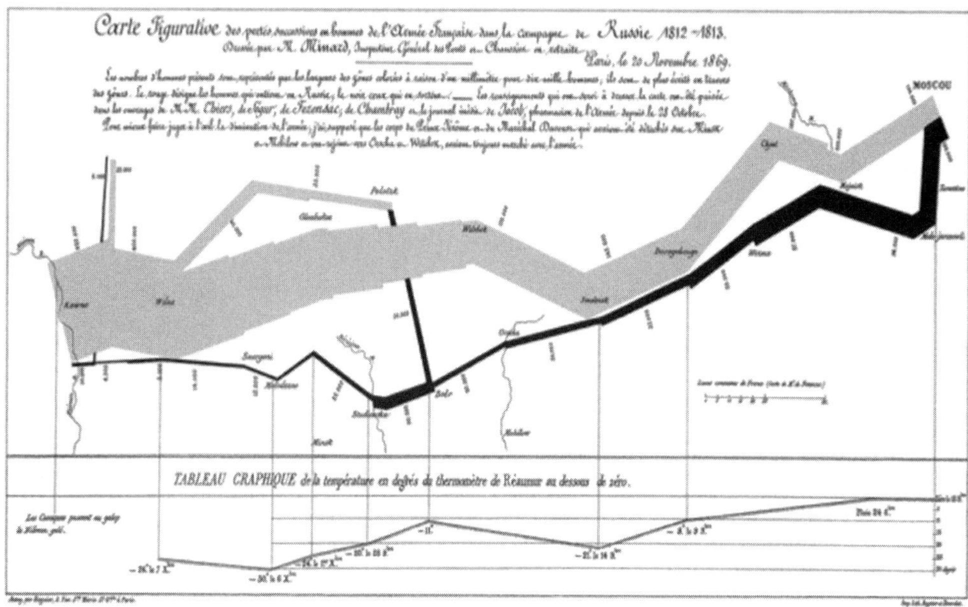

FIGURE 16.9 Minard's depiction of Napoleon's March to Moscow 1812–1813.

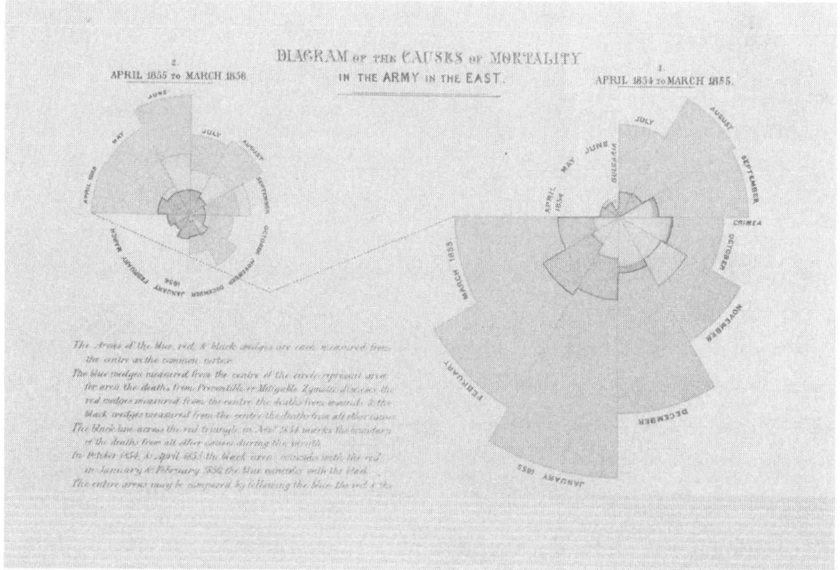

FIGURE 16.10 Florence Nightingale's Rose Diagram.

The following are excellent examples of healthcare analytic–centric infographics sites and the software used to create them.

The following sites exemplify great healthcare infographics:

- **Paul Sonnier:** www.pinterest.com/paulsonnier/digital-health-infographics-paul-sonnier/
- **Pinterest:** www.pinterest.com/search/pins/?q=healthcare%20infographics&rs=ac&len=10
- **HIT Consulting:** http://hitconsultant.net/2014/01/31/best-healthcare-technology-infographics-of-2013/
- **HHS.gov:** https://www.flickr.com/photos/hhsgov/sets/72157633968047018/

Infographics software organizations include:

- **Inbound:** http://blog.hubspot.com/blog/tabid/6307/bid/34223/5-infographics-to-teach-you-how-to-easily-create-infographics-in-powerpoint-templates.aspx?source=hspd-promoted-tweet-5-infographics-blog-post-20140601
- **Infogr.am:** http://infogr.am
- **Creative Bloq:** www.creativebloq.com/infographic/tools-2131971
- **Visually:** http://visual.ly/learn/infographics-software

Big Data

The real-time management of patients hospitalized, seen in clinics, transferred to specialty facilities, as well as those seen in the home will require us to look at analytics through a new lens. Delivering the required analytics functionality to manage patients 24/7, regardless of the setting, necessitates the adoption of Big Data technologies into our practice. Figure 16.11 demonstrates a modern healthcare data platform that not only considers current needs but also allows for the eventuality of new data sources.

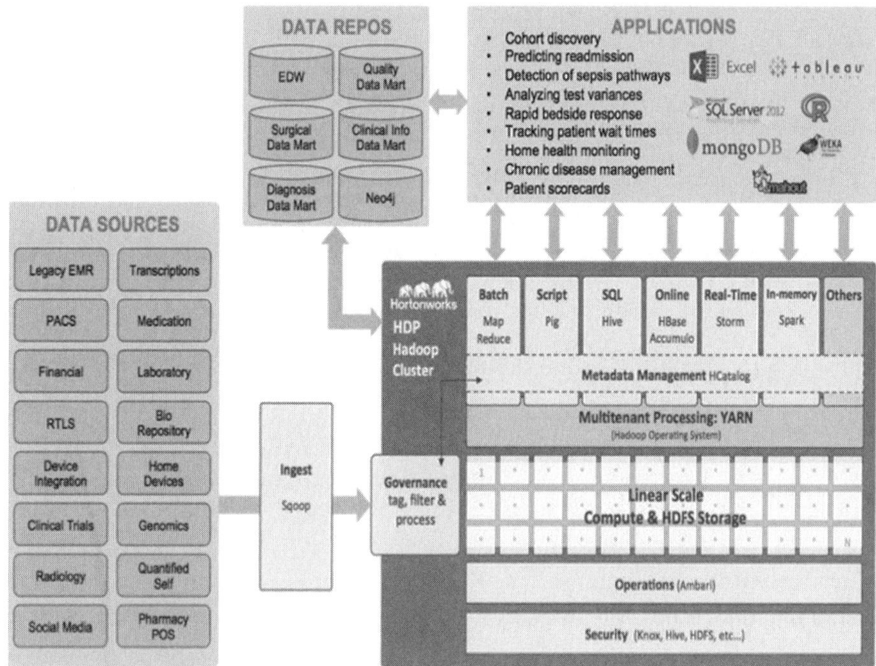

FIGURE 16.11 Modern healthcare data platform (Sears & Boicey, 2014).

Healthcare data sources can include:

Data from wearable devices

Device data (physiological monitors)

EHR–initiated data

EMR source system data: Radiology, Laboratory, Pathology, Images

Financial data

Genomics, proteomics, and metabolomics data

Health Language 7 (HL7) feeds from EHR source systems

Home monitoring

Legacy systems

Medication adherence

Open data sources

Quantified Self data

Real-time location systems

Smart pumps

Social media data

Ventilators

Newer analytics technologies such as R, Hadoop, MapReduce, and Pig require a deeper understanding than is possible in a single chapter. Visit the following references for these emerging technologies:

- **Demystifying Apache Hadoop in Five Pictures:** www.youtube.com/watch?v=xJHv5t8jcM8#t=706
- **Hadoop 101:** The Most Important Terms, Explained: www.plottingsuccess.com/hadoop-101-important-terms-explained-0314/
- **R Explained:** www.youtube.com/watch?v=M2u7kbcXI_k

Newer analytics technologies also bring with them their own set of acronyms and terminology. The following list contains Big Data terms and definitions:

- **Algorithm:** A step-by-step of instructions for caring out a process for problem-solving.
- **Hadoop:** An open source framework for the storage and processing Big Data across a distributed file system.
- **HBase:** Column-oriented data store allowing for fast access to data stored in HDFS. *See HDFS.*

- **HDFS:** Hadoop Distributed File System. A file system for the storage of data across many computers.
- **Hive:** A Hadoop data system that facilitates the interrogation of data stored in HDFS using Structured Query Language (SQL)–like queries.
- **In-memory:** A database management system that stores data in memory not on a disk, resulting in fast processing.
- **Machine learning:** A process in which software learns during data processing and becomes more accurate over time.
- **MapReduce:** The processes of breaking up problems into pieces that are then distributed across multiple computers on the same network or cluster.
- **Metadata:** Data about data. Information about stored data elements.
- **MongoDB:** An open source, reliable, high performance, scalable document database.
- **Natural language processing:** Extracting information from text.
- **NoSQL:** Databases that do not use the relational model, such as databases that store documents, tweets, and so on.
- **Open data:** A data movement in which data sets are made available to the public for use without charge.
- **Open source:** Applications in which the source code is available to the general public for use or modification.
- **Pattern recognition:** Identification of patterns in data via algorithms.
- **Pig:** A programing language used in the Hadoop framework.
- **Quantified Self:** A movement to incorporate data acquisition about self into all aspects of a person's daily living.
- **R:** An open source programing language used for statistical computation. Most commonly used to develop statistical software.
- **Recommender systems:** A system in which treatments, therapies, and medications are recommended based on patient data.
- **Sentiment analysis:** The use of algorithms to understand human feelings.
- **Structured data:** Data that is organized in a predetermined structure.
- **Unstructured data:** Data that does not prescribe to a predetermined structure, such as free text.

We must also consider the application of analytics in non–location-dependent environments. People are mobile. With the advent of wearable technology, we now have the capability to transmit healthcare-centric data irrespective of location. This is exciting because wearable technology offers us a non–location-dependent bidirectional pathway for data. Data from wearable devices, transmitted to a cloud environment with analytics applied, allows feedback to be presented directly to the patient.

For more on wearable technology, see Chapter 14.

Future Directions

I am often asked, "What can I do to stay relevant and keep up to date?" My answer is to stay informed and continue your education. As stated earlier, healthcare analytics technology is changing exponentially, and it is difficult to stay on top of these changes. Table 16.1 shows online graduate certificate and master of science programs offering analytic-centric programs. For the social media–conscious, Table 16.2 shows healthcare analytics LinkedIn groups you can join and Twitter handles you can follow. Additionally, you can join a healthcare informatics–centric association and attend as many conferences as you can. Look for conferences from industries outside the healthcare industry that have matured their analytics programs. There is much to be learned about analytics from other industries, and much of it carries over to healthcare.

Table 16.1 Online Analytics Certificate and Graduate Programs

Academic Organization	*Web Site*
University of California, Irvine (Certificate)	http://unex.uci.edu/areas/it/predictive_analytics/
University of California, Davis (Certificate)	https://extension.ucdavis.edu/unit/health_sciences/certificate/healthcare_analytics/
Northwestern (Master of Science)	http://sps.northwestern.edu/program-areas/Graduate/predictive-analytics/index.php

Academic Organization	*Web Site*
DePaul (Master of Science)	http://www.cdm.depaul.edu/academics/Pages/Current/Requirements-MS-In-Predictive-Analytics-Health-Care.aspx
North Carolina State University (Master of Science)	http://analytics.ncsu.edu/

Table 16.2 Social Media for Healthcare Analytics

LinkedIn Groups	*Twitter Handles*
Digital Health	@amit_p, @geek_nurse
Precision Medicine & Big Data in Life Science	@drsanders, @YvesMulkers
Big Data Visualization	@KirkDBorne, @Paul_Sonnier
Advanced Business Analytics, Data Mining and Predictive Modeling	@wareFLO, @Doug_Laney
Healthcare Analytics & Informatics	@dr_morton, @travisigood

Now that we have the technology, we can truly drive wellness and population health. By monitoring all aspects of wellness and applying analytics, we have the potential to minimize the chronic illness population by keeping the population informed as to their level of wellness.

Making the transition from EHR implementation to healthcare analytics is an exciting one. There is much work to be done, with many secondary uses for the data we worked so hard to place in the EHR. Please stay informed and have fun exploring and visualizing the petabytes of healthcare data out there.

References

Boicey, C. M. (2014, April 14). *Saritor: A big data ecosystem to advance research and clinical practice.* Lecture presented at Big Data in Health in Revere Hotel Boston Common, Boston, MA.

Feldman-Stewart, D., Kocovski, N., McConnell, B. A., Brundage, M. D., & Mackillop, W. J. (2000). Perception of quantitative information for treatment decisions. *Medical Decision Making, 20*(2), 228–238.

Few, S. (2009). *Now you see it: Simple visualization techniques for quantitative analysis.* Oakland, CA: Analytics Press.

Kahneman, D. (2011). *Thinking, fast and slow.* New York, NY: Farrar, Straus and Giroux.

Sears, J., & Boicey, C. (2014, February 2). Healthcare does Hadoop. Retrieved from http://hortonworks.com/industry/healthcare/

Xie, J. Z., Tarczy-Hornoch, K., Lin, J., Cotter, S. A., Torres, M., & Varma, R. (2014). Color vision deficiency in preschool children. *Ophthalmology, 121*(7), 1469–1474. doi:10.1016/j.ophtha.2014.01.018

Recommended Reading

Börner, K., & Polley, D. E. (2014). Visual insights: A practical guide to making sense of data. Cambridge, MA: MIT Press.

Card, S. K., Mackinlay, J. D., & Shneiderman, B. (1999). Readings in information visualization: Using vision to think. San Francisco, CA: Morgan Kaufmann.

Few, S. (2013). Information dashboard design: Displaying data for at-a-glance monitoring. Burlingame, CA: Analytics Press.

Few, S. (2013). Data visualization for human perception. Retrieved from http://www.interaction-design.org/encyclopedia/data_visualization_for_human_perception.html

Fluck, D. (2010, February 23). Color blind essentials | Colblindor. Retrieved from http://www.colorblindness.com/2010/02/23/color-blind-essentials/

Howson, C. (2014). Successful business intelligence: Unlock the value of BI & big data (2nd ed.). New York, NY: McGraw Hill.

Jones, B. (2014). Communicating data with tableau. Beijing, China: O'Reilly Media.

Redmond, E., Wilson, J. R., & Carter, J. (2012). Seven databases in seven weeks: A guide to modern databases and the NoSQL movement. Dallas, TX: Pragmatic Bookshelf.

Sears, J. (2013, November 21). Modern healthcare architectures built with hadoop. Retrieved from http://hortonworks.com/blog/modern-healthcare-architectures-built-with-hadoop/

Tufte, E. R. (2001). The visual display of quantitive information. Cheshire, CT: Graphics Press.

Tufte, E. R. (1997). Visual and statistical thinking: Displays of evidence for making decisions. Cheshire, CT: Graphics Press.

Wong, D. (2013, February 26). 5 infographics to teach you how to easily create infographics in PowerPoint. Retrieved from http://blog.hubspot.com/blog/tabid/6307/bid/34223/5-infographics-to-teach-you-how-to-easily-create-infographics-in-powerpoint-templates.aspx?source=hspd-promoted-tweet-5-infographics-blog-post-20140601

"The potential for mHealth to lead to the complete re-engineering of healthcare is limited by only two things: our imagination, and more immediately pressing, the need for direct evidence to guide its implementation."

–Steven Steinhubl

17

Connected and Mobile Health's Promise for the Triple Aim

Susan C. Hull, MSN, RN

OBJECTIVES

- Describe how mobility and connectivity are the new context for care.
- Preview opportunities for mobile health solutions to lower healthcare costs.
- Describe how mobile health technologies are converging with the fields of systems biology, genetics, and genomics to support co-producing precise, individualized, and personalized health.
- Identify current practices and challenges for adoption and scale of mobile health solutions, for consumers, nursing, and collaborative care teams.

Our mobile lifestyle is the new context of care for patients, families, care team providers, diverse care settings, and payers. Connected and mobile health innovations are catalyzing rich and alternative care-delivery models to complement the place-based care model around which we have organized so much of our workplace, technology, clinical practices, and education. These innovations offer promise within an individual care setting and its reach, and among care settings, providers, consumers, and community resources.

A growing cadre of U.S. patients—alternatively called "consumers," "caregivers," or "health citizens"—are engaging in their own health and healthcare, as well as the health of people that they care for, in historically unprecedented ways through the use of personal health information technology (PHIT). Adoption of PHIT is enabled by the convergence of social and economic forces including the following:

- A growing dependency on digital and mobile technologies in everyday life
- Expectations for real-time access to traditional place-based and virtual health services

- Increased clinical and financial responsibilities for patients
- Pressure on providers to transition from episodic to value-based and population health focus
- Significant regulatory and legislative mandates

Experience with these mobile and personal health technologies is early, yet we are catalyzing a multidimensional and relational collaborative care ecosystem. We are engaging patients, caregivers, and families as equal partners within the care team, at not only the health home but also where they work and live. We recognize that health is social and a function of participation. Outcomes are realized when patients and their family caregivers can incorporate health self-care into daily activities and are empowered to share care planning, decision-making, and outcomes evaluation with transparency. Mobile health and connected care solutions offer a tapestry of options to connect and support consumers in more active choices about health services, location, and timing of care. Goldstein and Masters (2014) described the mobile phone as a life management tool—a computer in our pocket—that can support fitness, health, and healthcare anywhere and anytime a person has his or her device activated.

Connecting care, caring, and healthcare interventions comprises one of our fundamental accountabilities as nurses. We are experts in coordinating care and advocating for continuity across settings, communities, and lifetimes. Mobile and connected health innovation now offers us the opportunity to step into leadership to bring this legacy into a timely and valued reality. "Smart" technology, consumers, and nurses will support us to practice to our full scope and strengthen our role in disruptive and more sustainable models of care. Predictions from a recent mobile health report from Compass Intelligence (2014) estimated that remote diagnostics, telecare, intuitive mHealth products, and green and intelligent infrastructure will become the norm by 2020, with 2014 being the tipping point in this trajectory. The promise of impacting Triple Aim outcomes—by simultaneously improving health and healthcare experiences, demonstrating significant health outcomes, and bending the cost curve in healthcare, enabled by mobility—has never been more available.

Mobile Health

The Global Observatory for eHealth (GOe) within the World Health Organization (WHO) defines mobile health (or mHealth) as "medical and public health practice supported by mobile devices, such as mobile phones, patient monitoring devices, personal digital assistants and other wireless devices" (p. 6). mHealth involves the use of voice and short message service (SMS) as well as more complex functionalities, such as 3G systems, global positioning system (GPS), and Bluetooth technology (WHO, 2011).

The background and opportunity of mobile health in the context of connected health, nursing, and the collaborative care team will be explored in this chapter, highlighting current practices, and challenges for adoption and scale.

Mobile Health Is a Disruptive Innovation

Multiple terms and adjectives—such as *mobile* (m-), *digital*, *wireless*, and *electronic* (e-)—describe the technology that is pervasive in our everyday lifestyles as well as how modern enterprises are managed.

Mobile Health—mHealth—as defined by Steinhubl (2014) is a wide-ranging term most commonly used to describe the usage of a wide variety of therapeutic interventions, from something as straightforward as text messaging appointment reminders to novel, standalone diagnostic and monitoring tools that can identify health concerns in real time, virtually anywhere in the world with access to a wireless network.

Telemedicine—literally "healing at a distance" (from the Latin *medicus* and the Greek *tele*)—is the use of technologies to remotely diagnose, monitor, and treat patients. Telehealth is the application of technologies to help patients manage their own health and illnesses through improved self-care and access to education and support systems, often combined with mHealth to create new ways to deliver care (Kvedar, Coye, & Everett, 2014).

Connected health is the umbrella term that has arisen to lessen the confusion of the definitions and distinctions among this family of technologies and services, and predicts the wide reach of expanding care and health data exchange across settings, communities, and geography (Iglehart, 2014).

Industry predictions from research2guidance (2014) estimated that mHealth will develop into a $26 billion market by 2017, partially due to the remarkable growth in wireless connectivity in general. In a world with more than 7.1 billion people, market research indicated that at the end of 2012, there were 6.8 billion mobile subscriptions, with an estimated 3.2 billion unique mobile users. In the United States, with 91% of Americans now owning a cellphone, 56% owning a smartphone, and 34% owning tablet computers (Pew, 2013), we are experiencing the equivalent of having an Internet-enabled computer of sorts in our hands: one of the most powerful health tools.

Steinhubl, Muse, and Topol (2013) postulated that the level of exuberance for mHealth is driven by the convergence of three powerful forces:

- Unsustainable healthcare spending and the need for disruptive solutions
- Rapid growth in wireless connectivity and the capability for bidirectional instantaneous transfer of information
- More precise and individualized medicine requiring a refinement in phenotypes that mandates novel, personal data streams beyond the occasional vital sign or laboratory data retrieved from intermittent clinic visits

Mobile health is a disruption whose time has arrived.

Mobility Is a New Care Model

As Thornberry (2014, p. 175) described in a case study, "[T]rue mobility for both patients and providers unleashes freedom that escalates throughout each aspect of the health continuum."

Thornberry (2014) further describes how the influence of mobile health is likely to be so pervasive that it may be the underlying solution for how many innovations in the Affordable Care Act (ACA) become sustainable. He believes mHealth solutions, in particular virtual visits, are a significant answer to opening access and liberating unnecessary waste in the system. A recent pilot study of providing online care in a primacy care clinic (Mayo Clinic), conducted by Adamson and Bachman (2010), estimated that the use of the e-visit prevented an office visit in at least 999 patients (40%). Topol (2012, p. 234) predicted, "in years ahead, some 50-70% of office visits [will become] redundant, replaced by remote monitoring, digital health records and virtual house calls." Kaiser Permanente predicted in 2014 that by 2016, with the expanded use of video, the number of virtual visits including secure email, telephone and video encounters, in the northern California region, would surpass the number of in-person office visits, which has remained flat since 2008 (Pearl, 2014, p. 254). A recent podium presentation in July 2014, by Kaiser Permanente Chief Information Officer Phil Fasano, confirmed the virtual visits now exceed in-person visits by 3:1, with only a modest effort to promote these (Fasano, 2014).

Virtual Healthcare Services

Delivering synchronous or asynchronous healthcare services through Internet-enabled mobile devices outside of a hospital, clinic, or medical practice to anywhere a person might be.

Examples may include:

- Two-way video visit for complex medication reconciliation by a nurse and pharmacists working with a patient in their home
- A series of email communications for test results clarification questions and answers between a patient and provider
- Structured questionnaires for medication adherence and mood tracking, triggered by a pharmacist on a set schedule after a new anti-depression medicine is started, with results going to pharmacist and/or nurse case manager/provider
- Sleep study conducted at home by a downloadable app with results transmitted via mobile phone
- Shared care plan goal updates sent by any member of a collaborative care team (including the patient) through mobile phone care plan

A new care delivery model that is consumer- and community-based, enabled by mobile and connected health technologies, is predicted to save hundreds of billions of dollars annually and can be instituted for pennies on the healthcare dollar. We have a significant opportunity to bend the mythical healthcare cost curve downward (Thornberry, 2014). The healthcare system, like the culture it serves, is transitioning from the model of renting a movie DVD to using streaming video services, from hailing a corner taxi cab to finding a precise cab and pre-paid driver arrangement on the mobile phone, and more.

Consumer health advocates, policy makers, providers, and payers are voicing agreement that the time is right for implementing a consumer-driven collaborative care model. Care for the empowered and mobile consumer can be received from any provider, anytime, anywhere, on demand, as mobile and connected health technologies mature. mHealth solutions can be tailored and personalized to the individual, while at the same time mass-customized to a larger group. A mobility model fits into the natural way we all live and work. A mobility model also saves time, travel, and money, thus lessening disruption in family and work life. Many of the innovations are keeping patients and family caregivers at home, bringing care teams virtually to patients. mHealth services complement traditional face-to-face services, and together can bring new value and deeper engagement.

For collaborative care teams, mHealth services increase communication opportunities across the professional care team and improves access to services for patients. Teams can engage patients virtually before and/or after face-to-face visits, providing greater capabilities to maintain persistent engagement across time and diverse care settings. Most of the mHealth innovations are device agnostic, meaning that solutions will work on any web-enabled device (e.g., a laptop, a mobile phone, a smart phone, a tablet). Solutions are also on a continuum from simple text messaging to downloadable apps to video technology. Providers will continue to need approaches for engaging patients without access to devices or who live/work in locations that may not be electronically connected.

New models of care such as Primary Care Medical Homes (PCMH), Health Homes, and Accountable Care Organizations (ACOs) are experimenting with how to drive value instead of volume, and mHealth solutions offer great promise. Clinicians can securely connect with other clinicians and with patients. Mobile services are predicted to lower liability through new forms of provider documentation including developing and updating longitudinal care plans, tracking adherence and outcomes, and capturing device and patient-generated health data (PGHD). New e-commerce tools support providers to obtain compensation for out-of-clinic visits. Mobility will support new forms of health information exchange through provider and consumer-mediated exchange, with new benefits of bidirectional instantaneous transfer of information (Hull, 2014).

For researchers, as Collins (2012) described, mobile devices offer low-cost, real-time ways to assess disease, movement, images, behavior, social interactions, environmental toxins, metabolites, and a host of other physiological variables. Many mHealth technologies could be put to highly innovative uses in biomedical research; at the same time, biomedical research could help build the foundation of evidence that many mHealth applications lack. Patient recruitment, engagement, participation, and results/outcomes reporting can all be enabled through a growing number of mHealth platforms, significantly improving the efficiency of trial completion time and new benefits to trial participants and sponsors. From simple HIPAA–compliant text messaging to FDA–endorsed patient reported outcomes (e-PRO) to device- and sensor-generated health and physiological data, we now have the power to bring the research laboratory to the patient in ways never before possible. Real-time, continuous biological, behavioral, and environmental data can greatly improve understanding of the underlying causes of disease. Combining mHealth data with GPS and other Big Data could also lead to early detection and warning systems for outbreaks of illnesses related to environmental exposures or infectious agents.

Payers and policy makers are working to consider new approaches to billing for e-visits and understanding the connected nature of the mHealth customer ecosystem. Krohn and Metcalf (2014) recognized that the number one issue that must be addressed for the mobile health ecosystem to come to fruition is defining, attracting, and retaining the customer. Unlike traditional buyers of healthcare, the mHealth market is largely a retail market, and will be sold on the strength of qualities of connectivity, clinical collaboration, convenience, and cost. It will take a wholesale restructuring of healthcare delivery, including culture change on the part of payers, providers, and patients; a new definition of clinical value based on mass personalization of the care experience; and partnerships that deliver collaborative, coordination, team-based care.

Additionally, employers can benefit from less absenteeism and more presenteeism from increased access to care with lower cost. Minor and moderately acute care and routine chronic illness follow-up becomes possible for employees in the workplace, at home, or virtually. Employers as self-insurers are investing in onsite work clinics and mHealth wellness solutions.

mHealth Enables Co-producing Individualized and Personalized Health

Leroy Hood (2010), well known as the inventor of the first automated DNA-sequencing machine and founder of the Biology Systems Institute at University of Washington, and for his work with the Ohio State University Idea Studio, is credited for his definition in the late 1990s of P4 Medicine (Prediction, Personalization, Prevention, Participation).

- **Prediction:** Using two new sources of health-related diagnostic data—genetic makeup and protein biomarkers—care providers can generate comprehensive predictions about a patient's health future, including the current effects of any abnormal genes and the current reactions to any environmental toxins or infectious pathogens.
- **Personalization:** Understanding each individual's genetic makeup and differences is supporting new approaches to personalization of care. On average, each human differs from another by less than 1% of his or her genetic makeup. These genetic differences give rise to our physical differences, including our potential predisposition to various diseases.
- **Prevention:** Approaches based on each individual's genetic makeup and current blood protein markers will help us determine the probability of an individual contracting certain diseases, as well as reveal how an individual may respond to various treatments, thereby providing guidance for developing customized therapeutic drugs and other prevention strategies.
- **Participation:** Because of prediction, personalization, and prevention, Hood predicts that patients will more actively participate in their health and well-being. However, participatory medicine will require the development of powerful new approaches for securely handling enormous amounts of personal information, including that generated from mHealth solutions, and for educating patients, physicians, nurses, and the entire collaborative care team.

Most of us realize that today's medicine is rather impersonalized, given that we use only a few measurements to diagnose disease and are generally unable to make fine distinctions among individuals' values, beliefs, preferences, health behaviors, and determinants of health, or between subtle variations of the same disease. This is a concern for care providers, and consumers themselves, who have few tools to understand their unique individuality, and the effectiveness of health interventions over time. Topol (2012) has begun to codify the "science of individuality": that is, being able to reveal and move data previously unavailable to patients, providers, and collaborative care teams. For example, as we develop tools for an individual's biologic and DNA sequence data inside the electronic health record (EHR) and the patient's personal health record (accessible from a mobile phone), indicating all pharmacogenomics interactions, our ability to share and exchange this information with pharmacists as consumers start a new plan offers us promise of a new precision in care. We are truly on the verge of understanding how each person in our universe is unique, and in the near future, we will have the capability to understand our digital health map in new ways. The "individualome", as Topol (2012) speaks about, will be the remarkable convergence of digital health tools that map individual differences in the epigenomic markings, bringing a window into understanding how every organ system responds with the environment. Many of these scientific breakthroughs are being established in the field labeled the "-omics" and include the:

- **Proteome:** for proteins, their structures, and functions
- **Transcriptome:** for the genetic material transcribed into RNA
- **Metabolome:** for molecules and how they are metabolized in our bodies, such as hormones
- **Glycome:** for sugars
- **Lipidome:** for lipids
- **Interactome:** for how proteins relate to one another
- **Exposome:** for how an individual's environment influences their health

Topol (2012, p. 229) predicted that "the entire classification system of medical conditions and diagnosis is about to be rewritten." Advances in understanding systems biology, genetics, and genomics are bringing new tools into the health domain of providers and patients; these will combine in powerful ways, enabled by mHealth innovation. There is a need and opportunity for nursing expertise to join and develop this emerging field.

mHealth's Potential to Impact the Triple Aim

Although there is a great need for clinical trials and solid evidence on the usability and clinical care integration of mHealth, there is a growing body of results and predictions on its promise to impact the Institute for Healthcare Improvement Triple Aim Initiative. mHealth's potential to improve patient healthcare experiences, demonstrate significantly improved health outcomes, and lower the per capita cost of healthcare has never been more promising.

The Triple Aim

The Triple Aim is a framework developed by the Institute for Healthcare Improvement (IHI) that describes an approach to optimizing health system performance. It is IHI's belief that new designs must be developed to simultaneously pursue three dimensions, called the "Triple Aim":

Improving the patient experience of care (including quality and satisfaction);

Improving the health of populations; and

Reducing the per capita cost of healthcare.

Preconditions to achieve the Triple Aim include the enrollment of an identified population, a commitment to universality for its members, and the existence of an organization (a macro-integrator) that accepts responsibility for all three aims for that population. The integrator's role includes at least five components: partnership with individuals and families, redesign of primary care, population health management, financial management, and macro system integration (Berwick, Nolan, & Whittingham, 2008). Starting with 15 health systems in the United States, England, and Sweden, in 2007, 60 sites from all over the world are participating in the IHI's Triple Aim Initiative (McCarthy & Klein, 2010).

In a recent 30-month study in collaboration with the University of Kentucky, one PCMH clinic's focused mobile health intervention improved capacity 19%, adding more than one hour per day of increased capacity, decreasing per capita cost of care 15%, and growing patient satisfaction (Thornberry, 2014). The study examined consecutive mobile encounters with well-established patients in a rural setting including five Appalachian counties, representing 15% of the state's geographic area. The team found that minor care, moderate acute care, and stable chronic disease care could be provided safely online. Additionally, 79% of care requests were submitted after hours, with fewer than 5% after 10 p.m. Patients were naïve to online care, yet 97% of the requests were deemed as appropriate. The average patient age was 41, with a distribution between 16 and 89 years. No safety issues were reported. The physicians included telephone conversations in the online encounters 17% of the time, and options for face-to-face video interaction were found to be unnecessary at any point during the study. In-office no-show rates evaporated, showing that patients do not miss appointments they can control.

Thornberry (2014) estimated that a single provider using mHealth to displace one uncompensated readmission and one emergency department (ED) encounter will save a healthcare system about $10,000 annually, while adding direct and indirect clinic revenue of $32,000 per provider. With implementation costs considered modest, the team extrapolated this study, applying it to primary care in the United States, and found the after-hour savings alone (related to increasing access to more cost-effective online after hours care by having the patient's encounter and care plan on a smart phone) represents $9.4 billion annually by Year 2.

"Applied to the larger health system, we estimated $28.8 billion annual savings for the 40% of outpatient care alone that could be mobilized online over time – greater than 1 percent of the total healthcare budget of the United States. Our finding, confirmed by a Deloitte Center for Health Solutions January 2013 independent study estimated that mHealth would save the U. S. healthcare industry $30.5 billion annually" (Thornberry, 2014, p. 177; Greenspun & Coughlin, 2012). Another study by PricewaterhouseCoopers (2013) for the global telecom community postulated that the European Union (EU) could save nearly €100 billion in spending, increase gross domestic product (GDP) by another €93 billion, and care for 24.5 million more lives with the same medical workforce.

Others acknowledged that, at least for the present, mHealth has the capacity to reduce provider revenue. One of the chief obstacles facing mHealth innovation is the complex arrangement of incentives that reinforce our current system. The prevailing model of healthcare reimbursement remains fee-for-service. mHealth is not particularly well suited to this reimbursement environment because its use may actually cause some revenue to disappear (e.g., traditional fee-for-service revenue) and may also interfere with the freedom of providers to determine which services will be delivered and with what frequency. As Krohn and Metcalf (2014) described, mHealth will become economically rational only when the calculus of healthcare includes a significant reliance on value-based revenue; a process reorientation toward patient-centered care; an integrated, standards-defined data-sharing environment; and the creation of a true mHealth ecosystem.

Another way to estimate projected value and savings for mHealth is to establish assumptions of benefit based on reversing expenses that we already are incurring for both acute and chronic care. Tables 17.1 and 17.2 outline potential impact. During an average month, for every 1,000 men, women, and children living in the United States, it is estimated that 800 experience some symptom of acute conditions, 327 consider seeking medical care, and 217 are seen in a physician's office (Green, Fryer, Yawn, Lanier, & Dovey, 2001). One-third (34%) of all physician office visits are related to an acute condition, and up to one-quarter of all ED visits could be managed in urgent care centers and retail clinics (CDC, 2010; Wieneck, Burns, & Mehrota, 2010).

Chronic conditions in the United States account for more than 90% of healthcare spending, limited to 50% of individuals who have at least one chronic medical condition. One-third of adults older than age 65 have four or more chronic conditions, and account for 74% of the $300 billion that Medicare spent in 2010. Hypertension and diabetes are two of the most common conditions for adults, with asthma and diabetes most common in children. About one-fourth of people with chronic conditions have one or more daily activity limitations (ADL). mHealth solutions are growing rapidly for these conditions. The Centers for Disease Control (CDC, 2013) estimates that improved self-management of chronic diseases results in an approximate cost-to-savings ratio of 1:10.

Additionally, patients with chronic diseases are incurring significant avoidable costs to our health system related to non-adherence to treatment. Poor medication adherence is a growing public health concern, and addressing the problem is especially critical as the number of Americans affected by at least one chronic condition requiring medication therapy is expected to grow from 133 million to 157 million by 2020. According to findings from the National Consumers League Script Your Future national campaign, nearly three of four Americans report that they do not always take their medication as directed. This problem causes more than one-third of medicine-related hospitalizations, causes nearly 125,000 deaths in the United States each year, and adds $290 billion in avoidable costs to the healthcare system annually (Script Your Future, 2011).

A recent IMS Institute for Healthcare Informatics report on Patient Apps for Improved Healthcare (Aiken & Gauntlett, 2013) demonstrates that the following six disease areas account for $105 billion dollars annually in avoidable cost from non-adherence to medication treatment:

- Hypercholesterolemia, $44B
- Diabetes, $24.6B
- Hypertension, $18.6B
- Osteoporosis, $15.5B
- HIV, $1.8B
- Congestive heart failure, $1B

IMS concludes that of the nearly 2,000 (as of this writing) mHealth applications (apps) related to specific therapy areas, those dedicated to chronic conditions dominate. However, according to the IMS study, the focus of these apps is *not* related to leading causes of mortality or non-adherence. There is opportunity for innovation here. The field is emergent, yet growing rapidly, as described in Tables 17.1 and 17.2.

Table 17.1 Impacting the Triple Aim for Acute Conditions

	mHealth Example	Bending Cost Curve, U.S. Healthcare	
		Prevalence	*Annual Cost*
Diagnosis and treatment	Scanadu Scout (https://www.scanadu.com/scout). A small portable scanner packed with sensors, easily placed on the forehead, bringing tools directly to patients' homes and living rooms for remote diagnosis and monitoring (including temperature, peripheral oxygen saturation, blood pressure, and heart rate). Usability clinical trial in progress at Scripps Health Translational Science Institute (http://clinicaltrials.gov/show/NCT02134145)		
Otitis Media in children	Remote image transmission and diagnosis with smartphone-based otoscope.	Recurrent ear infections are the most common acute complaint of children; one-half of all cases result in positive diagnosis.	$5 billion, not including lost work time by family caregivers (Bondy, Berman, Glazner, & Lezott, 2000)
Urinary Tract Infections (UTIs) in adults	Mobile devices for home urinalysis testing for signs of infection, with analytic, tracking & transmission capability may eliminate need for an office visit. Future advances detect both the presences of infection and the exact pathogen via mobile electrochemical biosensors (Mohan et. al. (2011).	UTIs are the most common bacterial infections in adults, accounting for 7M office visits, 1M ER visits and 100,000 hospitalizations/year. 50% of evaluations result in positive diagnosis	$2 billion annually Foxman (2002)

continues

Table 17.1 Impacting the Triple Aim for Acute Conditions *(continued)*

	mHealth Example	Bending Cost Curve, U.S. Healthcare	
		Prevalence	*Annual Cost*
Evaluating dizziness and other heart arrhythmia	Smartphone electrocardiographic (ECG) rhythm strips through case on phone, such as AliveCor (2014), or through wearable shirts or patches. Data recording, transmission, and evaluation can occur anywhere, any time. Automated algorithms support immediate diagnosis and feedback guiding next steps.	Nearly 4 million visit ED annually with complaint of dizziness	$4 billion for ED workup (Saber Tehrani et al., 2013)
Screening and early detection for atrial fibrillation	A single-lead iPhone electrocardiograph (iECG) with a validated atrial fibrillation (AF) algorithm could make systematic AF screening feasible, including earlier detection for treatment (Orchard, Freedman, Lowres, Peiris, & Neubeck, 2014). AF is often asymptomatic and substantially increases stroke risk. Lifetime risks are 1 in 4 for men and women 40 years of age and older and higher (1 In 6), even in the absence of antecedent congestive heart failure or myocardial infarction, underscoring the major public health burden posed by AF in general practice (Lloyd-Jones et al., 2004).	AF is the most common cardiac dysrhythmia seen in clinical practice, affecting an estimated 2 to 3 million Americans (Naccarelli, Varker, Lin, & Schulman, 2009). Prevalence is projected to increase to 15.9 million by the year 2050, with more than half of these patients 80 years or older, (Go et al., 2001; Miyasaka et al., 2006). Approximately 350,000 hospitalizations, 5.0 million office visits, 276,000 ED visits, and 234,000 outpatient visits (OPV) were attributable to AF annually within the U.S.	$6.65 billion, including $2.93 billion (44%) for hospitalizations $1.53 billion (23%) for outpatient treatment $235 million for prescription drugs (Coyne et al., 2006).

Table 17.2 Impacting the Triple Aim for Chronic Conditions

	mHealth Example	Bending Cost Curve, U.S. Healthcare	
		Prevalence	*Annual Cost*
Medication adherence	A recent IMS study (Aitken & Guantlett, 2013) evaluated 225 mHealth apps focused on medication compliance including pill reminders, medication trackers, and alert support networks. To date, no clinical trials or studies demonstrate effective use, other than results released by app developers.	Only 51% of Americans treated for hypertension are adherent to therapy (Yeaw et al., 2009). 25–50% of patients discontinue statins within one year of therapy (CDC, 2013). Non-adherence causes approximately 30% to 50% of treatment failures and 125,000 deaths annually (Script Your Future, 2011).	**$105 billion** in avoidable costs from medication non-adherence (Aiken, 2013). CDC (Aitken & Valkova, 2013) estimates direct cost estimated at $100 billion to $289 billion annually, with cost of $2000 per patient in physician visits annually.
Prescription filling	200 mHealth apps for finding a pharmacy, med availability, pricing, insurance coverage, refills, transfers, and accessing prescription history were reviewed by IMS. The U.S. market is the most advanced for chain pharmacy mobile apps, including Walgreens and CVS drugstores (Aiken, 2013).	20–30% of medication prescriptions are never filled; 50% are not taken as prescribed (CDC, 2013).	WHO estimates that by 2020, 157 million Americans will need prescription therapy for at least one chronic illness (CDC, 2013).

continues

Table 17.2 Impacting the Triple Aim for Chronic Conditions *(continued)*

	mHealth Example	Bending Cost Curve, U.S. Healthcare	
		Prevalence	*Annual Cost*
Home monitoring for Hypertension	Home monitoring is associated with small, yet statistically significant improvement in blood pressure (Uhlig, Patel, Ip, Kitsios, & Balk, 2013). When coupled with provider feedback and improved patient engagement, significantly greater BP control can be achieved (CDC, 2013). New non-invasive devices, which can measure beat-to-beat variability during daily activities, promise greater refinement in diagnosis and treatment (Chung, Chen, Alexander, & Cannesson, 2013). Novel mHealth solutions are needed.	32.5% of U.S. adults have hypertension; 38.9 million office visits have a primary diagnosis of essential hypertension, the most common diagnosed condition for an office visit, per CDC (2010). Less than one-half of patients with hypertension have their blood pressure (B/P) under control. And, only 51% of Americans treated for hypertension are adherent to their long-term therapy (Yeaw et al., 2009).	$93 billion in total costs (2010), $47.5 billion in direct costs (Heidenreich, et al., 2011; CDC, 2011a).

	mHealth Example	Bending Cost Curve, U.S. Healthcare	
		Prevalence	*Annual Cost*
Diabetes	Mobile transmission of glucose monitoring and bidirectional feedback, coupled with personalized engagement and feedback, complement traditional care services. Self-monitoring alone is of limited benefit in non-insulin–treated individuals (Clar, Banard, Cummins, Royle, & Waugh, 2010). Glooko Logbook, an FDA 510(k)-certified Diabetes Management System, can upload glucose readings from 19 FDA-approved glucose meters directly to a mobile device, costing only ~$40, with a built-in food database from more than 5,800 food manufacturers, 700 restaurants, and 250 supermarkets to encourage healthy habits. New advances in continuous glucose monitoring include a smartphone-based artificial pancreas (Kovatchev et al. 2013).	More than 25 million adults and children (8% of the U.S. population) have diabetes, with additional 79 million being pre-diabetic, reaching almost one-third of the U.S. population, (CDC, 2011b).	30 million office visits per year. Total cost of care in 2012 $245 billion, with $176 billion in direct costs (American Diabetes Association, 2013).

continues

Table 17.2 Impacting the Triple Aim for Chronic Conditions *(continued)*

	mHealth Example	Bending Cost Curve, U.S. Healthcare	
		Prevalence	*Annual Cost*
Obesity	Daily Carb by Maxwell Software, Glucose Buddy by Azumio, and Go Meals by Sanofi-Adventis were rated as top apps (Aitken & Gauntlett, 2013).	With rate of overweight children doubling and adults tripling in the last 30 years, 60 million adults are obese (about 30% of the adult U.S. population).	The estimated annual healthcare costs of obesity-related illness are a staggering $190.2 billion, or nearly 21% of annual medical spending in the United States (Cawley & Meyerhoefer, 2012).
Asthma and COPD	Propeller Sensor (formerly Astmapolis), smartphone-based technology, attaches to an inhaler and passively collects the exact time and location where used; and transmits with permission to provider and family/ friends. New low-energy sensor by Propeller Health eliminates charging, while enhanced analytics identify worsening patients. The FDA–cleared digital health solution and sensor wirelessly syncs with your smart phone using your phone's built-in Bluetooth technology and automatically captures the data from your sensor whenever it is nearby.	More than 20 million American adults and children have asthma. In 2011, 12.7 million U.S. adults (age 18 and older) were estimated to have COPD. However, close to 24 million U.S. adults have evidence of impaired lung function, indicating an under diagnosis of COPD (American Lung Association, 2013)	More than $37 billion dollars in direct medical costs plus additional $25 million lost work and school days (Kamble & Bharmal, 2009). Asthma and COPD are the fifth and sixth most costly conditions in the United States, estimated at $50 billion annually, each (Propeller Health, 2014).

Current Experience

The maturity and adoption of connected and mobile health solutions are in a nascent stage, and range from simple informational and way finding apps to FDA-regulated devices and sensors. Consumers, patients and family caregivers, healthcare providers, payers, health systems, and community-based healthcare organizations all each begin to have compelling use cases that are driving innovation. Because the work is early, nurses and nurse informatacists will be key to leading integration of these tools into clinical and care workflows and ensuring data standards and interoperability, often across care settings outside their primary domain.

Patient and Consumer Apps

Little is understood about the diverse array of mHealth apps available to the consumer, either consumer-directed apps or those prescribed by providers, and how they influence the patient's journey, their usage, and clinical integration into processes of care and coordination, within traditional and virtual care settings. A recent IMS study (Aitken & Gauntlett, 2013) showed 40,000 mHealth apps available for download from the Apple App Store. Overall wellness, diet, and fitness apps accounted for the majority of apps available. Assessment of their functionality reveals limited and simple functions, mostly providing information. Of interest, a significant skew was found in the download volume, with more than 50% of the apps studied achieving fewer than 500 downloads. Conversely, five apps accounted for 15% of all downloads. See Figures 17.1 and 17.2.

Patient journey stage	Description	No.	Functionality	Example
Prevention/Healthy Living 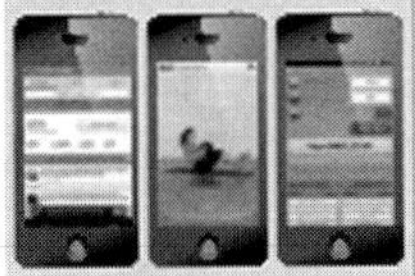	Focus on factors associated with overall wellness: • Healthy eating • Weight management • Fitness • Tips for healthy living • Smoking cessation • Stress management • Sleep	8,786 apps	• Display information • Display pre-loaded instructions for diet & fitness • Record and display user entered data • Track weight measurements over time	• CalorieCounter • NikeTrainingClub • OneSportsMan • Weight and BMI diary
Symptomatic/ Self-diagnosis 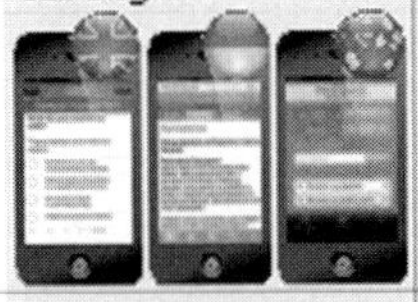	• Reference for common symptoms/conditions • Diagnosis based on data inputted/question answered • Communication with medical professionals	304 apps	• Display reference information • Record users answers and display appropriate guidance • Communication interface between patient and physician	• NHS Health and Symptom Checker • SingHealth Health Buddy • Medibank Symptom Checker • Melanoma Visual Risk Checker • Am I depressed? • HealthTap
Finding a Physician 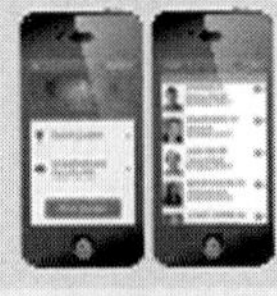	• Locate most appropriate physician or healthcare facility and find contact information • Rate and review physicians • Appointment reminders	931 apps	• Display search results • Display location information (and connect to GPS) • Connect to phone function • Display reviews • Remind appointments	• BetterDoctor • US Hospitals Lite • Patient fusion • Doctor visit manager
Education post-diagnosis 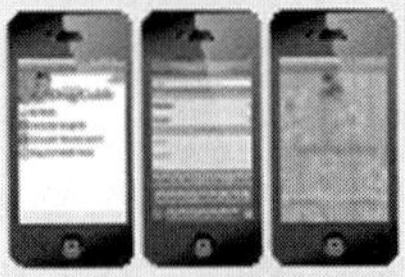	Provide health reference material: • Drugs/medication information • Emergency and first aid information • Condition management information	562 apps	• Display drug information • Display condition information • Record user entered data • Can connect to healthcare professionals or emergency services	• Drug Guide for Consumers • Family Drug Guide • Pill identifier by drugs.com • Health Handbook • Emergency Info 4Family • Medical Facts+
Filling prescription 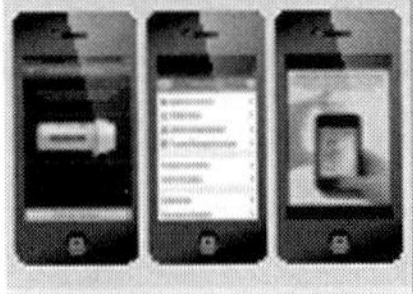	• Finding pharmacy • Price scans for medications/special offers • Refilling of prescriptions • Drug interactions and side effects	200 apps	• Display search results • Display location information (and connect to GPS) • Connect to pharmacy systems to register prescriptions • Offer discounts on medications	• CVS Pharmacy • Walgreens • LowestMed Mobile
Compliance 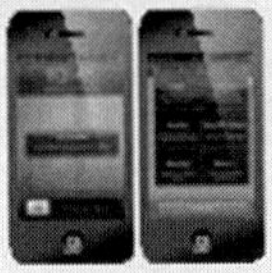	Assisting the patient to act within the prescribed interval and dose of a dosing regimen: • Pill reminders • Medication trackers • Alert support network if dose not recorded	225 apps	• Provide reminders • Display information • Record user entered data (e.g. register dose was taken) • Communicate with support network	• Medicine Reminder HD - with Local Notifications • MediSafe – virtual pillbox

Patient Apps for Improved Healthcare: From Novelty to Mainstream. Report by the IMS Institute for Healthcare Informatics

FIGURE 17.1 mHealth apps: Placement on the patient journey. Used with permission from IMS Health.

Patient Journey: Prevention/Healthy Lifestyles		
App Name	**Developer**	**Description**
Calorie Counter and Diet Tracker by MyFitnessPal HD	MyFitnessPal.com	Diet app featuring large calorie counting database and features such as food tracking, exercise and weight goals and links to friends
Calorie Counter PRO by MyNetDiary	MyNetDiary Inc.	Diet app featuring large calorie counting database and features such as food tracking, exercise and weight goals
Chest Trainer : powered by Fitness Buddy	Azumio Inc.	Weight training and fitness application which claims to mimic having a personal trainer in the home, requires no equipment
Cycle Tracker Pro - TrainingPeaks GPS	Peaksware, LLC	Converts phone into a GPS-enabled cycling computer, with a wide range of workouts, providing custom readouts and activity reports
Quit It 3.0 - stop smoking	Tommy Kammerer	A stop smoking motivational program, supporting and encouraging smokers to quit smoking, helping ex-smokers to stay quit; keeps track of the cigarettes not smoked and how much money saved as a result
Quit Smoking Now HD - Hypnotherapy with Max Kirsten	Max Kirsten	A four week quit smoking program with personal hypnotherapy sessions
Patient Journey: Finding a HCP or facility		
Healow	eClinicalWorks	Lets patients communicate with their doctor's office and access up-to-date health records, includes visit summaries and appointment reminders
Vitals - Your top 10 doctors!	Vitals	Provides customized lists of the best local doctors, as rated by their patients, allowing for searches by symptom, condition or medical specialty
ZocDoc - Doctor Appointments Online!	ZocDoc	Tool to find and book doctor's appointments based on zip code searches
Patient Journey: Diagnosis/Education		
App Name	**Developer**	**Description**
HealthTap - free doctor answers to medical and health questions	HealthTap	Provides health answers and healthy tips on any symptom, condition, medication, health concern, or even wellness topics from 47,000 U.S. doctors; provides current and vetted health information
iTriage	Healthagen LLC	Provides clear, concise, and useful information covering thousands of medical symptoms, diseases, conditions, procedures, medications and drugs
WebMD for iPad	WebMD	Provides mobile-optimized health information and decision-support tools including WebMD's Symptom Checker, Drugs & Treatments, First Aid Information and Local Health Listings
Patient Journey: Filling Prescription		
GoodRx	GoodRx	GoodRx compares prices for prescription drugs and provides prices, coupons and savings tips for more than 6,000 drugs at most pharmacies in the U.S.
MyRefill Rx	Intelecare Compliance Solutions, Inc.	Order medications straight from the phone and get them delivered to the door, as well as medication reminders and appointment reminders
Walgreens	Walgreen Co.	Refill by Scan function, Points for Refills, Pill Reminders, Transfer Prescription feature, Refill Reminders, Health Reference encyclopedia
Patient Journey: Compliance		
Dosecast	Montuno Software, LLC	Flexible medication reminder with customizable dose amounts and instructions, a large drug database and the ability to support multiple users
Pill Monitor Free – Medication Reminders and Logs	Maxwell Software	Prescription reminder that alerts the user every time they need to take a prescription. Allows user to enter all prescriptions, set up reminders, and track when they have been taken
RxmindMe Prescription / Medicine Reminder and Pill Tracker	RxmindMe, LLC	Prescription reminder that alerts the user every time they need to take a prescription. Allows user to enter all prescriptions, set up reminders, and track when they have been taken

FIGURE 17.2 mHealth apps: Top apps by placement on the patient journey. Used with permission from IMS Health.

Clinical Care and Coordination

Many cloud-based platforms for mHealth solutions are emerging to support the patient engagement and population health needs of payers and providers, Health Homes, Primary Care Medical Homes, community-based interventions, and Health Information Exchanges (HIEs). Creative solutions are emerging to populate and synthesize different streams of health data, including e-PROs, PGHD, physiological, device, sensor, and wearable data.

Patient-Generated Health Data

"Patient-generated health data (PGHD) is the 'now' of health care and the future of healthcare. Health happens every day, not just when you are in a clinical setting. We need ways to collect it, make sense of it, and make it actionable for individuals and clinicians. PGHD needs to be widely accessible now!" encouraged Katherine Kim (2014) at a recent Stanford Med X Google Hangout. Although EHR adoption has matured and efforts continue to make sense of its health data, predictions are that a much larger set of data will be tracked outside the healthcare system.

PGHD and rich content in the ecosystem is adding a new category and dimension to how we engage patients. Consumers are not just creating information but also helping to make it meaningful and navigable: first, by organizing themselves and the information into knowledge communities; and second, by individuals creating or interacting with the data to stratify it with relevancy and abstraction layers. Health social networks could become a key quantitative indicator and independent barometer of both the demand for medical research and the execution of research.

A recent PatientsLikeMe study (Wicks, Vaughan, Massagli, & Heywood, 2011) spoke to the value of collecting patient-reported outcome data online. Each represents a significant movement forward in getting new knowledge regarding therapies to patients and caregivers:

- **Speed:** It took only 9 months from initiation of the PatientsLikeMe tool (March 2008) to the first public sharing of preliminary results (December 2008).
- **Cost:** Online studies have lower marginal costs per patient as compared with thousands of dollars per patient in traditional clinical trials.

- **Patient access:** There is a potential to rapidly recruit widely dispersed patients with rare conditions and to overcome selection bias favoring patients living near specialist centers.
- **Availability of control participants:** Clinical outcome data were passively collected from thousands of patients who served as potential matched controls.
- **Patient engagement:** Patients who submitted data using the PatientsLikeMe website (www.patientslikeme.com) were connected with other patients, which increased their investment in their disease; true participatory medicine.

These solutions are highly dependent on new understandings of how to engage and sustain participation with consumers in health solutions, getting into the science and psychology of relationships, visual analytics, and patient activation. For example, Better—the Mayo Clinic–backed, Palo Alto, California–based company—recently launched a personal health assistant service, building on learning from launching Health Hero back in the late 1990s (Dolan, 2014). Believing that the time is right for a consumer-driven care coordination model, Better offers a 24/7 personal assistant to take the complexity out of health care for the consumer, with basic tasks (such as appointments, prescriptions, or finding a new doctor) all the way to high-end clinical work (such as, "Something is wrong. Help me find a specialist, doctor, or nurse."). Yet, the new tools are focused on relationship building. With a goal of reaching 200 million lives by 2020, Mayo is interested in ways to extend its brand through technology and mobile.

Pilots, Interoperability, Clinical Trials, Research, and FDA Regulation

The evidence for mHealth is an emerging field, driven in part by needs for greater synergy in app maturity, adoption, and clinical integration based on the evidence. The 2013 report from the IMS Institute for Healthcare Informatics (Aitken & Gauntlett) suggests that this maturing process will by driven by stakeholder collaboration, including:

- Payer and provider recognition of the potential role of apps in healthcare management
- Creation of standard benchmarks for security/privacy guidelines that protect personal health information (PHI) globally
- Curation and evaluation of healthcare apps
- Integration of apps with other healthcare information technology (IT) systems

End-to-End, Plug-and-Play Interoperability Standards for Personal Connected Health

- A recent PricewaterhouseCoopers study commissioned by the West Health Institute identified more than $30 billion of annual costs to the U.S. healthcare system because of the lack of medical device interoperability, or simple connectivity between devices.
- The focus is on relevant standards that enable the integration of data and technology used by clinicians and caregivers to help patients live active and independent lives.
- The standards will enable greater implementation of interoperable personal health devices for disease management, health and fitness, and independent living.
- This collaboration follows the announcement of 12 IEEE 11073 standards that were recognized by the U.S. Food and Drug Administration that are relevant to interoperability of medical devices.

www.businesswire.com/news/home/20131111006293/en/IEEE-Standards-Association-Continua-Health-Alliance-Join#.U-2XcKCh25o

Many vendors are conducting and documenting results of pilots and collaborations that are establishing credible results in terms of patient engagement and health outcomes. The Health Information Management Systems Society (HIMSS) announced in 2014 a new collaboration among the Continua Health Alliance, HIMSS, and the mHealth Summit. Increasing consumer engagement and recognition that health delivery is occurring outside the traditional care settings is the catalyst for what the three founding members are naming the "Personal Connected Health Alliance." The overarching mission of the Alliance is to promote the adoption of technology designed to produce highly informed and integrated solutions, described as personal health tools that meet lifestyle needs. The Design Guidelines from Continua, as well as certification processes for global interoperability, will encourage vendors toward end-to-end plug-and-play connectivity in personal connected health. The HIMSS mHealth Roadmap is another example of guidance and collaboration.

Concurrently, systematic development of credible evidence of the value derived from using mHealth apps is also necessary. Clinical trials range from proof of concept to clinical trials focused on usability or device development/effectiveness, and/or FDA device regulatory. With more than 4,000 mHealth apps in the market place, the FDA reports that it has reviewed only 100 of them (Aiken & Gauntlett, 2013).

Building on the July 2012 Food and Drug Administration Safety and Innovation Act of 2012 (FDASIA) passed by the U.S. Congress, the FDA has developed a risk-based regulatory framework pertaining to health IT that promotes innovation, protects patient safety, and avoids regulatory duplication. The FDASIA report (April 2014) includes guidelines that regulate mHealth apps based on the FDA's assessment of potential to harm patients. Under these guidelines, an app that only records your diet and exercise information would not rise to the level of a regulated device. However, an app that tells you to adjust your insulin dose based on a reading from a glucometer will likely be regulated, given the diagnostic nature of its intent.

Scripps Health, through its Clinical Translational Science Institute, has recently added a focus on digital health, with five trials initiated in July 2013 and 15 in the planning stages. Dr. Steve Steinhubl, Director of Digital Medicine, reports that one-third of these trials are specific to a device requiring clinical data primarily for regulatory purposes; the other two-thirds of the trials involve payers looking for technology solutions (personal interview, January 30, 2014).

mHealth Evaluation

Assessing mHealth app functionalities for wellness, prevention, treatment, care coordination, access, and cost for use in improving health status for acute and chronic conditions is also in the early stage (Brown, Yen, Rojas, & Schnall, 2013; Evans, Abroms, Poropatich, Nielsen, & Wallace, 2012; Kumar et al., 2013). All acknowledge that there are few evaluation frameworks for assessing the utility of mobile health technology. Performance speed, information needs, and convenience are some of the focal points studied. This is an emerging body of work where nursing and collaborative care teams can learn more about measuring patient engagement in a mobile and connected ecosystem, including distinctions with types of mobile devices and use with different conditions and age groups.

Future Directions

The future for mobile, smart, and connected health innovations are predicted to come sooner than perhaps our ecosystem of care, infrastructure, and health policy can prepare for. Smart diagnostics, such as AliveCor mobile heart monitor (an FDA cleared device) is now available over the counter, direct to consumer. In addition to being able to use it anywhere, including on an airplane, consumers can record their heart rhythms, learn more with personalized analytics, and contribute if desired to their data anonymously to heart health research to help others at risk. It is not just the device or app: It is the meaningful data and sense-making we have access to, as both consumers and providers. With access to unprecedented feedback loops with patients, providers are encouraging new models of more transparent sense-making with patients.

The consumer eHealth community and other advocates are talking about promising notions (such as individuals being the "CEO" of their own health), as well as innovations (such as using Dropbox [an online cloud storage app] for health and health record banking, where a lifetime of health data can be securely stored, accessed, and exchanged as directed by the consumer).

Our success will be to integrate these new care technologies and modalities into today's nursing and collaborative care practice, while also rethinking how care and health engagement can be achieved more easily to meet the Triple Aim.

A Global, Immersive, Invisible, Ambient Networked Sensing Environment

A 2014 Pew Research Center Internet and American Life Project report predicted that health data connectivity will be widespread by 2025, and the use of embedded and wearable computing devices that share and transmit data will become widespread and fully immersed into consumer's daily routines. The report, marking the 25th anniversary of the World Wide Web, was developed after surveying 1,600 individuals about the Internet of the future, its impact on their social environment, and specifically about wearable devices. Participants in the study agreed that technology in the future will be a "global, immersive, invisible, ambient networked computing environment built through the continued proliferation of smart sensors, cameras, software, databases, and massive data centers in a world-spanning information fabric known as the Internet of Things" (Pew, 2014, p. 2).

Companies like Scanadu (https://www.scanadu.com/) are bringing sensors and platforms to the market, which can conduct lab test at home automatically transmitting results to the point of care, enabling digital checkups from anywhere, and fundamentally changing the nature of the doctor-patient visit and the health data available. New technologies are in development for home dialysis that is monitored and web-connected. Artificial intelligence, intelligence augmentation, and cognitive computing (like Watson, from IBM) will bring new decision support tools to both the consumer and provider. Data will be in diverse layers, streams, and cloud-based analytics to make sense of the patterns. Many are predicting that within 5 years, more than one-half of all doctor visits will be virtual.

As Topol (2012) stated, the quest to provide individualized medicine, knowing the biology of a person via genomics (including proteomics, metabolomics, epigenomics, and "biomarkers") is one essential step. The other goal is to know about an individual's physiology, through non-invasive wireless sensors, which are wearables that can continuously collect data on metrics such as blood pressures, heart rhythm and rate, oxygen saturation, blood glucose, and more. By coupling genomics and wireless technologies, we are bringing together exceptionally powerful tools to define the unique biological and physiological picture and digital map of each individual to improve health prevention and preservation.

Portable High Resolution Diagnostics

Topol (2012, p. 124) described "pocket-size, high-resolution ultrasound is one of the most significant advances in medical imaging in decades and is replacing the stethoscope, which has been around since 1816." In a recent Forbes Magazine interview (2013), John Nosta asked Eric Topol, What "home runs" have you seen in digital health that exemplify the future? Topol describes, "I believe the portable high-resolution ultrasound (Vscan or Mobisante) represents a home run to replace the stethoscope for heart, abdominal and fetal examinations. We validated the Vscan compared with the standard hospital lab echocardiogram (Leibo et al., 2011). To have such high-quality imaging done anywhere "flattens the earth"—not just all over the planet, but from a paramedic in the field or an emergency room doctor—to simply acquire the image and transmit the video loop to a radiologist or cardiologist expert with a rapid read and text back.

Embedded Nanosensors with Signals to Smart Phones

Embedded nanosensors in our blood streams will support continuous surveillance and capturing of bio-signals, transmitting these to our smartphones. Signals could alert us to preventable autoimmune, cancer, and heart attacks. Google has recently announced progress on efforts for wearable contact lenses for patients with diabetes to measure blood sugar levels in their tears, and then sending this information to a smartphone. And, as Tate (2014) described, the Apple Healthbook is 'huge," a body-monitoring app—tracking everything from sleep to nutrition to exercise to vital signs, a tipping point for Apple to move into the market of digital infrastructure for sensing and other technologies. The new app is designed to track your blood sugar, heart rate, breathing rate, weight, hydration, physical movement, and health tests, bringing device and sensor information into a portable mobile personal health record. Tate (2014, ¶ 3) contended that "Pundits are already speculating that it will be a key selling point for Apple's forthcoming iOS 8 mobile operating system or its long-rumored 'iWatch' smartwatch or both."

The Intelligent Home

The Lake Nona (http://learnlakenona.com) Medical City has inspired a Well Home living laboratory and model for Ambient Health, seeking to shift a paradigm to put the home as the center of personal and family wellness (Metcalf, 2014). The learning lab is following the lives of the family in a model home, designed to bring in inexpensive and easy-to-implement solutions and tools that encourage healthy choices and easy access to healthy portions/foods: for example, fitness equipment that is pervasive throughout the home, including 7-minute workouts and healthy games that are simple and may or may not rely on technology.

Conclusion

One of the primary characteristics of the evolving healthcare delivery models inspired by mobile and connected health is that of collaboration and a learning health system, a core competency for nursing to lead into the future. We are creating a strong foundation for the co-production of health and care, moving to a co-diagnosis/co-care model among patients and family caregivers, nurses, collaborative care team members, physicians, and the health ecosystem. Patients and family caregivers are shifting from being a minimally informed advice recipient to an active participant, instigating collaborator, information sharer, peer leader, and self-tracker engaged in owning and improving their health. New definitions are emerging for the concept of health and healthcare, including the role that resilience and well-being play for health at individual, family, neighborhood, community, and national levels. Peer-based and community health networks are poised to become a powerful member of the healthcare ecosystem with an expanding role, possibly having influence in policy, ethics, regulation, research, and finance.

References

Adamson, S. C., & Bachman, J. W. (2010). Pilot study of providing online care in a primary care setting. *Mayo Clin Proc, 85*(8), 704–710.

Aitken, M., & Gauntlett, C. (2013). Patient apps for improved healthcare: From novelty to mainstream. *IMS Institute for Healthcare Informatics.* Retrieved from http://www.imshealth.com/deployedfiles/imshealth/Global/Content/Corporate/IMS%20Health%20Institute/Reports/Patient_Apps/IIHI_Patient_Apps_Report.pdf

Aitken, M., & Valkova, S. (2013). Avoidable costs in US healthcare: The 200 billion opportunity from using medicines more responsibly. *IMS Institute for Healthcare Informatics.* Retrieved from http://www.imshealth.com/deployedfiles/imshealth/Global/Content/Corporate/IMS%20Institute/RUOM-2013/IHII_Responsible_Use_Medicines_2013.pdf

AliveCor. (2014). FDA cleared mobile device monitor. Retrieved from http://www.alivecor.com/home

American Diabetes Association. (2013). Economic costs of diabetes in the US in 2012. *Diabetes Care,* April 2013;36(4):1033-1046.

American Lung Association. (2013). *Trends in COPD (chronic bronchitis and emphysema): Morbidity and mortality,* March 2013 report. Retrieved from http://www.lung.org/finding-cures/our-research/trend-reports/copd-trend-report.pdf

Berwick, D., Nolan, T., & Whittington, J. (2008). The triple aim: Care, health, and cost. *Health Affairs, 27*(3), 759–69.

Bondy, J., Berman, S., Glazner, J., & Lezotte D. (2000). Direct expenditures related to Otitis Medica diagnoses: Extrapolations from a pediatric medical cohort. *Pediatrics, 105*(6), e:72.

Brown, W., Yen, P., Rojas, M., & Schnall, R. (2013). Assessment of the Health IT Usability Evaluation Model (Health-ITUEM) for evaluating mobile health (mHealth) technology. *Journal of Biomedical Informatics, 46*(6), 180–87.

Cawley, J., & Meyerhoefer, C. (2012). The medical care costs of obesity: An instrumental variables approach. *Journal of Health Economics, 31*(1), 219–230.

Centers for Disease Control and Prevention. (2010). National ambulatory medical care survey: 2010 summary tables. Retrieved from www.cdc.gov/nchs/data/ahcd/namcs_summary/2010_namcs_web_tables.pdf

Centers for Disease Control and Prevention. (2011a). Vital signs: Prevalence, treatment, and control of hypertension—United States, 1999–2002 and 2005–2008. Washington, DC: U.S. Department of Health and Human Services, Centers for Disease Control and Prevention. Retrieved from http://www.cdc.gov/mmwr/preview/mmwrhtml/mm6004a4.htm.

Centers for Disease Control and Prevention. (2011b). *National diabetes fact sheet: National estimates and general information on diabetes and pre-diabetes in the United States, 2011.* Washington, DC: U.S. Department of Health and Human Services, Centers for Disease Control and Prevention.

Centers for Disease Control and Prevention Education Conference. (2013). *Medication adherence* [PowerPoint presentation]. Retrieved from http://www.cdc.gov/primarycare/materials/medication/docs/medication-adherence-01ccd.pdf

Chung, E., Chen, G., Alexander, B., & Cannesson, M. (2013). Non-invasive continuous blood pressure monitoring: a review of current applications. *Frontiers of Medicine, 7*(1), 91–101.

Clar, C., Banard, K., Cummins, E., Royle, P., & Waugh, N. (2010). Self-monitoring of blood glucose in Type 2 Diabetes: Systematic review. *Health Technology Assessment, 14*(12), 1–140.

Collins, F. (2012, July 1). The real promise of mobile health apps. *Scientific American, 307*(1). Retrieved from http://www.scientificamerican.com/article/real-promise-mobile-health-apps

Coyne, K. S., Paramore, C., Grandy, S., Mercader, M., Reynolds, M., & Zimetbaum, P. (2006). Assessing the direct costs of treating nonvalvular atrial fibrillation in the United States. *Value in Health, 9*(5), 348–356.

Evans, W. D., Abroms, L. C., Poropatich, R., Nielsen, P. E., & Wallace, J. L. (2012). Mobile health evaluation methods: The Text4baby case study. *Journal of Health Communication, 17*(Suppl 1), 22–29.

Fasano, P. (2014). Keynote address. 2014 Summer Institute in Nursing Informatics. Baltimore, Maryland.

FDASIA Health IT Report (2014). Proposed strategy and recommendations for a risk-based framework. April 2014. Retrieved from http://www.fda.gov/downloads/aboutfda/centersoffices/officeofmedicalproductsandtobacco/cdrh/cdrhreports/ucm391521.pdf

Go, A. S., Hylek, E. M., Phillips, K. A., Chang, Y. Henault, L. E., Selby, J. V., & Singer, D. E. (2001). Prevalence of diagnosed atrial fibrillation in adults: National implications for rhythm management and stroke prevention: The AnTicoagulation and Risk Factors in Atrial Fibrillation (ATRIA) Study. *Journal of the American Medical Association, 285*(18), 2370–2375.

Goldstein, D., & Masters. G. (2014). Innovation cure for mHealth barriers. In R. Krohn & D. Metcalf (Eds.), *mHealth Innovation: Best practices from the mobile frontiers* (chapter 35). Chicago, IL: Health Information and Management Systems Society (HIMSS).

Green, L. A., Fryer, G. E., Jr., Yawn, B. P., Lanier, D., & Dovey, S. M. (2001). The ecology of medical care revisited. *The New England Journal of Medicine, 344*(26), 2021–2025.

Greenspun, H., & Coughlin, S. (2012). *mHealth in an mWorld: How mobile technology is transforming healthcare.* Deloitte Center for Health Solutions. Retrieved from http://www.deloitte.com/assets/Dcom-UnitedStates/Local%20Assets/Documents/us_chs_2012_mhealth_HowMobileTechnologyIsTransformingHealthCare_032213.pdf

Heidenreich, P. A., Trogdon, J. G., Khavjou, O. A., Butler, J., Dracup, K., Exekowitz, M.D., . . . Woo, Y. J. (2011). Forecasting the future of cardiovascular disease in the United States: A policy statement from the American Heart Association. *Circulation, 123*(8), 993–944.

Hood, L. (2010). *Personalized medicine: A shift from reactive to proactive medicine.* Cambridge, MA: MIT Tech Review.

Hull, S. C. (2014). Blue button: Empowering consumers for shared decision making and improved health. In R. Krohn & D. Metcalf (Eds.), *mHealth Innovation: Best practices from the mobile frontiers* (chapter 7, pp. 57-76). Chicago, IL: Health Information and Management Systems Society (HIMSS).

Iglehart, J. K. (2014). Connected health: Emerging disruptive technologies. *Health Affairs, 33*(2), 190.

Kamble, S., & Bharmal, M. (2009). Incremental direct expenditure of treating asthma in the United States. *The Journal of Asthma: The Official Journal for the Association for the Care of Asthma, 46*(1), 73–80.

Kim, K. (2014, May 6). Stanford Medicine X Live! Patient-generated data: Is it the future of healthcare? [Video file]. Retrieved from http://www.youtube.com/watch?v=XGWXJvqueYU&feature=share

Kovatchev, B. P., Renard, E., Cobelli, C., Zisser, H. C., Keith-Hynes, P., Anderson, S. M., ... Doyle, F. J. (2013). Feasibility of outpatient fully integrated closed-loop control: First studies of wearable artificial pancreas. *Diabetes Care, 36*(7), 1851–1858.

Krohn, R. and Metcalf, D. (2014) mHealth Innovation: Best practices from the mobile frontiers, Chicago, Health Information and Management Systems Society (HIMSS). Retrieved from http://ebooks.himss.org/product/mhealth-innovation

Kumar, S, Nilsen, W. J., Abernethy, A., Atienza, A., Patrick, K., Pavel, M., ... Swendeman, D. (2013). Mobile health technology evaluation: The mHealth evidence workshop. *American Journal of Preventive Medicine, 45*(2), 228–236.

Kvedar, J., Coye, M. J., & Everett, M. (2014). Connected health: A review of technologies and strategies to improve patient care with telemedicine and telehealth. *Health Affairs, (33)*2, 194–199.

Liebo, M. J., Israel, R. L., Lillie, E. O., Smith, M. R., Rubenson, D. S., & Topol, E. J. (2011). Is pocket mobile echocardiography the next-generation stethoscope? A cross-sectional comparison of rapidly acquired images with standard transthoracic echocardiography. *Annals of Internal Medicine, 155*(1), 33–38.

Lloyd-Jones, D. M., Wang, T. J., Leip, E. P., Larson, M. G., Levy, D., Vasan, R. S., . . . Benjamin, E. J. (2004.) Lifetime risk for development of atrial fibrillation: The Framingham Heart Study. *Circulation, 110*, 1042–1046.

McCarthy, D., & Klein, S. (2010). *The triple aim journey: Improving population health and patient's experience of care, while reducing cost.* Retrieved from http://www.commonwealthfund.org/~/media/files/publications/case-study/2010/jul/triple-aim-v2/1421_mccarthy_triple_aim_journey_overview.pdf

Miyasaka, Y., Barnes, M. E., Gersh, B. J., Cha, S.S., Bailey, K.R., Abhayaratna, W. P., ... Tsang, T. S. (2006). Secular trends in incidence of atrial fibrillation in Olmsted County, Minnesota, 1980 to 2000, and implications on the projections for future prevalence. (Published correction appears in *Circulation, 114*(11), e498). *Circulation, 114*(2), 119–125.

Mohan, R., Mach, K. E., Bercovici, M., Pan, Y., Dhulipala, L., Wong, P. K., & Liao, J. C. (2011). Clinical validation of integrated nucleic acid and protein detection on an electrochemical biosensor array for urinary tract infection diagnosis. *PlOS One, 6*(10), e26846.

Naccarelli, G. V., Varker, H., Lin, J., & Schulman, K. L. (2009). Increasing prevalence of atrial fibrillation and flutter in the United States. *American Journal of Cardiology, 104*(11), 1534–1539.

Nosta, J. (2013, January). The STAT Ten: Eric Topol, MD speaks out on digital health. *Forbes*. Retrieved from http://www.forbes.com/sites/johnnosta/2013/01/30/the-stat-ten-eric-topol-md-speaks-out-on-digital-health

Orchard, J., Freedman, S. B., Lowres, N., Peiris, D., & Neubeck, L. (2014, May). iPhone ECG screening by practice nurses and receptionists for atrial fibrillation in general practice: The GP-SEARCH qualitative pilot study. Australian Family Physician: *Cardiology, 43*(5), 315–319.

Pak, H., & Hull, S. (2013). Mobile health wallet as an enabler for patient engagement. Healthcare Industry Perspective. Retrieved from http://www.diversinet.com/whitepapers/Mobile_Health_Wallet_as_an_Enabler_for_Patient_Engagement.pdf

Pearl, R. (2014). Kaiser Permanente Northern California: Current experiences with Internet, mobile and video technologies. *Health Affairs, 33*(2), 251–257.

Pew Research Center. (May 2014). The Internet of things will thrive by 2025. Retrieved from http://www.pewinternet.org/2014/05/14/internet-of-things/

PricewaterhouseCoopers. (2013, June 18). Socio-economic impact of mHealth: An assessment report for the Europeon Union. Presented for the Global System for Mobile Communications Association.

PRNewswire. (April 2014). mHealth market poised for increased investment in various levels of the ecosystem says compass intelligence. Retrieved from http://www.bioportfolio.com/news/pdf/1899966/mHealth-Market-Poised-for-Increased-Investment-in-Various-Levels-of-the-Ecosystem.pdf.

Propeller Health. (2014). http://propellerhealth.com. Accessed May 20, 2014.

research2guidance. (2014). Mobile Health Market Report 2013–2017. Retrieved from http://research2guidance.com/shop/index.php/downloadable/download/sample/sample_id/262

Saber Tehrani, A. S., Coughlan, D., Hsieh, Y. H., Mantokoudis, G., Korley, F. K., Kerber, K. A., … Newman-Toker, D. E. (2013). Rising annual costs of dizzinesss presentations to U.S. emergency departments. *Academic Emergency Medicine, 20*(7), 689–696.

Script Your Future. (2011). November 2 press release; Retrieved from http://scriptyourfuture.org/wp-content/themes/cons/m/release.pdf

Steinhubl, S.R. (2014). Where mobile technologies are needed in healthcare. In R. Krohn & D. Metcalf (Eds.), *mHealth innovation: Best practices from the mobile frontiers* (chapter 32, pp. 287-295). Chicago, IL: Health Information and Management Systems Society (HIMSS).

Steinhubl, S. R., Muse, E. D., & Topol, E. J. (2013). Can mobile health technologies transform health care? *Journal of the American Medical Association, 310*(22), 2395–2396.

Tate, R. (2014, March 17). Apple's upcoming health app is the start of something huge. *Wired.* Retrieved from http://www.wired.com/business/2014/03/apple-healthbook-is-just-the-beginning/

Thornberry, W. C. (2014). *Implications or a Mobile-to-Mobile Online Delivery Model: A Case Study.* Chapter in mHealth Innovation: Best Practices from the Mobile Frontiers (pp. 173-179). Chicago, IL: Health Information and Management Systems Society (HIMSS).

Topol, E. J. (2012). *The creative destruction of medicine: How the digital revolution will create better health-care.* New York, NY: Basic Books.

Uhlig, K., Patel, K., Ip, S., Kitsios, G. D., & Balk, E. M. (2013). Self measured blood pressure monitoring in the management of hypertension: A systematic review and meta-analysis. *Annals of Internal Medicine, 159*(3), 185–194.

Wicks, P., Vaughan, T. E., Massagli, M. P., & Heywood, J. (2011). Accelerated clinical discovery using self-reported patient data collected online and a patient-matching algorithm. *Nature Biotechnology Advance Online Publication, 29,* 411–414. doi:10.1038/nbt.1837

Wieneck, R. M., Burns, R. M., & Mehrotra, A. (2010). Many emergency department visits could be managed at urgent care centers and retail clinics. *Health Affairs, 29*(9), 1630–1636.

World Health Organization (WHO). (2011). *mHealth: New horizons for health through mobile technologies.* Global Observatory for eHealth Series, Volume 3.

Yeaw, J., Benner, J. S., Walt, J. G., Sian, S., & Smith, D. B. (2009). Comparing adherence and persistence across 6 chronic medication classes. *J Manag Care Pharm, 15*(9), 728–740.

Index

A

ABMS (American Board of Medical Specialties), 6
Abstract section, IT evaluation reports, 177–178
ACA (Affordable Care Act), 382
Accountable, RACI diagram, 188
ACOs (Accountable Care Organizations), 351, 384
AD (active directory)
  definition of, 218
  system administrators' roles, 218
adaptive maintenance, 133–135
ADDIE training model
  analysis, 92–95
    learner analysis, 94
    organizational analysis, 93
    task analysis, 94–95
  design
    delivery methods, 96
    learning objectives, 96–97
  development
    content based on learning objectives, 97
    subject matter experts, 98
    training materials, 98
  implementation
    delivering training materials, 98
    evaluation types, 99–104
ADLs (daily activity limitations), 390
ADT (Admission, Discharge, and Transfer), 274
adult learning theory, 91–92
AHIMA (American Health Information Management Association), 9
AHRQ (Agency for Healthcare Research and Quality), 297
  common formats, 300–301
  EHR (electronic health record), alert effectiveness, 56-57
  Five Rights model, CDS (clinical decision support), 238–240
  Guide to Reducing Unintended Consequences of Electronic Health Records, 299–300
  Health Information Technology Evaluation Toolkit
    plans for IT evaluations, 161–162
    sample sizes, 175
  Health IT Hazard Manager, 301–302
alarm fatigue, EHRs (electronic health records), 56
alerts, EHRs (electronic health records), 56–57
ambulatory care, 343–345
Ambulatory EHR Optimization Check List, 146–150
American Academy of Orthopedic Surgeons, 328
AMIA (American Medical Informatics Association)
  Clinical Informatics
    Board Review Courses, 6
    definition of, 6

subspecialty, 6
10 X 10, distance learning programs, 6
EHRs (electronic health records), usability assessment, 42
project failures, reasons for, 183
ANA (American Nurses Association)
ANCC (American Nurses Credentialing Center), 5
CNPII (Committee for Nursing Practice Information Infrastructure), 259–261
informatics
board certification, 3
definition of, 4
Standards of Practice, 4
Nursing Informatics: Scope and Standards of Practice, 352
recognition of, 4
training issues, 87–88
nursing
processes, 185
terminology standards, 255–256
recognition of terminology standards, 272
analysis phase, ADDIE training model, 92–95
learner analysis, 94
organizational analysis, 93
task analysis, 94–95
analytics, 361
assessment, 361-363
Big Data, 372-376
data visualization, 364–370
infographics, 370–372
Apple App Store, 397
Apple Macintosh user interface, influence on usability, 43
application evaluations, ADDIE model, 101, 103–104
architecture/authentication mechanisms
technical security safeguards, 217
testing process, 83
ARRA (American Recovery and Reinvestment Act), 321
EHRs (electronic health records), 181
EMRs (electronic medical records), 181
HITECH (Health Information Technology for Economic and Clinical Health) Act, 2–3
ASHIM (American Society of Health Information Managers), 10–11
ASHP (American Society of Health-System Pharmacists), Medical Informatics, 7
ASQ (After Scenario Questionnaire), 152
assessment, 273, 278
asynchronous CDS reports, 235
Atlassian Jira, 81
auditory learning preference, 92
authentication procedures
technical security safeguards, 217
testing process, 83

B

bar charts, data display, 176–177
barcode systems, testing, 69
BAU (business as usual) changes, 137
BCMA (Bar Code Medication Administration), 181
behaviorist learning theory, 91
Big Data, 179, 363, 372–376, 385
biometrics, 218
Blue Button Initiative, 329–330
BMI (body mass index), 277
Borland
Caliber, 81
Silk Performer, 82
bullet point lists, data display, 176–177
business results evaluations, ADDIE model, 101, 104

C

CAHs (critical access hospitals), 321
Caliber, Borland, 81
California Hospital Association, business continuity toolkit, 142
care presentations, planning of, 276
case studies, 174
CCC (Clinical Care Classification System), 260–261
nursing process, 281. *See also* nursing process
RNDx items of, 275
standard nursing terminology in, 283–287
CCHIIM (Commission on Certification for Health Informatics and Information Management), 9
CDC (Centers for Disease Control), 390
CDS (clinical decision support)
background
DXplain, 232
HELP (Health Evaluation through Logical Processing) system, 232–233
RMRS (Regenstrief Medical Record System), 230, 232

definition of, 229
design worksheet, 243–244
development committees, 242–243
Five Rights model, 238–240, 245, 247
implementation tasks checklist, 245–248
overview, 16–17, 229–231
point of care, 229, 235
system optimization, 154
Ten Commandmentss of, 240–242
types
appointment alerts/reminders, 234, 236
clinical documentation support, 236
diagnostics recommendations, 235
documentation, 234-235
drug/lab alerts, 236
knowledge tool access, 235
medication alerts, 234
order sets, 230, 233–234, 236
real-time dashboards, 235
reminders, 237
reports, 235, 237
treatment recommendations, 235–237
uses of, 233–234
CEHRT (certified electronic health record technology), 323
Centers for Medicare and Medicaid Services Partnership for Patients initiative, 297
change management, 134–138
"Characteristics of a Good Nursing Nomenclature from an Informatics Perspective", 258
CHaRM™, 335–336
charts, data display, 176–177
CHISP (Certified Health Informatics Systems Professional), 10–11
chronic care, 341
CINAHL (Cumulative Index to Nursing and Allied Health Literature), 171
Citrix printing, 67
clinical care and coordination, mobile health, 400–401
Clinical Informatics
aid with design/workflow of electronic systems, 5–6
AMIA (American Medical Informatics Association)
Board Review Courses, 6
10 X 10, distance learning programs, 6
definition of, 6
overview, 5–7
clinical information systems, implementation of
readiness assessment, 32
success measurements, 36
system selection, 30–31
workflow, 32–36
Clinical Translational Science Institute, 403
closure phase, project management, 186–187
Cloud
testing process in, 84
CMS (Centers for Medicare and Medicaid Services), 181, 345, 354
CCC (Clinical Care Classification System), 260–261
Meaningful Use program, 181, 292, 297–298
PA (Privacy Act), 206, 212, 227
CNPII (Committee for Nursing Practice Information Infrastructure), 259
Cochrane Reviews, 171
Code of FIPP (Fair Information Practice Principles), 210–212
cognitive learning theory, 91
collection of nursing information, 273, 274
colors
in EHRs (electronic health records), 54
vision deficiency, 367
Colour Contrast Analyser tool, 54–55
communication, project management, 199
Community College Consortia Program, informatics training, 9
Conclusion section, IT evaluation reports, 177–178
configuration management, 134–136
connected health, 381
connectivity, 404–405
constructivist learning theory, 91
Consulted, RACI diagram, 189
consumer and patient apps (mobile health), 397–399
controlled trials of EHRs (electronic health records), 292
control phase, project management, 186
corrective maintenance, 134–135
COTS (commercial off-the-shelf) applications, testing, 78–79
CP/DR (contingency plan/disaster recovery), 219
CPHIMS (Certified Professional in Healthcare Information & Management Systems), 9–10
CPOE (computerized provider order entry), 5, 292
CDS, drug/lab alerts or order sets, 236
design and usability, 43
Design Checklist, 309–310
IOM (Institute of Medicine) recommendations, 181
Pick-list Checklist, 310–312

"Crossing the Quality Chasm: A New Health System for the 21st Century," 254
CSUQ (Computer System Usability Questionnaire), 152
current state, descriptive evaluations of, 174
custom applications, testing, 79–80
CyberSecurity 10 Best Practices for the Small Healthcare Environment, 222–225

D

dashboards, 199–201
data marts, 363
data visualization, 363, 364–370
decision making, 273. *See also* nursing process
"Defining and Testing EMR Usability: Principles and Proposed Methods of EMR Usability Evaluation and Rating" (HIMSS), 44
density of information, EHRs (electronic health records), 49–50
Dental Informatics, overview of, 8
design and usability
  cognitive loads, minimizing, 49–50
  consistency
    examples of, 47–48
    GUIs (graphical user interfaces), 47
  content preservation, 55–56
  Digital Communications Division, HHS (tools), 44
  EHRs (electronic health records), 41
  Electronic Health Record Usability Task Force report, 44
  forgiveness and feedback, 51–53
  information presentation, effectiveness of, 54–55
  interactions, efficiency of, 50–51
  language, effective use of, 53–54
  naturalness, 47–48
  overview, 12–13
  simplicity
    80/20 rule, 47
    stackable content, 45–47
  versus software testing, 62
  usability
    assessment, 42–43, 58
    checklists, 56–57
design phase, ADDIE training model
  delivery methods, 96
  learning objectives, 96–97
development phase, ADDIE training model
  content based on learning objectives, 97
  subject matter experts, 98
  training materials, 98
diagnosis, 273, 278
dietitians, 8
Digital Communications Division, design and usability tools, 44
directors/managers, governance models, 25
Discussion section, IT evaluation reports, 177–178
DMZ (demilitarized zone)
  definition of, 219
  risk reduction, 208
DoD (Department of Defense), PA (Privacy Act), 206, 212, 227
downtime
  best practices, 142–143
  scheduled and unscheduled, 138, 140–143
drift, 151
driving forces
  health consumer, 324–325
  providers, 320–323
DR plans. See CP/DR
DXplain systems, 232

E

ECRI Institute, 307–308
  health technology hazards, 154
  safety hazards, 154
EDs (emergency departments), 321, 389
education, 319. See also patient engagement
EHRs (electronic health records)
  adoption of, 321, 342
  AHRQ *Guide to Reducing Unintended Consequences of Electronic Health Records,* 299–300
  history of, 292–293
  HITECH (Health Information Technology for Economic and Clinical Health) Act, 3
  informatics
    early role of, 1–2
    gaming industry influence on, 43
  lifecycles, 309
  Meaningful Use program, 3, 160, 181
  percentage use in U.S., 159

personal data inside, 386
SAFER (Safety Assurance Factors for EHR Resilience) guides, 304
safety of, 291
Electronic Health Record Usability Task Force report, 41
e-manuals, training, 97
embedded nanosensors, 406
EMRs (electronic medical records)
"Defining and Testing EMR Usability: Principles and Proposed Methods of EMR Usability Evaluation and Rating," 44
"EMR Usability: Bridging the Gap between Nurse and Computer," 44
encryption
PKI (public key infrastructure), 217, 221
WPA (Wi-Fi Protected Access), 207
engagement, 317. *See also* patient engagement
enterprise architecture, testing, 85
EP (Eligible Provider), 322
ePHI (electronic protected health information), 215–217
e-PRO (endorsed patient reported outcomes), 385
errors
in EHRs (electronic health records), 291
medication, 293
MERP (Medication Errors Reporting Program), 303
EU (European Union), 389
evaluation, 282
of informatics, 15–16
as step of nursing process, 273
evolution of healthcare analytics, 362
execution phase, project management, 186
executives/senior leaders, governance models, 25
experiential learning preference, 92

F

Facebook, 328
Fair Credit Reporting Act of 1970, 227
FCC (Federal Communications Commission), 298
FDA (Food and Drug Administration), 206, 212, 227, 298
FDASIA (Food and Drug Administration Safety and Innovation Act), 403
feedback, 376. *See also* Big Data
FIPP, Code of (Fair Information Practice Principles), 210–212
FISMA (Federal Information Security Management Act) of 2002, 206, 212
Five Rights model, CDS (clinical decision support), 238–240, 245, 247
formative evaluations, implementation stage, ADDIE model, 99
FRCA (Fair Credit Reporting Act), 206
function testing, 14, 64–68
HL7 (Health Level Seven) interface, 65
scripts, 64
SQL (Structured Query Language) database queries, 65–67

G

GDP (gross domestic product), 389
GOe (Global Observatory for e Health), 381
Google Glass, 335–336
GPO (group policy object)
definition of, 219
system administrators' roles, 208
GPS (global positioning system), 381
granularity, 258–259
graphs, data display, 176
Guidelines for Standard Order Sets (ISMP), 302–303
A Guide to EHR Adoption: Implementation Through Organizational Transformation
governance models, 25
A Guide to the Project Management Body of Knowledge, 183–184

H

Harvard Business Review, projects, failures and overruns, 183
Harvard Medical School Laboratory of Computer Science, 232
HCFA (Health Care Financing Agency). See CMS
healthcare analytics. See analytics
"Healthcare IT and Patient Safety: Building Safer Systems for Better Care," 161

healthcare IT systems. See also IT (information technology)
climate of, 160–161
network administrators, 207–208
outcome evaluations, considerations, 160–161
Big Data, 179
data collection, 174–177
data requirements, 172–173
literature searches, 171–172
questions to ask, 169–171
reports, 177–178
study types, 173–174
topics, priority of, 164–169
system administrators, 208
health consumer driving forces, 324–325
Health Information Technology Evaluation Toolkit
plans for IT evaluations, 161–162
sample sizes, 175
Health Insurance Marketplace, 194
"Health IT and Patient Safety: Building Safer Systems for Better Care," 293–296, 310
HealthIT.gov website, 336
Health IT Hazard Manager, 301–302
Health IT Implementation toolbox, 226
Health IT Patient Safety Action & Surveillance Plan, 296–298
Health IT Safety Program, 298
Health IT Value Suite, 162
Health On the Net Foundation, 328
HELP(Health Evaluation through Logical Processing) system, 232–233
HFES (Human Factors and Ergonomics Society), 54
HHS (Department of Health and Human Services), 292
CDS (clinical decision support), definition of, 229
CyberSecurity 10 Best Practices for the Small Healthcare Environment, 222–225
Digital Communications Division, design/usability tools, 44
FCRA (Fair Credit Reporting Act), 212
OCR (Office of Civil Rights), 213–214, 227
HIDS (host-based intrusion detection system), 220
HIE (health information exchange), 363, 400
HIMSS (Health Information and Management Systems Society), 402
CAHIMS (Certified Associate in Healthcare Information & Management Systems), 10
CPHIMS (Certified Professional in Healthcare Information & Management Systems), 9–10
EHRs (electronic health records), 44
"Defining and Testing EMR Usability: Principles and Proposed Methods of EMR Usability Evaluation and Rating," 44
Electronic Health Record Usability Task Force report, 41, 44
A Guide to EHR Adoption: Implementation Through Organizational Transformation
stop, start, continue example, 35
three-tiered governance model, 25
Health IT Value Suite, 162
HIMSS Health IT Value STEPS, 162–163
HIPAA (Health Insurance Portability and Accountability Act), 206, 385
CP/DR (contingency plan/disaster recovery), 219
ISO (information security officer), 209
privacy officials, 210
Privacy Rule, 213, 227
Security Rule, 227
HIRS (health information record systems)
controlled medical vocabularies, 257–258
data interoperability, 255
implementation of, 254
incorporating nursing process, 272
ANA (American Nurses Association), 273–274
data collection, 274
data management, 276
data tree build, 274–276
MEDCIN® Engine, 274–278, 281–284
Nursing Plan of Care, 277–287
incorporating nursing terminology, 269–272
incorporating terminology into nursing processes, 272
ontology frameworks, 255–256
structured data, 254–255
system nomenclature, 255
versus traditional medical records, 253
HIT (Health Information Technology), 300
HITECH (Health Information Technology for Economic and Clinical Health) Act, 292, 344
EHRs (electronic health records), Meaningful Use program, 3, 160, 181
informatics
Electronic Health Record Usability Task Force report, 41
training and information to colleges, 8
HL7 (Health Level Seven), 65
HPI (human performance improvement) models, 88, 90–91

HP LoadRunner, 82
HPSA (Health Professional Shortage Area), 352
HP Unified Functional Testing, 82
HQRP (Hospice Quality Reporting Program), 349
HRSA (Health Resources and Services Administration), 350
HTTPS (HyperText Transfer Protocol Secure), 207, 219

I

IaaS (infrastructure as a service) Cloud services, 84
IBM
  ASQ (After Scenario Questionnaire), 152
  CSUQ (Computer System Usability Questionnaire), 152
  PSSUQ (Post Study System Usability Questionnaire), 151–152
IDS (intrusion detection system), 208
  definition of, 220
  traffic monitoring, 208
IEEE 11073 standards, 402
IHI (Institute for Healthcare Improvement), 388. *See also* Triple Aim Initiative
implementation of systems, 280
  activation, 110–112, 127
    checklists, 122–124
    communication issues, 112–115
    contingency plans, 125
    documentation, 115–116
    lessons-learned meetings, 126
    Operational Readiness Review documents, 116–121
    post-live meetings, 126
    rehearsals, 125–126
    resource schedules, 124–125
    support staff roles, 127–128
  planning and analysis
    readiness assessment, 32
    success measurements, 36
    system selection, 30–31
    workflow, 32–36
  as step of nursing process, 273
implementation phase, ADDIE training model
  delivering training materials, 98
  evaluation levels
    application, 101, 103–104
    business results, 101, 104
    formative and summative, 99
    learning, 101, 103
    reaction, 100, 102–103
    ROI (return on investment), 102, 104
Improving Outcomes with Clinical Decision Support: An Implementer's Guide, 245
infographics, 370–372
informaticists
  need for, 2–3
  roles of, 22
informatics
  certifications available
    AHIMA (American Health Information Management Association), 9
    ASHIM (American Society of Health Information Managers), 10–11
    HIMSS (Health Information and Management Systems Society), 9–10
  core elements of
    CDS (clinical decision support), 16–17
    design and usability, 12–13
    evaluation, 15–16
    implementation, 15
    maintenance, 15
    planning and analysis, 11–12
    project management, 16
    security and privacy, 16
    testing, 13–14
    training, 14
  definition of, ANA (American Nurses Association), 4
  disciplines
    Clinical Informatics, 5–7
    Dental Informatics, 8
    Nursing Informatics, 4–5
    Pharmacy Informatics, 7
  emerging trends, 17–18
  history of, 2
  IT (information technology) in non-acute settings, 343–354
  in non-acute care settings, 341–343
  origins of, 1
  training opportunities, 8–9
information security, 206–208
  application administrators, 209
  basic safeguards, 214–215
    administrative, 215–216
    physical, 216
    technical, 217
  best practices/checklist, 222–225
  defense in depth, 205

FCRA (Fair Credit Reporting Act), 211–212
FIPP, Code of (Fair Information Practice Principles), 210–212
FISMA (Federal Information Security Management Act) of 2002, 206, 212
frameworks, 210–214
HIPAA (Health Insurance Portability and Accountability Act), 206
CP/DR (contingency plan/disaster recovery), 219
Privacy Rule, 213, 227
Security Rule, 213–214, 219, 227
ISO (information security officer), 209
network administrators, 207–208
organizations mandating security, 206
PA (Privacy Act) of 1974, 206, 212, 227
privacy officials, 210
resources, 227
systems administrators, 208
Information Security—An Overview. Appendix A: Information Security Checklist for Healthcare Professionals, 226
Informed, RACI diagram, 189
initiation phase, project management, 185
inpatient rehabilitation facilities, 353–354
instructor-led training, 96, 98
integration testing, 14, 68–70
Intelligent PromptingTM, MEDCIN® Engine, 278
interventions
planning, 280
pre-post evaluations, 174
Introduction section, IT evaluation reports, 177–178
An Introductory Resource Guide for Implementing the Health Insurance Portability and Accountability Act (HIPAA) Security Rule (SP 800-66 Revision 1), 214
IOM (Institute of Medicine), 291, 317
To Err is Human, 181
"Healthcare IT and Patient Safety: Building Safer Systems for Better Care," 161
"Health IT and Patient Safety: Building Safer Systems for Better Care," 293–296
recommendations, 181
IRFs (inpatient rehabilitation facilities), 342
ISMP (Institute for Safe Medication Practices), 302–304
ISO (International Organization for Standardization), 256
IT (information technology), 291
"Health IT and Patient Safety: Building Safer Systems for Better Care," 293–296
Health IT Patient Safety Action & Surveillance Plan, 296–298
meaningful use of, 321–323
in non-acute care settings, 343–354
ambulatory care, 343–345
home care, 348–350
long-term care and skilled nursing facilities, 345–348
LTACHs (long-term acute care hospitals), 353–354
LTPAC (Long-Term and Post-Acute Care), 354–359
telehealth technologies, 350–353
patient engagement, 317. See also engagement
patient-provided data, 330–336
CHaRM™, 335–336
Google Glass, 335–336
hardware and software, 331–332
PulsePoint, 334–335
wearable devices, 332–334
resources and tools, 298–312
ITIL (IT Infrastructure Library), change management, 134, 136

J–K

Jira, Atlassian, 81
job aid documents, training, 97
Journal of the American Medical Association, 293
just-in-time training, 96

Keywords section, IT evaluation reports, 177–178
kinesthetic learning preference, 92
KPMG and projects
failures, 183
success factors, 184

L

LDS Hospital, Salt Lake City, Utah, 232
learner analysis, ADDIE training model, 94
learning evaluations, ADDIE model, 101, 103
learning preferences, 92
learning theories, 91–92

lifecycles of EHRs (electronic health records), 309
List of Error-Prone Abbreviations, Symbols, and Dose Designations (ISMP), 304
listservs, 325
LoadRunner, HP, 82
logical learning preference, 92
LTACHs (long-term acute care hospitals), 342, 353–354
LTPAC (Long-Term and Post-Acute Care), 342, 354–359

M

Macintosh user interface, influence on usability, 43
maintenance of systems
  adaptive maintenance, 133–135
  business continuity, 141–142
  change management, 134–138
  configuration management, 134–136
  corrective maintenance, 134–135
  downtime
    best practices, 142–143
    scheduled and unscheduled, 138, 140–143
  implementation cutover steps, 139–140
  optimization, 133, 145–146
    CDS (clinical decision support), 154
    check lists, 146–150
    goals of, 150–151
    resource use, 155–156
    safety evaluations, 153–154
    usability questionnaires, 151–153
  overview, 15, 130–133
  perfective maintenance, 134–135
  predictive maintenance, 134–135
  redundancy of network/infrastructure components, 141
  request management, 136–137, 143–144
malware, 220
Massachusetts General Hospital, 232
Mayo Clinic, 382
MDS (Minimum Data Set), 346
Meaningful Use program, 281, 295–297
MEDCIN® Engine
  HIRS (health information record systems)
    incorporating nursing process, 274–278, 281–284
    incorporating nursing terminology, 269–270, 272
  Intelligent PromptingTM, 278
medical informatics, post-doctoral fellowships, 6
medical technicians, informatics, 8
medication
  errors, 293
  ISMP (Institute for Safe Medication Practices), 302–304
  MERP (Medication Errors Reporting Program), 303
MERP (Medication Errors Reporting Program), 303
Methods section, IT evaluation reports, 177–178
Microsoft Windows
  NT systems, GPO (group policy object), 219
  Windows registry, 221
MITM (man-in-the-middle) attacks, 220
mobile devices, testing, 84–85
mobile health, 381–396
  clinical care and coordination, 400–401
  consumer and patient apps, 397–399
  evaluation, 403
  impact on Triple Aim Initiative, 387–396
  maturity of, 401–403
  mobility as care model, 382–385
  personalized health, 385–387
mobility as care model, 382–385
monitoring software, 71, 330
MSA (metropolitan statistical area), 352
multifactor authentication, 221

N

nanosensors, embedded, 406
narrative text, data display, 176–177
National Consumers League Script Your Future, 390
National Council of State Boards of Nursing, 328
National Quality Forum (2008), 317
National Quality Strategy, 297
networks, connectivity, 404–405
NI (Nursing Informatics). See Nursing Informatics
NIDCR (National Institute of Dental and Craniofacial Research), 8
NIDS (network-based intrusion detection system), 220
Nightingale, Florence, 2
NIH (National Institutes of Health), PA (Privacy Act), 206, 212, 227
NIST (National Institute of Standards in Technology), 212, 214

NLM (National Library of Medicine)
Dental Informatics training programs, 8
Medical Informatics, support and funding for, 6
nominal group prioritization technique, 166–167
non-acute care settings, IT (information technology) in, 341–343, 343–354
ambulatory care, 343–345
home care, 348–350
long-term care and skilled nursing facilities, 345–348
LTACHs (long-term acute care hospitals), 353–354
LTPAC (Long-Term and Post-Acute Care), 354–359
telehealth technologies, 350–353
Nursing Home Compare, 347
nursing informatics
certification requirements, 5
Master's and post-Master's programs, 4
overview, 4–5
Nursing Informatics: Scope and Standards of Practice, 343, 352
Nursing Plan of Care, 277–287
nursing process, incorporating terminology into, 272–287
data collection, 274
data management, 276–277
data tree build, 274–276
Nursing Plan of Care, 277–287
nursing terminology standards
ABC (Alternative Billing Codes), 265
benefits of, 267
CCC (Clinical Care Classification System), 260–261, 283–287
characteristics of, 256
CNPII (Committee for Nursing Practice Information Infrastructure), 259–261
definition of, 259
ICNP (International Classification for Nursing Practice), 261–262
incorporating into HIRS (health information record systems)
CCC into MEDCIN® Engine, 269–272
CCC Nursing Diagnoses and Nursing Interventions, 267–269
incorporating into nursing process, 272–287
LOINC (Logical Observation Identifiers Names and Codes), 265–266
NANDA International, 262
NIC (Nursing Interventions Classification), 262
NMDS (Nursing Minimum Data Set), 263–264
NMMDS (Nursing Management Minimum Data Set), 264–265
NOC (Nursing Outcomes Classification), 263
Nursing Informatics: Scope and Standards of Practice, 260
Omaha System, 263
PNDS (Perioperative Nursing Data Set), 260, 263
recognized standards, 255–256
SNOMED CT (Systematized Nomenclature of Medicine Clinical Terms), 257, 266

O

observational studies, 174
OCR (Office of Civil Rights), 213–214
ONC (Office of the National Coordinator for Health Information Technology), 292, 321, 342
EHRs (electronic health records)
Health IT Implementation toolbox, 226
Meaningful Use program, 3, 160, 181
usability assessment, 58
Health IT Patient Safety Action & Surveillance Plan, 296–298
informatics training, 8–9
LTPAC (Long-Term and Post-Acute Care), 354–359
SAFER (Safety Assurance Factors for EHR Resilience) guides, 226
on-the-job training, 96
Open Notes, 330
open source software, 83
optimization of systems, 133, 145–146
CDS (clinical decision support), 154
check lists, 146–150
goals of, 150–151
resource use, 155–156
safety evaluations, 153–154
usability questionnaires, 151–153
organizational analysis, ADDIE training model, 93
outcome identification, 273, 279

P

P4 Medicine (Prediction, Personalization, Prevention, Participation), 385–386
PaaS (platform as a service) Cloud services, 84
Paciello Contrast Analyser tool, 55
PA (Privacy Act) of 1974, 206, 212, 227
paper-based training, 96
patient engagement, 317
  assessment of, 320–325
  definition of, 318–319
  patient-provided data, 330–336
  social media and, 327–330
  tools, 326–327
patient-provided data
  CHaRM™, 335–336
  Google Glass, 335–336
  hardware and software, 331–332
  PulsePoint, 334–335
  wearable devices, 332–334
patient safety, 291
  "Health IT and Patient Safety: Building Safer Systems for Better Care," 293–296
  Health IT Patient Safety Action & Surveillance Plan, 296–298
  resources and tools, 298–312
PatientsLikeMe study, 400
PCMHs (patient-centered medical homes), 351, 384, 388
performance testing, 14, 70–71
personalized health, 385–387
Pew Research, 318
PGHD (patient-generated health data), 384, 400
Pharmacy Informatics
  board certification not available, 7
  Master's degree in Healthcare Informatics, 7
  Medical Informatics' role, 7
  overview, 7
  training programs, 7
phases of project management
  closure, 186–187
  control, 186
  execution, 186
  initiation, 185
  planning, 185–186
PHIT (personal health information technology), 379–380
physical therapists, 8
PICOT method, 170
pie charts, data display, 176–177, 366
PIV (personal identity verification) cards, 221
PKI (public key infrastructure) encryption
  definition of, 221
  ePHI (electronic protected health information), 217
Plain Writing Act, 53
planning and analysis
  analysis principles, 23–24
  benefits measurement, 27
  bidirectional communication, 26
  of care presentations, 276
  end-user engagement, 26–27
  executive sponsorship, 24
  goals/vision principles, 22–23
  governance models, 24–25
  implementation
    readiness assessment, 32
    success measurements, 36
    system selection, 30–31
    workflow, 32–36
  leadership engagement, 24
  ongoing support and optimization, 29–30, 37–38
  overview, 11–12
  planning success factors, 22
  versus software testing, 62
  as step of nursing process, 273, 280
  value realization, 27–28
  workflow-based training, 28–29
planning phase, project management, 185–186
PMBOK Guide, 183–184
PMI (Project Management Institute), *A Guide to the Project Management Body of Knowledge,* 183–184
PMS (population management system), 363
PNDS (Perioperative Nursing Data Set), 260, 263
portable high resolution diagnostics, 405
portals, 324
POS (place of service), 321
PricewaterhouseCoopers, 183
printing, testing of, 67
processes, incorporating terminology into, 272–287
project charters
  approaches, 192
  assumptions, 192
  purpose and goals, 191
  reporting structure, 192
  roles and responsibilities, 192–194
  scope, 191
project management/projects
  communication, 199
  dashboards, 199–201

definition of, 182
failures of, 183
guidelines, 184, 187, 190
overview, 16
phases
closure, 186–187
control, 186
execution, 186
initiation, 185
planning, 185–186
PMBOK Guide, 184
project charters, 191–194
resources, 182
scope
decision documents, 195–197
management plans, 194–197
necessity of, 182–183
stakeholders
analysis of, RACI diagram, 188–190
identifying, 187–188
project governance, 190
versus standard operations, 183
status reports, 201–202
timelines, 197–199
WBS (work breakdown structure), 197–199
proprietary software, 83
provider driving forces, 320–323
PSOPPC (PSO Privacy Protection Center), 300, 301
PSOs (Patient Safety Organizations), 297
PSSUQ (Post Study System Usability Questionnaire), IBM, 151–152
PubMed, 171
PUEU (Perceived Usefulness and Ease of Use), 153
PulsePoint, 334–335

Q

QAPI (Quality Assurance and Performance Improvement), 347
QIS (Quality Indicator Survey), 348
Quality of Health Care in America 2001 report, 254
quantitative perception, 368
Quippe, 284
QUIS (Questionnaire for User Interaction Satisfaction), 152

R

RACI diagram, 188–190
RAI (Resident Assessment Instrument), 347
RCTs (randomized controlled trials), 173–174
reaction evaluations, implementation stage, ADDIE model, 100, 102–103
REALM (Rapid Estimate of Adult Literacy in Medicine), 326
RECs (Regional Extension Centers), 344
regression testing, 14, 72–74, 127
rehabilitation, inpatient facilities, 353–354
reports
CDS (clinical decision support), 235
transparency of, 295
resources
IT (information technology) safety, 298–312
AHRQ common formats, 300–301
AHRQ *Guide to Reducing Unintended Consequences of Electronic Health Records,* 299–300
CPOE (computerized provider order entry) Design Checklist, 309–310
CPOE (computerized provider order entry) Pick-list Checklist, 310–312
ECRI Institute, 307–308
Health IT Hazard Manager, 301–302
ISMP (Institute for Safe Medication Practices), 302–304
SAFER (Safety Assurance Factors for EHR Resilience) guides, 304–306
project management, 182
respiratory therapists, 8
Responsible, RACI diagram, 188
Results section, IT evaluation reports, 177–178
retrospective studies, 174
RMRS (Regenstrief Medical Record System), 230, 232
RN-BC (Registered Nurse–Board Certified) title, 5
Robert Wood Johnson Foundation, 6, 330
ROI (return on investment) evaluations, ADDIE model, 102, 104
run charts, data display, 176–177

S

SaaS (software as a service) Cloud services, 84
SAFER (Safety Assurance Factors for EHR Resilience) guides, 226, 304–306
safety evaluations, 153–154. *See also* patient safety
scenario testing. *See* integration testing
Scientific American, 335
scope of projects
  management plans, 194–197
  necessity of, 182–183
security and privacy, overview of, 16
Serena Business Manager, 81
Silk Performer, Borland, 82
Six Sigma Black Belts, workflow processes, 35
smart phones, embedded nanosensors and, 406
SMEs (subject matter experts), governance models, 25
SNFs (skilled nursing facilities), 342
SNOMED CT (Systematized Nomenclature of Medicine Clinical Terms), 257, 266
social learning preference/theory, 91–92
social media and patient engagement, 327–330
sociotechnical model, workflow, 34
software
  consumer and patient apps (mobile health), 397–399
  infographics, 370–372
  testing
    open source software, 83
    proprietary software, 83
solitary learning preference, 92
sources of Big Data, 372. *See also* Big Data
SQL (Structured Query Language) database queries, 65–67
stakeholders, project management
  analysis of, RACI diagram, 188–190
  identifying, 187–188
  project governance, 190
standard operations *versus* projects, 183
STARE-HI (Statement on Reporting of Evaluation Studies in Health Informatics), 171–172, 177
status reports
  project management, 201–202
STEPS. *See HIMSS Health IT Value STEPS*
S-TOFHLA (Shortened Test of Functional Health Literacy in Adults), 327
stop, start, continue example, workflow, 35
store-and-forward imaging, 351
STSI (Scripps Translational Science Institute), 333
Study Context section, IT evaluation reports, 177–178
subject matter experts, 98
SUMI (Software Usability Measurement Inventory), 152–153
summative evaluations, ADDIE model, 99
super users. *See* SMEs
SUS (System Usability Scale), 151
synchronous CDS reports, 235
systems software testing
  clinical systems, 62–63
    architecture/authentication mechanisms, 83
    in Cloud, 84
    COTS (commercial off-the-shelf) applications, 78–79
    custom applications, 79–80
    enterprise architecture, 85
    function testing, 14, 64–68
    goals, 62
    integration testing, 14, 68–70
    for mobile devices, 84–85
    overview, 13–14
    performance testing, 14, 70–71
    regression testing, 14, 72–74, 127
    unit testing, 14, 63–64
    user acceptance testing, 71–72
    web-based applications, 80
  testing process
    assessing completion, 77–78
    debugging, 76
    key requirements, 75
    preparation for, 73–74
    reporting metrics, 77
    script criteria, 76
    timelines, 77
  tools
    automating processes, 82
    defining requirements and mapping, 81
    performance testing, 82
    tracking and reporting issues/incidents, 81

T

tables, data display, 176–177
TAM (Technology Acceptance Model) questionnaire, 151

task analysis, ADDIE training model, 94–95
telehealth technologies, 350–353
telemedicine, 350, 381
Ten Commandments of CDS (clinical decision support), 240–242
testing. See systems software testing
Thinking, Fast and Slow, 364
time/motion studies, 174
Title section, IT evaluation reports, 177–178
TJC (The Joint Commission), 53
To Err is Human, 181, 291, 317
tools
  IT (information technology) safety, 298–312
    AHRQ common formats, 300–301
    AHRQ *Guide to Reducing Unintended Consequences of Electronic Health Records,* 299–300
    CPOE (computerized provider order entry) Design Checklist, 309–310
    CPOE (computerized provider order entry) Pick-list Checklist, 310–312
    ECRI Institute, 307–308
    Health IT Hazard Manager, 301–302
    ISMP (Institute for Safe Medication Practices), 302–304
    SAFER (Safety Assurance Factors for EHR Resilience) guides, 304–306
  patient engagement, 326–327
  systems software testing
    automating processes, 82
    defining requirements and mapping, 81
    performance testing, 82
    tracking and reporting issues/incidents, 81
training for informatics
  ADDIE model
    analysis, 92–95
    design, 96–97
    development, 97–98
    evaluation, 100–104
    implementation, 98–99
  versus education, 88
  focus areas for improvement, 104–106
  HPI (human performance improvement) models, 88, 90–91
  lack of information about, 87–88
  learning
    preferences, 92
    theories, 91–92
  overview, 14
transparency of reports, 295
Triple Aim Initiative, impact on mobile health, 387–396
Twitter, 328

U

Unified Functional Testing, HP, 82
unit testing, 14, 63–64
University-Based Training Program, informatics training, 9
University Hospitals, Cleveland, Ohio, 184
University of Maryland, Nursing Informatics graduate education, 4
University of Utah, Nursing Informatics graduate education, 4
UPA (Usability Professionals' Association) assessment tools, 43
usability testing, questionnaires for optimization, 151–153
user acceptance testing, 14, 71–72

V

VA (Veterans Administration)
  EHRs (electronic health systems), 42
  PA (Privacy Act), 206, 212, 227
verbal learning preference, 92
virtual healthcare services, 383. *See also* mobile health
visual learning preference, 92
VPNs (virtual private networks)
  definition of, 221
  network administrators' roles, 207

W–X–Y–Z

WAMMI (Website Analysis and Measurement Inventory), 153
WBS (work breakdown structure), 185, 197–199
wearable devices, 332–334, 376
web-based applications, testing, 80

web-based training, 96
Well Home living laboratory, 406
WHO (World Health Organization), 381
WNL (within normal limits), 277
workflow, 362
workforce, system optimization, 155
WPA/WPA 2 (Wi-Fi Protected Access and II) protocols, 207, 221

Xerox, informatics system usability, 43

FROM THE HONOR SOCIETY OF NURSING, SIGMA THETA TAU INTERNATIONAL

The *Nurse's Advantage* Series

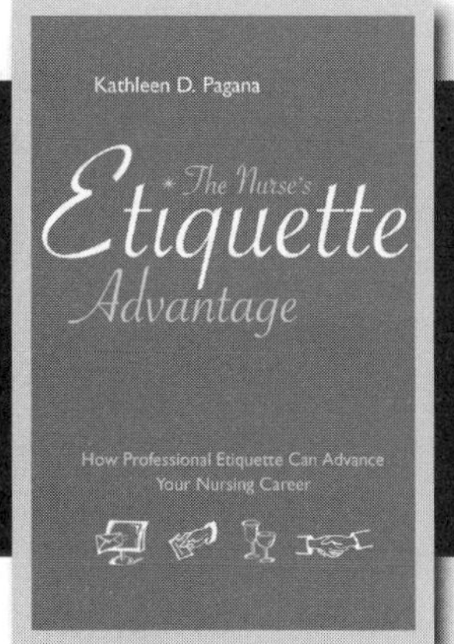

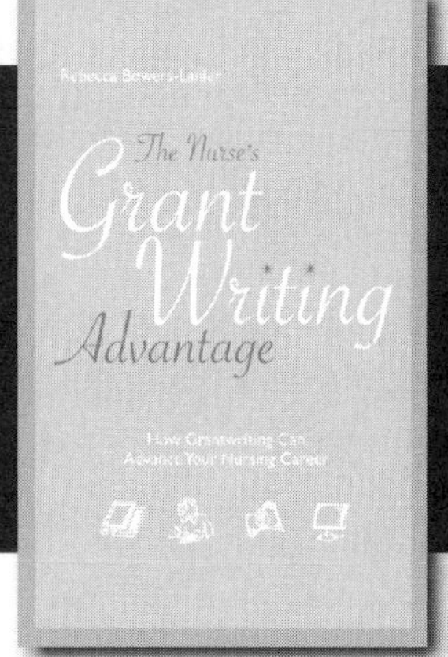

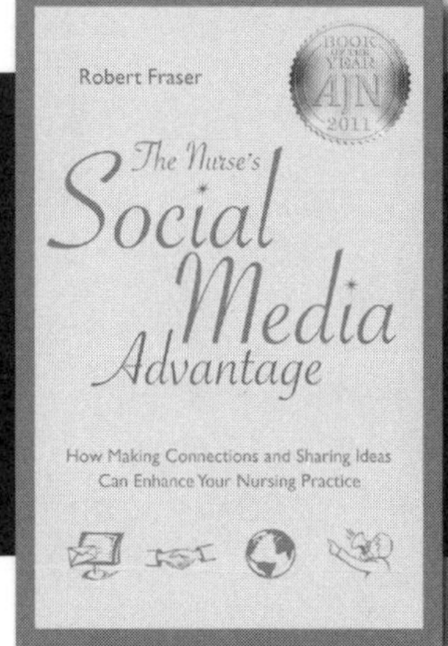

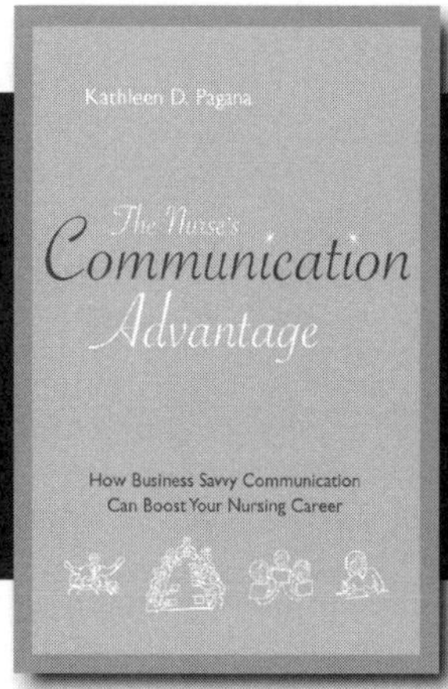

The Nurse's Etiquette Advantage
Kathleen D. Pagana

The Nurse's Grantwriting Advantage
Rebecca Bowers-Lanier

The Nurse's Social Media Advantage
Robert Fraser

The Nurse's Communication Advantage
Kathleen D. Pagana

To order, visit **www.nursingknowledge.org/sttibooks.**
Discounts are available for institutional purchases.
Call **888.NKI.4YOU** for details.

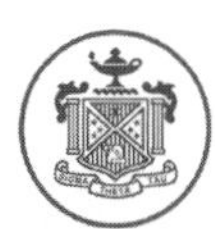

Sigma Theta Tau International
Honor Society of Nursing®

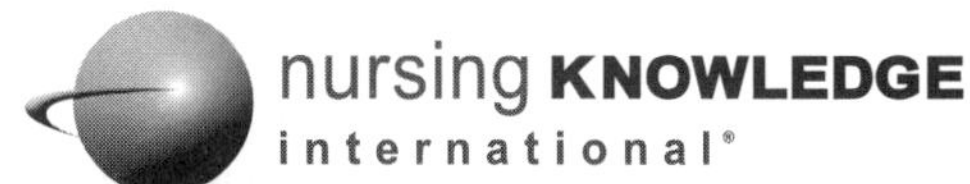

From the Honor Society of Nursing, Sigma Theta Tau International

Handbooks for Success

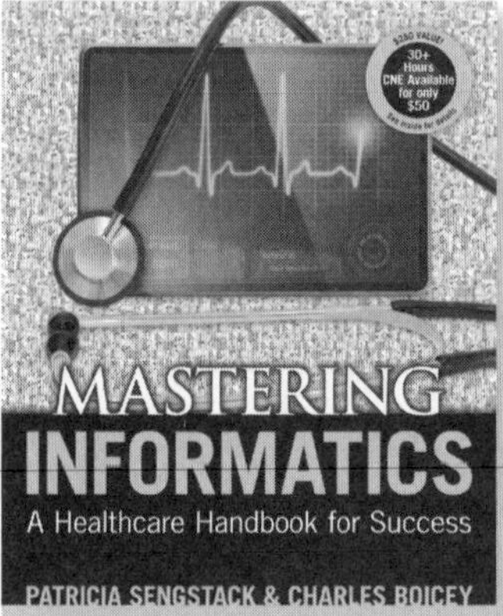

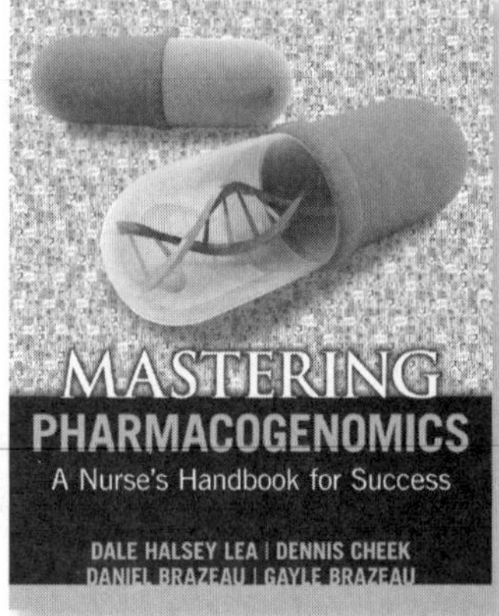

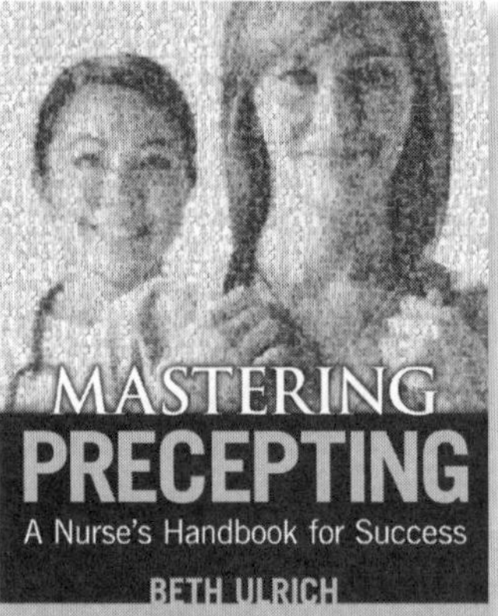

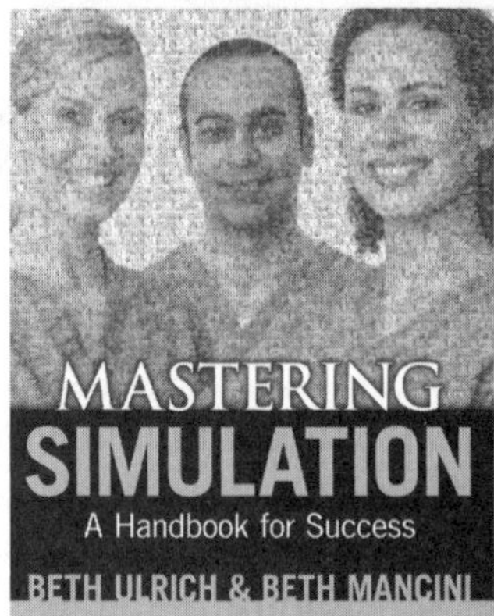

Mastering Informatics
Patricia Sengstack and Charles Boicey

Mastering Pharmacogenomics
Dale Halsey Lea, Dennis Cheek, Daniel Brazeau, and Gayle Brazeau

Mastering Precepting
Beth Ulrich

Mastering Simulation
Beth Ulrich and Beth Mancini

To order, visit **www.nursingknowledge.org/sttibooks.**
Discounts are available for institutional purchases.
Call **888.NKI.4.YOU** for details.

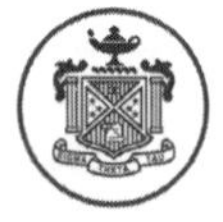

Sigma Theta Tau International
Honor Society of Nursing®

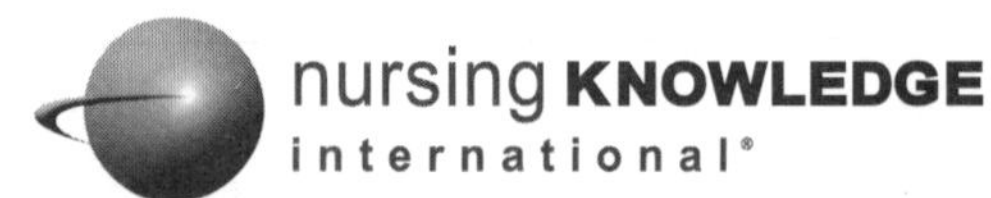